Psychology and Psychiatry

Psychology and Psychiatry

Integrating Medical Practice

Edited by

Jeannette Milgrom
Graham D. Burrows

University of Melbourne, and Austin & Repatriation Medical Centre,
Melbourne, Australia

Forewords by

Frederick K. Goodwin
John Weinman

JOHN WILEY & SONS, LTD

Chichester • New York • Weinheim • Brisbane • Singapore • Toronto

Other Wiley Editorial Offices

John Wiley & Sons, Inc., 605 Third Avenue,
New York, NY 10158-0012, USA

WILEY-VCH Verlag GmbH, Pappelallee 3,
D-69469 Weinheim, Germany

John Wiley & Sons Australia, Ltd., 33 Park Road, Milton,
Queensland 4064, Australia

John Wiley & Sons (Asia) Pte, Ltd., 2 Clementi Loop #02-01,
Jin Xing Distripark, Singapore 129809

John Wiley & Sons (Canada), Ltd., 22 Worcester Road,
Rexdale, Ontario M9W 1L1, Canada

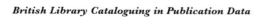

British Library Cataloguing in Publication Data

A catalogue record for this book is available from the British Library

ISBN 0-471-98108-7

Typeset in 10/12pt Baskerville by Kolam Information Services Pvt. Ltd, Pondicherry, India
Printed and bound in Great Britain by Biddles Ltd, Guildford and King's Lynn
This book is printed on acid-free paper responsibly manufactured from sustainable forestry,
in which at least two trees are planted for each one used for paper production.

Contents

About the Editors

Jeannette Milgrom, BSc (Hons), PhD

Departments of Psychology, University of Melbourne and Austin & Repatriation Medical Centre, Building 1, Repatriation Campus, Banksia Street, Heidelberg West, Victoria, 3081, Australia

Jeannette Milgrom is Professor of Psychology at the University of Melbourne and Director, Department of Psychology, at the Austin & Repatriation Medical Centre in Melbourne, Australia. She completed her PhD in 1977 and obtained a postdoctoral Harkness Fellowship in 1983 for study in the United States. She has pioneered extensive psychological services in a medical setting over the past 20 years and established a department that is held in high regard as a model for integrating clinical services, research and teaching in health psychology. Clinical health psychology services operate alongside consultation-liaison psychiatry. Professor Milgrom has developed a number of training programs, including the Doctor of Psychology (Health), University of Melbourne. She has a significant track record of research and publications and is at the forefront of international developments in the area of postnatal depression, focusing on its etiology, its psychological management, and disturbances of the early mother–infant interaction. This has resulted in innovative interventions, ongoing research and a recent Wiley publication *Treating Postnatal Depression* with co-authors P. R. Martin and L. M. Negri. Her current research in health psychology is in the areas of breaking the bad news, coping with surgery and cardiology and depression.

Professor Milgrom has also been active professionally and had long-term involvement with the Australian Psychological Society (APS), beginning in 1979 as President of the Victorian Section of the Division of Clinical Psychologists, a position she held for three years. More recently, she has been Secretary (1997) and Course Approval Convenor (1998) of the newly formed National Executive of the College of Health Psychologists (APS). She has also acted on the Advisory Group of the (APS) Directorate of Scientific Affairs for the past two years, and is now a Fellow of the Australian Psychological Society.

Graham D. Burrows, AO, KSJ, MD, ChB, BSc, DPM, FRANZCP, FRCPsych, MRACMA, Dip. M. Hlth Sc (Clinical Hypnosis)

Departments of Psychiatry, University of Melbourne and Austin & Repatriation Medical Centre, Austin Campus, Studley Road, Heidelberg, Victoria, 3084, Australia

Graham Burrows is Professor of Psychiatry at the University of Melbourne and Director of the Psychiatry and Psychology Clinical Service Unit at the Austin & Repatriation Medical Centre, Heidelberg, Victoria, Australia. Professor Burrows has published more than 650 scientific articles in peer-reviewed journals. He is the author or editor of more than 91 books, including the *Handbook of Anxiety Disorders* and the *Handbook of General Hospital Psychiatry*, and has contributed chapters to approximately 190 other scientific books. He serves on the editorial boards of 30 International and Australian journals.

Professor Burrows serves on a number of advisory boards to Australian, International, Governmental and Scientific Organisations, including the World Psychiatric Association and the World Health Organisation. He was President of the First and Second World Congress on Stress, Chairman of the International Congress in Melbourne Collegium International Neuropsychopharmacologicum (CINP), Chairman of the Australian Society of Hypnosis and Mental Health Foundation of Australia.

Professor Burrows has been honoured with the following awards for distinguished service to medicine: the Order of Australia (AO) in 1989, Knight of The Order of Saint John of Jerusalem (KSJ) in 1996 and the Paul Harris Fellowship, Rotary International in 1997.

About the Authors

Felicity Allen, BSc, MSc, PhD
Department of Psychology, Monash University, 246 Clayton Road, Clayton, Vic 3168, Australia

Felicity Allen is an Associate Professor of Psychology at Monash University. She obtained her BSc and MSc from the University of Melbourne in 1971 and 1973 respectively and her PhD from Monash University in 1988. In 1998, she wrote Australia's first book on health psychology. Her other major research area is equal opportunity and the assessment of merit, especially in large organizations like universities. Her teaching areas include multivariate statistics, social psychology and the encouragement of scepticism in students.

Andrew Baum, BS, PhD
405 Iroquois Building, Pittsburgh, PA 15213, USA

Andrew Baum is Professor of Psychiatry and Psychology, University of Pittsburgh, and Deputy Director of the University of Pittsburgh Cancer Institute (UPCI) where he is responsible for Cancer Control and Population Sciences. He is also Director of the UPCI's Behavioral Medicine Program. Dr Baum earned a BS in psychology at the University of Pittsburgh (1970) and PhD from the State University of New York at Stony Brook (1974). Before returning to the University of Pittsburgh in 1993, Dr Baum served on the faculty of Trinity College (1974–1978) and the Uniformed Services University of the Health Sciences (1978–1993) where he was Professor of Medical Psychology, Psychiatry, and Neuroscience and Assistant to the President for Sponsored Programs. His interests and expertise include stress, psychoneuroimmunology, trauma, and biobehavioral aspects of cancer. He has received awards from several professional societies, including the American Psychological Association and its Division of Health Psychology.

Cynthia Belar, PhD
APA, 750 First St NE, Washington DC 20002-4242, USA

Cynthia D. Belar is Executive Director of the Education Directorate of the American Psychological Association. Until 2000 she was director of the clinical psychology doctoral program and associate chair for academic affairs in the Department of Clinical and Health Psychology at the University of Florida Health Science

Center. She has served as the president of the APA Division of Health Psychology, chair of the Council of University Directors of Clinical Psychology, and president of the American Board of Clinical Health Psychology.

Chris Borthwick, BA (Hons), LLB
VicHealth, 333 Drummond St, Carlton Vic 3053, Australia

Chris Borthwick is Managing Editor of *Health Promotion Journal of Australia*, the journal of the Australian Health Promotion Association. He has a BA (Hons) in History from the Australian National University (1969) and an LLB from the University of Melbourne (1990). He has lectured and published widely on disability studies, the history of professional attitudes, psychological belief systems, and health promotion theory and practice.

David Copolov, MD
The Mental Health Research Institute of Victoria, Locked Bag 11, Parkville, Victoria, Australia 3052

David Leon Copolov is Director of the Mental Health Research Institute of Victoria, Professor of Psychiatry at the University of Melbourne and Honorary Professor in the Department of Psychological Medicine at Monash University.

He graduated in medicine from The University of Melbourne (1974) and completed a PhD in neurochemistry at Monash University (1983). He also holds postgraduate qualifications in psychiatry and internal medicine. He is Chief Investigator of the Australian National Health and Medical Research Council's Network for Brain Research into Mental Disorders and was co-Director of the Australian National Health and Medical Research Council's Schizophrenia Research Unit (1988–1996). His research interests have focused on the phenomenology, neuroendocrinology and neurochemistry of schizophrenia, with a particular interest in the pathophysiology of auditory hallucinations. He has written more than 160 research papers and chapters, mainly in the field of schizophrenia research.

Jane Duff, BSc (Hons), DClinPsychol
National Spinal Injuries Centre, Stoke Mandeville Hospital, Mandeville Road, Aylesbury, Buckinghamshire HP21 8AL, UK

Dr Jane Duff is a Clinical Psychologist at the National Spinal Injuries Centre, Stoke Mandeville Hospital. She obtained her BSc Honours degree in Psychology at the University of Plymouth in 1991 and her Doctorate in Clinical Psychology from the University of Southampton in 1997.

Dr Duff developed her interest in spinal cord injury rehabilitation during training, and has continued this into her current post. Her research interests include:

post-traumatic stress disorder, coping and adjustment to chronic health conditions, and coping effectiveness training.

Rhonda Galbally, AO, BEc, DipEd, D.SC (h.c.)
Australian International Health Institute, The University of Melbourne, Melbourne, Victoria, 3010, Australia

Rhonda Galbally, AO, BEc, DipEd (Monash University, Melbourne), D.SC (h.c.), La Trobe University, is Managing Director, Australian International Health Institute, The University of Melbourne (AIHI). The AIHI is the Australian Institute developing leadership programs for equity-based health reform. It is the hub for the Bill and Melinda Gates Foundation's child vaccination program for South East Asia. Rhonda is the Independent Chair of the Review of Drugs, Poisons and Controlled Substances Legislation; Technical Advisor/Consultant to the World Health Organization and the World Bank and Trustee of the Lance Reichstein Foundation since 1985. She was previously the founding CEO of Victorian Health Promotion Foundation 1988–1997. In that role she led the development of the strategy for mental health promotion. Other roles played by Rhonda include Trustee of the National Gallery of Victoria 1985–1995; Founding Director of Commission for the Future 1985–1988 and Executive Director of the Myer Foundation and the Sidney Myer Fund 1982–1985.

John P. Garofalo, PhD
UPCI—Behavioral Medicine, 405 Iroquois Bldg, 3600 Forbes Ave., Suite 405, Pittsburgh, PA 15213, USA

John P. Garofalo is an Assistant Professor at the University of Pittsburgh. He obtained his Bachelor of Arts in Psychology at the University of Wisconsin (1991) and his PhD in Clinical Psychology from the University of Texas Southwestern Medical Center at Dallas (1997). The majority of Dr Garofalo's research is conducted at the University of Pittsburgh Cancer Institute. His main areas of interest include psychological adjustment in medical populations, psychological comorbidity, quality of life in cancer populations, and adherence to medical treatment.

Mal Hopwood, BS, MB
Department of Psychiatry, Austin & Repatriation Medical Centre, Repatriation Campus, Banksia Street, Heidelberg West, Victoria 3081, Australia

Dr Hopwood is currently Director of the Austin and Repatriation Medical Centre Statewide Brain Disorders Program and Veterans Psychiatry Unit. He obtained his MB, BS from the University of Melbourne (1986) and his Doctor of Medicine from the same institution (1998). He became a member of the Royal Australian and New Zealand College of Psychiatrists in 1993. His clinical and research areas of interest are neuropsychiatric disorders including the psychiatric aspects of Acquired Brain Injury, Mood and Anxiety disorders, particularly Post Traumatic Stress and Disorder.

David J. de L. Horne, BA (Hons), MPhil, PhD
Department of Psychology, Charles Connibere Building, Royal Melbourne Hospital, Parkville, Victoria 3052, Australia

David James de Lancy Horne is Associate Professor and Reader in Medical Psychology at The University of Melbourne. He obtained his BA (Hons) in psychology from The University of Adelaide (1963); his MPhil from The University of London, at The Institute of Psychiatry (1968); and his PhD from The University of Melbourne (1974). He holds an academic/clinical position at The Royal Melbourne Hospital and has been there for over 30 years. His interests and expertise include neuropsychology, the psychology of coping with medical and surgical procedures, cognitive-behaviour therapy for anxiety and depression following traumatic accidents, and teaching medical and other health-care students about the relevance of psychology to their own professional and clinical work.

Jack E. James, BSc (Hons), PhD
Department of Psychology, National University of Ireland, Galway, Newcastle Road, Galway, Ireland

Jack James is Professor and Head of the Department of Psychology at the National University of Ireland, Galway, where he has been since 1998. He completed a BSc (Applied Psychology) degree with First Class Honours at the University of New South Wales in 1971 and a Masters degree in clinical psychology at the same University. In 1976, he completed a PhD on the clinical management of stuttering at the University of Western Australia. Subsequently, he held academic appointments in the Psychology Departments of the University of Queensland and Flinders University. During the 1980s, his teaching and research activities broadened to include the emerging specialisms of behavioural medicine and health psychology. In 1991, he was appointed Foundation Professor of Behavioural Health Sciences at La Trobe University, and in 1997, he was elected Founding National Chair of the College of Health Psychologists of the Australian Psychological Society. His main academic interests are in the fields of applied behaviour analysis and health psychology. Currently, his research is mainly in the field of cardiovascular behavioural health, with specific reference to the effects of habitual caffeine consumption on blood pressure and cognitive performance, stress-induced patterns of hemodynamic reactivity, and the moderating influences of social support on psychophysiological responses to stress.

Caren Jordan
University of Florida, Department of Clinical & Health Psychology, PO Box 100165, Gainesville, FL 32610-0165, USA

Caren Jordan is a Doctoral Candidate in the Department of Clinical and Health Psychology at the University of Florida Health Science Center. Her interests include the psychological aspects of women's reproductive health from both clinical and research viewpoints.

Paul Kennedy, BSc Hons, MSc, DPhil, FBPsS

Department of Clinical Psychology, Stoke Mandeville Hospital, Mandeville Road, Aylesbury, Buckinghamshire HP21 8AL, UK

Dr. Paul Kennedy gained his Honours degree (BSc) in Psychology at the University of Ulster and completed his Clinical Psychology training (MSc) at Queen's University, Belfast. In 1995 he was awarded his DPhil by the University of Ulster for his research into the behavioural, emotional and coping aspects of spinal cord injury.

His first post was at the Royal National Orthopaedic Hospital, London in 1984. He moved to the National Spinal Injuries Centre, Stoke Mandeville Hospital in 1988, where he now works in a part-time capacity as Consultant Clinical Psychologist. He is also Academic Director on the Oxford Doctoral course in Clinical Psychology.

Dr Kennedy has published widely on the psychological aspects associated with spinal cord injury and chronic conditions. His main research themes include: adjustment and coping following spinal cord injury; chronic pain; self-harm; rehabilitation and goal planning; coping effectiveness training; and post traumatic stress disorder.

Stan Maes, PhD

Clinical, Health and Personality Psychology, Faculty of Social & Behavioural Sciences, Rijks University, Pieter de la Court Building, Wassenaarseweg 52, Leiden, The Netherlands

Stan Maes is Professor in Health Psychology at Leiden University, the Netherlands, and Dean of the Faculty of Social and Behavioural Sciences. He studied psychology and educational sciences, obtaining a doctor's degree in 1976 at Ghent State University (Belgium). He has held academic positions at Ghent State University, at Antwerp University, and at Tilburg University in the Netherlands (1981–1990) where he became Professor in Health Psychology, the first such chair outside the US. He was co-founder and first president of the European Health Psychology Society (1986–1992), is president of the Health Psychology Division of the International Association of Applied Psychology and since 1998 president of the International Society on Health Psychology Research. He is co-editor of two health psychology journals and editorial board member of eight others. He is author of over 150 scientific publications and five books concerning health promotion in school and work settings, doctor–patient communication and psychological aspects and interventions in chronic diseases. His current work focuses on developing a new model for predicting health behaviour and extending traditional stress coping models applied to chronic illnesses. He specializes in coronary heart disease, asthma and chronic obstructive pulmonary diseases.

Paul R. Martin, DipClinPsych, DPhil
School of Psychology, University of New England, Armidale, NSW 2351, Australia

Paul R. Martin is Professor of Psychology and Head of the School of Psychology at the University of New England. He is also Director of Scientific Affairs of the Australian Psychological Society and was National President of the Australian Behaviour Modification Association. He has previously held positions in the University of Oxford, Monash University and the University of Western Australia, including being Director of the Adoption Research and Counselling Service at the latter university. Authored and edited books include *Clinical Psychology* (with J.S. Birnbrauer), *Psychological Management of Chronic Headaches*, *Handbook of Behavior Therapy and Psychological Science*, and *Treating Postnatal Depression* (with J. Milgrom and L. Negri). In addition to his research and teaching roles, he is a practicing clinical and health psychologist.

Peter E. Nathan, AB, PhD
Department of Psychology, The University of Iowa, 11 Seashore Hall E, Iowa City, Iowa 52242-1407, USA

Peter E. Nathan is University of Iowa Foundation Distinguished Professor of Psychology. He obtained the PhD in Clinical Psychology from Washington University (1962) and the AB in Social Relations from Harvard College (1957). He has been at the University of Iowa for 10 years, first as Provost for six years, more recently as a member of the Department of Psychology. Prior to that, he spent 20 years at Rutgers University, in the Department of Psychology and as Director of the Center of Alcohol Studies. His research interests have focused on the etiology, course, and treatment of alcoholism, syndromal diagnosis and decision-making, and empirically supported treatments for psychopathology.

Michael K. Nicholas, MSc (Hons), MPsychol, PhD
Pain Management and Research Centre, Royal North Shore Hospital, St Leonards, NSW 2065, Australia

Michael Kenneth Nicholas is a Senior Lecturer in the Department of Anaesthesia and Pain Management at the University of Sydney, based at the Royal North Shore Hospital, Sydney. He has been working in the pain field since 1980 as a clinical psychologist, educator, and researcher. His PhD, from the University of Sydney, was based on an evaluation of cognitive behavioural treatment for low back pain. Between 1988 and 1990 Michael was the inaugural director of the inpatient pain management program (INPUT) at St Thomas' Hospital in London where he and his colleagues developed and evaluated an intensive program for people with persisting pain. Michael took up his present position in 1994 after three years of post-graduate teaching in clinical psychology at the University of New South Wales. Since then he has established and continues to direct the multidisciplinary ADAPT pain management program and he remains heavily involved in clinical, teaching and research activities. To date, Michael has published over 30 papers in books and scientific journals on the management of pain. He has lectured on the field in Australia and internationally and is a founding member of the faculty for the postgraduate degree and diploma courses on pain management conducted at the University of Sydney.

Nick Paoletti, MB BS, DPM, MPH FRANZCP, MRCPsych

Consultation-Liaison Psychiatry, Austin & Repatriation Medical Centre, Austin Campus, Studley Road, Heidelberg West, Victoria 3084, Australia

Nick Paoletti is Principal Fellow/Associate Professor in the Department of Psychiatry at The University of Melbourne. He obtained his MB BS (1973) and DPM (1979), both from The University of Melbourne. In 1979, he also obtained Membership of the Royal Australian and New Zealand College of Psychiatrists (MRANZCP) and he was elected to Fellowship (FRANZCP) in 1983. In 2000, he became a Member of the Royal College of Psychiatrists in the United Kingdom (MRCPsych). He holds a Master of Public Health (MPH–Clinical Epidemiology) at Monash University, Melbourne. He holds the clinical positions of Head of Consultation-Liaison Psychiatry and Head of the Drug Dependence Clinic at the Austin & Repatriation Medical Centre, Melbourne. His interests and expertise include depression in the medically ill, delirium, somatization, psychosomatic medicine, drug dependence, anorexia nervosa, post-partum disorders and transcultural psychiatry. He is an enthusiast of evidence-based medicine/psychiatry. He is actively involved in teaching and supervision, both at undergraduate and postgraduate levels.

Ellen Redinbaugh, MA, PhD

University of Pittsburgh School of Medicine, 3600 Forbes Ave. Suite 405, Pittsburgh, PA 15213, USA

Ellen Redinbaugh is a research instructor at the University of Pittsburgh's School of Medicine. She obtained her Bachelor of Music degree from Baldwin Wallace College (1982), and she worked for several years as a music therapist before initiating her graduate work in clinical psychology (MA 1991 from Cleveland State University; PhD 1996 from Ohio State University). Dr. Redinbaugh holds a clinical appointment at the University of Pittsburgh Medical Center where she provides behavioral medicine interventions for patients and families enrolled in the Palliative Care Service. Her research interests include stress, coping, family caregiving, and palliative care.

Steven Schwartz, BA, MSc, PhD

Murdoch University, Murdoch, WA. 6150, Australia

Steven Schwartz is Vice Chancellor and President of Murdoch University, Perth, Western Australia. He obtained his BA in psychology from the City University of New York in 1967 and his MSc and PhD in clinical psychology from Syracuse University in 1970 and 1971, respectively. He has held academic positions at the University of Texas, The University of Queensland and was Executive Dean of Medicine and Dentistry at the University of Western Australia. He is a fellow of the Academy of Social Sciences in Australia and has held fellowships from WHO, NATO, the Royal Society, and the Australian Academy of Science. His interests and expertise include clinical psychology, cost-effectiveness analysis, and medical decision-making. He is the author of 12 books and more than 100 scientific articles and has received more than $1 million in research grants and prizes.

Lucio Sibilia, MD

*Neurology and Psychiatry Department of Clinical Sciences, Università degli Studi di Roma "La Sapienza",
Policlinico Umberto I - 00161 ROMA (Italy)*

Lucio Sibilia is Confirmed Researcher and Reader in Psychiatry at the Department of Clinical Sciences of the University of Roma "La Sapienza". He obtained his degree in Medicine at the University of Roma "La Sapienza" (1972); his Specialty Diploma in Neurology and Psychiatry at the same University, Clinic of Nervous and Mental Diseases (1975). He has held his academic position since 1981. His research interests are concentrated in the Medicine–Psychology interface, with particular focus on conceptual models in psychiatry, effectiveness of psychotherapy, doctor–patient interaction, risk perception, and the applications of cognitive-behavioural assessment and intervention methods in prevention and reduction of chronic diseases, psychosocial risk factors for cardiovascular diseases, such as stress and stress management.

Bruce S. Singh, MB, BS (Syd), FRACP, FRANZCP, PhD

Department of Psychiatry, The University of Melbourne, Melbourne, Victoria 3084, Australia

Bruce S. Singh is Cato Professor and Head of the Department of Psychiatry of the University of Melbourne since 1991; Associate Dean (International), Faculty of Medicine, Western Health Care Network Mental Health Program since 1996. He has been Foundation Professor of Psychological Medicine, Royal Park and Alfred Hospitals, Co-director of the NHMRC Schizophrenia Research Unit, Chief Policy Adviser to the Health Department of Victoria Psychiatric Services, Chairman of the Fellows Board of the RANZCP. He was NHMRC Travelling Fellow in Clinical Science at Rochester University NY and Kellogg Travelling Fellow in Medical

Education at Maudsley Hospital, London. His publications include *Foundations of Clinical Psychiatry* (S. Bloch, coeditor) and *Understanding Troubled Minds* (with S. Bloch).

Susan Stollings, PhD
UPCI–Behavioral Medicine, 405 Iroquois Bldg, 3600 Forbes Ave., Suite 405, Pittsburgh, PA 15213, USA

Susan Roberta Stollings is a Senior Clinician in Behavioral Medicine and Oncology at the University of Pittsburgh Cancer Institute (UPCI). She obtained a BA in psychology from Chatham College (1988) and a PhD in Counselling Psychology from the University of Pittsburgh (1997). She then completed a post-doctoral fellowship at UPCI. Her interests include psychosocial interventions for cancer patients, smoking cessation, and post-traumatic growth.

James Strain, MD
731 Ladd Road, Riverdale, NY 10471, USA

James J. Strain is Professor and Director of the Division of Behavioral Medicine and Consultation Psychiatry at the Mount Sinai School of Medicine (New York City) and a former chairperson of ethics at that Institution. He received his medical degree from Case Western Reserve University School of Medicine and did his postgraduate training in psychiatry at University Hospitals of Cleveland, and the New York Psychoanalytic Institute. He has been President of the Society of Liaison Psychiatry and the first recipient of the Outstanding Award for Contributions to that subdiscipline. He is Chairman of the MICROCARES Consultation-Liaison Consortium for computerized data management systems and international collaborative studies. Dr Strain was awarded three National Institutes of Mental Health Contracts to develop a taxonomy of mental health training programs for primary care house officers. He has been involved in cost-offset evaluations for psychiatric interventions in the medical setting. His chapter provides information of how to access the novel MICROCARES systems and details of its assistance in clinical database management, and assembling literature databases at the interface of psychiatry and medicine.

Diane Thompson, BA, MD
Western Psychiatric Institute and Clinic, Rm 141A, 3811 O'Hara St., Pittsburgh, PA 15213, USA

Diane S. Thompson is an Assistant Professor at Western Psychiatric Institute and Clinic, Medical Director of Behavioral Health at Magee-Women's Hospital and Medical Director of Behavioral Medicine Clinical Services and the University of Pittsburgh Cancer Institute. She obtained her BA from Washington and Jefferson

College in Washington, PA and her medical degree at Wright State School of Medicine in Dayton, Ohio. She completed a psychiatric residency at Western Psychiatric Institute and Clinic and finished a fellowship in women's issues in psychiatry during her last year of residency. She is board certified and has been in her current position for over three years. Her interests and expertise include the treatment of medically ill patients, women's issues in psychiatry, drug metabolism and psycho-oncology. She is engaged in several research projects and enjoys working with medical students and residents who are involved in her clinical rotations at Magee-Women's Hospital.

Thérèse van Elderen, PhD
Leiden University, The Netherlands

Thérèse van Elderen is Associate Professor in Health Psychology at Leiden University in the Netherlands. Her interests and expertise include psychosocial aspects of coronary heart disease, evaluation of psycho-educational programmes for coronary heart patients and the development of screening instruments.

Murray Wright, MBBS, FRANZCP
Pain Management and Research Centre, Royal North Shore Hospital, St Leonards, NSW 2065, Australia

Murray Wright is a Senior Staff Specialist in Consultation–Liaison Psychiatry at Royal North Shore Hospital in Sydney, and is also a conjoint Senior Lecturer in the Faculty of Medicine at The University of Sydney. He obtained his MBBS from the University of Sydney in 1981, and his FRANZCP in 1990. His interests include the management of psychiatric co-morbidity in people with medical conditions, particularly those with spinal injuries, traumatic brain injuries, and other conditions associated with chronic pain. Other interests include medical education, rural mental health service delivery, and impairment among health practitioners.

Forewords

TEAMWORK IN TODAY'S HEALTH CARE ENVIRONMENT— OVERLAPPING TRADITIONS OF LIAISON-PSYCHIATRY AND HEALTH PSYCHOLOGY

Frederick K. Goodwin
George Washington University, Washington DC, USA

In the broadest terms, this book addresses the ongoing struggle underway in our increasingly complex, mechanized, depersonalized, bureaucratic, and fragmented health care "systems" in the developed world. Fundamentally this uphill struggle is about finding ways to reconcile the fragmented health care in the age of specialization with the unalterable reality that the only justification for the entire enterprise is the well-being of individual patients; individual patients who will always remain a complex mix of psyche and soma.

As the disparate components of health care continue the fragmented approach to patients – as an eye, a liver, an MRI, a kidney, a heart, a tumor, a depression – how does one get and keep the whole person in focus?

In the "good old days" the individual doctor *was* that integration. With little in the way of technology, without modern surgical techniques or pharmacology, the knowledge base was small enough, and the treatment options few enough, that the physician could still be the generalist, dealing with the whole patient as an individual, quite naturally integrating the biomedical and psychosocial.

Today we face a paradox: medicine's stunning progress, its life-saving triumphs, its technological brilliance are all threatening to undermine the very foundation of the whole enterprise—the mission to heal. As sheer technological capacity and skill continue to accelerate, patient satisfaction with their health care continues to slip. Third-party control of the financing of health care further diminishes individual patients by depriving them of control of the health care dollars that ultimately come from them through insurance premiums or taxes.

So the bureaucratic system that has helped to foster this fragmentation is now faced with the consequences—one of which is the staggering cost of ignoring psychological factors in medicine. In the USA, mental health services account for only 10% of total health care cost, but the impact on general health of untreated mental illness and neglected psychological health on general health care costs is enormous. It is especially ironic in an era when we are just beginning to understand many of the complex

links between psyche and soma (the neuroendocrine systems, receptors and modulators shared by the brain and the immune system, etc.), the structure of health care is
making it more difficult to exploit this new knowledge in the service of patient
outcomes. The central player in health care—the physician—is not only too busy
to apply this knowledge at the bedside, but he often lacks the requisite training.

It should be obvious that any improvement in this area will have to involve teamwork. The doctor of the good old days must be replaced by a team. How does one
achieve such teamwork in today's health care environment? Confronting that question is essentially what this book is about. The inspiration for this book is itself a
product of teamwork between a psychiatrist and a psychologist who have woven
together two separate but overlapping traditions—psychosomatic medicine (liaison
psychiatry) and health psychology—each with its own history, traditions, language
and conceptual models.

The usual problem with multi-authored, edited books is the sense one gets of
people from different fields describing the same phenomenon from vastly different
perspectives, applying different terminology and concepts, with little or no effort to
harmonize or even acknowledge the dissonance and overlap.

However, in this book professors Milgrom and Burrows have neatly minimized
this problem by having each chapter co-authored by a psychiatrist and a psychologist, working together at the outset across conceptual and semantic boundaries.
The strategy allows the book to undertake a most challenging goal—to remain a
cohesive whole while covering a very large and disparate area comprehensively.
Professors Milgrom and Burrows pull it off to a remarkable degree.

REFERENCES

Conner M and Norman P: *Predicting Health Behaviour*. Open University Press: Buckingham, 1996.
Fitzpatrick R: Patient satisfaction. In Baum A, Newman S, Weinman J, West R and Mac-
    Manus IC (Eds), *Cambridge Handbook of Psychology, Health and Medicine*. Cambridge University
    Press: Cambridge, 1997.
McGinnis JM and Foege WH: Actual causes of death in the United States. *Journal of the
    American Medical Association*, **270**, 2207–2212, 1993.
Petrie KJ and Weinman, J (Eds): *Perceptions of Health and Illness: Current research and applications*.
    Harwood Academic Press: London, 1997.
Spilker B (Ed): *Quality of Life and Pharmacoeconomics in Clinical Trials*. Lippincott-Raven: Phila-
    delphia, PA, 1996.

A HEALTH PSYCHOLOGY PERSPECTIVE

John Weinman
GKT School of Medicine, University of London, UK

Health psychology is a recently developed field which is concerned with understanding human behaviour in the context of health, illness and health care. It is the

study of the psychological factors which determine how people stay healthy, why they become ill, and how they respond to illness and health care.

There are many reasons for its recent emergence and rapid development. An important background factor is the major change in the nature of health problems in industrialized societies during the twentieth century. Chronic illnesses such as heart disease and cancer have become the leading causes of death, and behavioural factors such as smoking, diet and stress, are now recognized as playing a major role in the aetiology and progression of these diseases (McGinnis & Foege, 1993). At the same time the provision of health care has grown enormously. There is an increased awareness that psychological processes such as good communication are a central ingredient of medical care and that factors such as patient satisfaction (Fitzpatrick, 1997) and quality of life (Spilker, 1996) are key outcomes in evaluating the efficacy of medical interventions.

As health psychology has established itself rapidly, it is still very much an emerging discipline. Greater insights are needed into the ways in which psychological processes can influence health and illness, and more comprehensive models are required to explain all aspects of health and illness behaviour. All of this will result in the increasing use of psychological interventions for preventing and managing health problems and for the effective delivery of health care. As such, this field will no doubt develop at an exciting pace to build on existing approaches, and use new psychological knowledge to improve patient care.

At the present time, health psychology is primarily a disciplinary area of psychology with an emphasis on research into health and illness behaviour. However, many interventions have been developed including those with a prevention focus for healthy individuals, as well as drawing from the field of clinical psychology for ill patients and health-care staff. Many of these are well illustrated in this comprehensive volume. An important sequela has been that this practitioner aspect of health psychology is now being accompanied by specific professional developments, and formal postgraduate training in health psychology is now available in many countries providing skilled graduates in both health promotion and clinical health psychology intervention.

Whilst health psychology has developed over a similar time period to general hospital/liaison psychiatry and shares some common areas of interest, there are some clear differences between these two fields. Liaison psychiatry appears to have retained its primary focus on hospital patients, particularly those experiencing psychological difficulties in the face of a physical health problem. In contrast, health psychology not only offers specialized treatment approaches to ill patients, such as those in pain, but also has a broader focus on both healthy and ill populations and on the psychological processes which influence their level of health or their degree of adaptation to disease. Whereas health psychology has been mainly concerned with developing theoretically-based explanations for health-related (Conner & Norman, 1996) and illness-related behaviour (Petrie & Weinman, 1997), liaison psychiatry has concentrated on the diagnosis and treatment of either unexplained symptoms or psychiatric disorders occurring in people with medical conditions.

This book provides an extensive and impressive account of developments in both health psychology and liaison psychiatry, as well as showing how the two fields link and relate to each other. It succeeds in offering a very comprehensive resource for understanding and intervening in the whole area of psychological aspects of physical health. In providing such a broad overview of the very wide range of clinical problems, contexts and interventions, it will undoubtedly be an invaluable source book not only for established practitioners but also for those entering this exciting and rapidly developing field.

Preface

Plato [427?–347 B.C.]

The cure of many diseases is unknown to the physicians of Hellas, because they are ignorant of the whole, which ought to be studied also; for the part can never be well unless the whole is well ... This ... is the great error of our day in the treatment of the human body, that the physicians separate the soul from the body.

Sir Robert Platt [1900–]

Future generations, paying tribute to the medical advances of our time, will say: "Strange that they never seemed to realize that the real causes of ill-health were to be found largely in the mind ...".

From Strauss MB: *Familiar Medical Quotations.*
Little, Brown & Co: Boston, 1968.

Successive generations have grappled with the mind–body interrelationship, and its relevance to medicine. The new millennium provides an opportunity to review the evolution of this concept and the practical implications that have resulted in the presence of the psychologist and psychiatrist in the medical centre. Whilst there is clearly still much to be desired to achieve an holistic approach to treatment of medical patients, this book describes the current status, exciting advances and the future of "integrated medical practice".

This book was conceived a number of years ago when, as Heads of separate Psychology and Psychiatry Departments in a large teaching hospital, we took stock of the rich interrelationship that had developed between our two disciplines. We were aware that it was uncommon to find psychologists and psychiatrists presenting their perspectives on assessing and treating psychological disorders in the medical setting in the same book. It was even more unusual to compare their respective roles and the complementary ways of working. The relationships and interchanges that have occurred between professionals during the development of this book have reflected the challenge involved in developing a framework which allows the strengths and differences of the two disciplines to combine to provide quality care to patients suffering from a variety of medical disorders. It is hoped that this book will be a stimulus to ongoing development of the joint contribution of psychology and psychiatry to medicine, as well as providing an authoritative text on this subject.

Jeannette Milgrom and Graham Burrows

Acknowledgements

This book would not have been possible without the patience of all contributors, as the evolution of this book was a lengthy, and at times a difficult process. Considerable thought, debate, justification of different positions held and academic research was involved in making explicit a collaborative relationship that has not often been written about: the psychology and psychiatry partnership. In addition, we are deeply indebted to Barbara Frazer and Gertrude Rubinstein who assisted in the manuscript, and never shied from tackling the many and varied demands. Their input has resulted in a text that is more cohesive, carefully referenced and with attention to detail. Our families have also been the quiet support, ready to provide whatever needed – from the stretches of time necessary to the internet reference at the right moment. Finally, this book is a product of the lessons we have learnt from our patients and colleagues as we have traversed the many corridors of the general hospital, and we hope we have captured the tremendous benefits that can arise when psychologists and psychiatrists become centrally involved in medical practice and improving healthcare.

Psychology and Psychiatry in the Medical Centre

Jeannette Milgrom and Graham D. Burrows

Departments of Psychology and Psychiatry, University of Melbourne, and Austin & Repatriation Medical Centre, Melbourne, Australia

INTRODUCTION

The health care system is undergoing dramatic and rapid changes. A number of factors contribute to these changes, and provide unprecedented opportunities for the application of psychology and psychiatry in the Medical Centre. Spiralling expenditure within the health system has placed an emphasis on cost containment and a broader approach to health care. At the same time, there is a growing acceptance of the biopsychosocial model of health and illness, and of the importance of psychosocial and psychopharmacological interventions. Medical practitioners and managers in health care settings are becoming aware of the prospect of using psychological interventions to control runaway health-care costs effectively (Groth-Marnat & Edkins 1996; Strain et al 1994). These interventions include strategies for improving patient adherence to treatment, preparing patients for surgery, and treating disease-specific difficulties, such as chemotherapy-related nausea. The potential benefits of a wider application of the skills of the psychologist and psychiatrist to medical patients are enormous. Up to 60% of physical disorders have been estimated as somatized or with a significant contribution from psychological factors (Ludwigsen & Albright 1994). Behaviourally related problems such as obesity represent about 50% of all consultations with doctors. Furthermore, concomitant psychological symptoms, such as anxiety or depression, and more serious psychiatric co-morbidity increase length of stay in hospitals and result in repeat visits (Saravay & Lavin 1994).

Typical roles for psychologists and psychiatrists in the Medical Centre include direct patient management with a focus on psychological or psychiatric factors affecting medical conditions, supporting staff with difficult patients and/or their

Psychology and Psychiatry: Integrating Medical Practice.
Edited by J. Milgrom and G. D. Burrows © 2001 John Wiley & Sons, Ltd.

own reactions, and addressing behavioural issues that arise in the health setting (e.g. poor information communication). In addition, patterns of illness and deaths are shifting from infectious disease to diseases such as cardiovascular disease, cancer and accidents, which have a significant stress and lifestyle-related component, amenable to psychological intervention. Health promotion is being recognized as a major approach to escalating health costs and increasing the health of the community, providing new opportunities for mental health professionals. Lifestyle management, such as weight reduction, to prevent the onset of or deterioration of medical conditions continues to be the target of novel methods of behaviour change in the community, with input from a variety of professions, including psychiatry and psychology. Intervention at the broader levels of the health care system is also the province of psychologists and psychiatrists through systems intervention, such as influencing policy direction or change management. Growing interest in mechanisms underlying the linkages between health and behaviour also provides important research opportunities for psychologists and psychiatrists to further elucidate the role of psychological factors in the maintenance of health and etiology of illness.

A historical overview of the development of the role of both the clinical health psychologist and the psychiatrist in the Medical Centre is provided in this chapter, to set the context for the following chapters of the book, which describe the state-of-the-art contribution of these two professions to medical practice.

HEALTH PSYCHOLOGY AND CLINICAL HEALTH PSYCHOLOGY

A Historical Perspective

Whilst psychological knowledge has its roots in philosophy, religion and literature, the use of the controlled experiment as a source of data for developing psychological concepts only began in the nineteenth century (Boring 1950). The discipline of psychology has subsequently evolved as the field of scientific study of behaviour and experience. From principles evolved, a professional psychology stream has developed, concerned with assessment and behaviour change. In response to this emphasis in psychology, of careful and specific measurement, a specialty area of "clinical psychology" made its beginning with the introduction of "mental tests". Clinical psychologists were initially limited to testing and educational work with children (Watson 1953, 1965). Albert Binet's intelligence test for children was published in 1905 in Paris and was instrumental in rapidly expanding the field of testing. World War I provided a further need to sort and classify recruits and this challenge was successfully met by psychologists with the development of group intelligence and personality tests. Over the next few years numerous tests appeared, initially in the area of adult intelligence tests and personality (mainly drawing on projective techniques such as Thematic Apperception Tests), but later with a burgeoning of structured and reliable tests of various aspects of functioning. However, despite the growing interest in academic psychology in human motivation, drives, and psychological processes, in response to the works of William James (1890, 1902), Hall (1911) and Sigmund Freud (1953), clinical psychologists early on in the evolution of the profession remained identified and valued mainly as psychodiagnosticians (Hersen et al 1984).

A dramatic change in the role of psychologists occurred with World War II. Thousands of psychological casualties of the war could not be dealt with by the existing mental health personnel. Psychologists, who had been drafted into the armed forces, were often thrust into clinical treatment roles. The United States federal government began hiring more mental health personnel and funding training. The American Psychological Association was asked by the Veterans Administration and the Public Health Service to develop a specialized training programme for clinical psychologists, to provide clinicians capable of treating psychological problems. The resultant 1947 Shakow Report (APA 1947; Shakow 1965), later known as the Boulder Model, has become the blueprint for training ever since, with its recommendation of scientist-practitioner training for psychologists. Ideally, clinical skills of the psychologist, combined with research skills, allow for on-going evaluation of clinical outcome, a critical analysis of new research and an ability to contribute to basic research. There is some debate around the benefits of training clinicians in both areas and the incompatibility of these orientations. The scientist, objective, dispassionate, often has a skeptical approach to the world. The clinician, humane, concerned, desiring to help is often sympathetic, responsive to suffering and distress, and introspective. Nevertheless, the Boulder model of scientist-practitioner predominates and provides the unique identity of the professional psychologist. "Thus far these attributes have been successfully combined to produce a unique, dynamic and vital profession" (Bellack & Hersen 1980).

In the past 50 years the field of professional psychology has expanded into many subspecialties, such as clinical and health psychology (the focus of this book) neuropsychology (see brief overview Chapter 12, but not the focus of this book), forensic psychology, and child psychology. Psychologists have moved from working as psychodiagnosticians, to work in a variety of settings: hospitals, universities, schools, dental schools, family law courts, business and industry, government, labor unions, prisons, private practice and mental health centers.

The Expansion of Clinical Psychology to Medical Settings

As the role of the clinical psychologist broadened, new opportunities and new settings became possibilities for practice. Growing national concern for improved health services led a small number of clinical psychologists to apply their skills and knowledge to the general medical setting. At the same time, health–illness research became a significant area for psychologists. Well-designed studies confirmed the age-old hypothesis of a high prevalence of psychological problems among individuals seeking medical care (Bakal & Kaganov 1977; Olbrisch 1977). Accumulating empirical literature established the role of psychological factors in the etiology, treatment and prevention of physical illness (Engel 1977; Leigh & Reiser 1977; Lipowski 1977a&b; Weiner & Walker 1977). Conferences in Behavioural Medicine and Health Psychology had psychologists as major participants. A number of text-books suggesting that clinical psychology broaden its field from the area of mental health to the medical setting appeared on the market, and suggested potential areas of application (e.g. Rachman & Philips 1975). The American Psychological Associ-ation in 1976 highlighted psychology's role "to encourage an ever-broadening realization that the individual's total functioning is threatened whenever either component of the interactive mind–body equation is impaired" (APA 1976; Sachar 1976). Ways of contributing to this equation increased as clinical psychologists continued to refine psychological interventions by constant evaluation of outcome, leading to a set of strategies and techniques, notably derived from cognitive-behav-ioural therapy, whose effectiveness are now supported by a significant body of literature (Clark & Fairburn 1997; Dobson & Craig 1996).

The Field of Health Psychology

At the same time, the field of health psychology started to develop with formal recognition as a field of specialization with the establishment in 1978 of the Division of Health Psychology (No. 38) within the American Psychological Association. Health psychology was defined as: *the aggregate of the specific educational, scientific, and professional contributions of the discipline of psychology to the promotion and maintenance of health, the prevention and treatment of illness, and the identification of etiologic and diagnostic correlates of health, illness and related dysfunction, and to the analysis and improvement of the health care system and health policy formation* (Matarazzo 1980 p 815). The scope of health psychology is very broad, encompassing both basic and applied research, and most theories and methods of psychology have been applied to health-related topics. Furthermore, health psychology draws from other disciplines such as public health, epidemiology, physiology, medical anthropology, and sociology.

Health psychology provides a rich body of knowledge, with its focus on biological, psychological and social determinants of health and illness. Models of health behaviour and behaviour change are used to explore the psychology of health risk factors, health beliefs and attitudes and concepts such as stress and coping. Epidemi-ological information is used to explore the prevalence of disease and contributing factors. Intervention approaches are broad, covering not only individuals but using health promotion strategies to intervene in communities. Public health marketing, communication, media advocacy, health service planning and consumer behaviour are all of interest in the context of health psychology.

This had led to a broadening of the biopsychosocial perspective of illness, a wellness and health promotion movement, and a great number of health psychology books (e.g. Baum et al 1997; Bernard & Krupat 1994; Sarafino 1994; Sheridan & Radmacher 1992; Taylor 1986).

Clinical Health Psychology

The term "clinical health psychology" describes the specialized field combining knowledge from clinical psychology and health psychology (Milgrom & Hardardottir 1995; Belar 1990). The clinical psychologist is an expert in the application of clinical assessment and treatment skills to change an individual's maladaptive behaviour, thoughts, and emotions. Health psychology provides an expanding knowledge base regarding psychological factors in health and illness within a biological and sociological context.

Historically, a number of competing terms have been used to describe the expanding contributions of psychology to health care, including "psychosomatic medicine", "medical psychology", and "behavioural medicine" (Taylor 1990; Bloom 1988). The term "medical psychology" historically preceded the term "clinical health psychology", but was criticized as old-fashioned, inferring a medical model, and in Great Britain was synonymous with psychiatry (Bishop 1994). Similarly, "behavioural medicine" and "behavioural health" referred more to the interdisciplinary professions, with psychology being but one of a number of contributing disciplines.

Whilst "professional health psychology" was initially proposed to refer to the applied area (Marks 1994), the term "clinical health psychology" is recognized in the United States of America, Europe and Australia and seems to best acknowledge the area where clinical psychology and health psychology overlap and combine to produce a specialty area of practice.

The practice of clinical health psychology is continually expanding, and this book covers current applications including psychological and behavioural strategies to manage:

- Responses to and recovery from physical illness
- Adherence to medical treatment
- Reactions to hospitalization and medical investigations
- Coping with specific health difficulties or medical procedures
- Pain both acute and chronic
- Health risk behaviours
- Concomitant psychological problems in individuals presenting with a medical complaint, and their families (this has traditionally been the domain of the clinical psychologist, e.g. depression)
- Adaptation to terminal illness or disability
- Organizational interactions in a health setting which influence management of a patient
- Provision of psychological guidance, education and training of other health professionals, as well as support for dealing with issues such as death and bereavement.

Additional areas of concern for clinical health psychologists, which were initially the mandate of the broader field of health psychology, include community or organizational interventions and the maintenance of health. Lifestyle behaviours such as smoking, insufficient exercise and diet, are tackled by population-based preventative interventions, which remain the most likely strategy to reduce health costs.

Similarly, clinical health psychologists are increasingly becoming involved in health psychology research to further our understanding of the contribution of psychological factors to disease onset, progression or susceptibility to illness. Health-related psychological research includes attempts to develop theoretical models and understand cognitive processes such as health beliefs, illness perception and perception of risk and attributions which mediate behaviour which influences health status (Sheeran & Abraham 1998; Weinman et al 1996). There is growing evidence for the role of cognitions and factors such as individual differences in personality, self-efficacy and negative affect on health-related outcomes such as pain tolerance, adherence to treatment, utilization of medical services and perhaps even survival. The relationship between individual differences, psychosocial factors, stress, health and disease is also understood to be mediated by and to influence physiological processes. Some of this research is elaborated in Chapter 2.

Central to clinical health psychology is research evaluating the effectiveness of interventions and how to create behaviour change. Despite the incomplete evidence for psychological and social factors associated with health status, psychological interventions in illness have been advocated for targeting outcomes ranging from improvement in quality of life, to delaying disease progression (Hutchinson 1997; Harrison, Mullen & Green 1992).

Current Status

The visibility of clinical health psychologists is still limited and no comprehensive data on their numbers are available. Physicians who are generally aware of the clinical signs that justify a psychiatric consultation are not always certain of the applicable skills of the psychologist. This book is designed to highlight the comparative roles of psychology and psychiatry in the medical centre.

In 1979, Stone et al predicted, "It is a reasonable expectation that in the not too distant future every major health care agency, hospital, extended care facility, or clinic, will include a health care psychologist (or department) on its resident of consultant staff and that this psychologist will be appropriately prepared by education, training and experience to provide clinical, consultative and research skills to the care of its patients." In addition, psychologists were predicted to become increasingly involved in formulation of mental health policy and in administration of health facilities as executive directors or ward administrators in mental hospitals (Fiester 1978). Whilst psychologists are not yet as much an integral part of the medical system as was predicted twenty years ago, hospital departments of psychology are emerging and facilitating the expanding role of psychologists (Milgrom, Nathan & Martin 1996). Particularly in the United States, medical specialties such as oncology are increasingly employing psychologists to be part of the multidisciplinary team. Further development requires psychologists to be better trained in the new field of clinical health psychology and to increase their contribution through health-related research.

CONSULTATION-LIAISON PSYCHIATRY: A HISTORICAL PERSPECTIVE

The Origins

Consultation-liaison (C-L) psychiatry developed as an outgrowth of general hospital psychiatric units, emerging first as a separate discipline in the United States. Schwab (1989), in his historical overview, notes that as early as 1751, the charter of the Pennsylvania Hospital in Philadelphia provided both for the care of indigents and for the treatment of persons disordered in their minds.

In the early 1800s, Pennsylvania Hospital still had its psychiatric wards, and Benjamin Rush, father of American Psychiatry and a signer of the Declaration of Independence, practiced there until the wards were moved in the 1840s to the Philadelphia General Hospital (Schwab 1989). Already in 1811, his published views coincide with the psychosomatic aspect that "... in the eyes of the physician, a patient's soul and body are so united that one cannot be moved, without the other. The actions of the former upon the latter ... are the causes of many diseases" (Rush 1811, cited by Schwab 1989).

The psychosomatic approach is the basis of liaison psychiatry. It is founded on the assumption that human health and disease result from an interaction of biological, psychological and social factors. The focus is on individuals whose psychiatric problems are related to physical illness and disability. Schwab (1989) points out that during the late nineteenth century, there were remarkable changes in medical practice following Lister's discovery of antisepsis, and progress in cellular pathology, bacteriology and surgery. Despite the great achievements of the new scientific medicine, it was also criticized for its loss of humanism. It was in the following decades that C-L psychiatry began, with its emphasis on the importance of the individual, together with his or her behaviour and environment, rather than on the illness alone.

When psychiatry was confined to the asylum, it was isolated from mainstream medicine (Lipowski 1992). This isolation was reduced as the early years of the twentieth century saw an increasing formation of psychiatric units in general hospitals. Moreover, as more psychiatry was taught in medical schools, research began to occur at the border between psychiatry and general medicine.

Development of Psychosomatic Medicine and C-L Psychiatry

Several principles still fundamental to C-L psychiatry were enunciated by Mosher (1909, cited by Schwab 1989). Among others, he noted that psychiatric consultations with other specialties in the general hospital could fill a need in treating mental symptoms which may complicate medical and surgical disease, as well as helping psychiatric patients, many of whom have physical abnormalities (Sweeney 1962).

Further development of psychosomatic medicine in the early years of the twentieth century came not from within the biomedical establishment, but from the psychodynamic approach of Sigmund Freud and the reaction to life stress approach of Adolph Meyer (Engel 1977).

Meyer's ideas were taken up by two of his students, George Henry, who published the first paper to appear on C-L psychiatry (Henry 1929), and Helen Flanders Dunbar who initiated research on the psychological aspects of physical illness. Flanders Dunbar's book published in 1943 presented the results of 12 years' research and clinical investigation at Columbia University, New York. Flanders Dunbar pointed out that while infectious disease still dominated medical teaching, diseases of unknown causes were responsible for increasing chronicity, disability and mortality. To confront this problem, basic concepts of a different type were needed in medical teaching. She commented that the question is not whether the basis of disease is physical or psychic, but how much is physical and how much psychic. Henry noted that while general physicians were insufficiently educated in emotional problems, consultant psychiatrists often overlooked the medical aspects of their patients' illnesses. Schwab (1989) in his fine overview of the history of C-L psychiatry, comments that Henry's case vignettes still remain worthwhile reading.

Starting in the early 1930s, university hospitals featured C-L educational programs. In 1936 Billings, in his paper "Teaching psychiatry in the medical school general hospital: a practical plan", outlined the obligations of the C-L psychiatrist in regard to his own role, to other physicians and to the patient.

Whereas to most psychoanalysts, psychosomatic disease was of only marginal interest, Franz Alexander was convinced that the exploration of the human mind should lead to more fulfilling lifestyles. In his opinion, the notion of mind–body interaction had a long history, from Descartes right back to Hippocrates. But the first really fundamental understanding came from the work of Breuer and Freud (1955). They stated that "specific unconscious events could be symbolically expressed in the 'body language' of somatic symptoms." This opened a new era in the scientific approach to psychogenesis in somatic illness (Alexander et al 1968, p 1). The research of Alexander and his colleagues over 14 years (1951–1965) at the Chicago Institute for Psychoanalysis provided a basis for early concepts of the specificity of psychosomatic diseases such as peptic ulcer (Alexander et al 1968). Alexander became President of the American Society for Research in Psychosomatic Medicine, and was one of the founding authors of the *Journal of Psychosomatic Medicine* in 1939.

During World War II the status of psychiatry advanced as psychiatrists worked alongside their medical colleagues with the armed forces. On the experimental side, the work of Cannon (1932) and later of Selye (1946) demonstrated how the intangible, stress, was clearly seen to produce physical changes in the body. As the concept of stress became popularized in the postwar decades, the psychosomatic concept expanded, and with it C-L psychiatry developed further.

Engel in 1967 published three papers on the psychosomatic approach to medicine and his experience with teaching this approach at the University of Rochester (Engel 1967a, b, c). A psychoanalytic aspect still prevailed, as most of the interns at whom the course was directed had some psychoanalytical training. Later Engel challenged the reductionistic approach to medicine with an influential article in the journal *Science*. He coined the term "biopsychosocial", a comprehensive approach to the treatment of the patient, which included physical, emotional and environmental aspects (Engel 1977).

C-L programs increased in number so that by 1966 Mendel reported that 75% of 202 psychiatry training sites provided C-L training. During the 1970s, The American Board of Psychiatry and Neurology made C-L training a requirement for residency accreditation. Over this period, a C-L team began to function in major medical centres; the team initially consisted usually of a psychiatrist, trainees, a psychiatric nurse and a social worker (Schwab 1989).

Funding for C-L programs by the National Institute for Mental Health in the 1970s stimulated expansion of C-L programs, but this was discontinued in 1985. In 1992 Noyes et al investigated the current status of C-L psychiatry. They reported that although 30–60% of patients admitted to general hospitals had notable psychiatric disorders, only 1% were currently being seen (Lipowski 1967; Strain 1982). Noyes et al noted that more C-L psychiatrists were needed to deal with the more difficult problems. This was unfortunate, not only from the humane aspect, but also "in view of the evidence that psychiatric consultation reduces morbidity, shortens length of stay, and decreases the cost of hospitalization." (Levitan & Kornfeld 1981; Cassem & Hackett 1983; Strain et al 1991). Lipowski, also writing in 1992, pointed out the dramatic development of C-L psychiatry over the final decades of the twentieth century.

Lipowski (1986) defined C-L psychiatry as the subspecialty of psychiatry concerned with clinical service, teaching, and research in non-psychiatric health-care settings, its main objective being to enhance the overall quality of patient care by taking into account all the psychosocial aspects of the patient. The chapters in this volume describes how the C-L team helps to achieve an optimal health-care program, and how the addition of the psychologist to the medical centre further enhances this development.

Collaborative Opportunities: The Experience of a Consultation-Liaison Psychiatry Team and a Medical Psychology Service in a General Hospital

The Austin Repatriation Medical Centre (formerly the Austin Hospital) in Melbourne, Australia is a 680-bed teaching hospital, treating approximately 66 800 patients per annum. A number of specialist units exist, one of which is for patients with acute traumatic spinal cord injuries. Patients are generally admitted within 24 hours of their injury and remain in the unit for their acute treatment and rehabilitation, and are then discharged to the community. A psychosocial team meets regularly and has a mixed membership consisting of consultant and trainees of the medical staff, psychiatry, clinical and health psychology, social work, chaplaincy and home-visiting nurses. All new patients are seen by the liaison psychiatrist/registrar and/or the psychologist at the earliest opportunity, generally within a week of admission. This assessment aims to identify individuals with major psychiatric disorder who require specific psychiatric intervention, and to determine each individual's personality and coping style in order to identify individuals' strengths and vulnerabilities, and which individuals are at particular risk (Judd & Brown 1992).

Following the initial assessment, patients identified as needing specific psychiatric treatment continue to be seen by the liaison psychiatrist. Patients with recognized vulnerabilities are individually followed up by other members of the psychosocial team, usually the social worker or psychologist.

Spinal cord injury may produce both immediate and long-term stress and disability. The role of the psychiatrist and psychologist is to deal with the problems of the patient, the family and the medical team. Problems which occur may be exacerbated by psychological difficulties (Judd & Burrows 1986). The psychosocial team at the Austin and Repatriation General Hospital was first established in 1985, and since then the psychological care of patients has progressively expanded. The experience of the team emphasizes that psychological health is an integral part of medical care in such a unit. Affective disorder is the most common psychiatric diagnosis, but a number of other disorders are also identified (Judd & Brown 1992).

The benefits of a collaboration between psychology and psychiatry and the formation of a therapeutic alliance with medical practitioners, nurses and other allied health professionals are further expanded in Chapter 4. Multidisciplinary issues are dealt with in Chapter 12.

THE AIM OF THIS BOOK: INTEGRATING MEDICAL PRACTICE

The scope of this book is to clarify the increasingly wide-ranging influence of psychology and psychiatry in a medical setting. It is expected that, in the near future, psychology and psychiatry will be considered essential for integrated medical practice. Medical students who routinely now have a behavioural science component in their curricula, and residents who are often taught by psychologists and psychiatrists in the evaluation and treatment of emotional components of illness, will have a better understanding of their role. In addition, if there is to be sound growth in this field, there must be provision for innovations in the standard training. Training must keep up with the rapidly expanding field of knowledge, seizing opportunities for new applications and evaluating outcome.

The contributions of clinical health psychology and psychiatry to health care have developed independently. This book provides a unique comparison of the rapidly growing practice of clinical health psychology and psychiatry in the medical centre and the complementary nature of this partnership. Both professionals contribute information and strategies to assist other clinicians to recognize and deal with psychological problems in medical settings. Various chapters highlight what specific expertise to expect when referring to the psychologist and the psychiatrist, common professional issues, and differences in areas of specialization. The book aims to provide information on behavioural, psychological and psychiatric aspects of health and illness and how physicians can work together to maximize synergistic mind–body processes and improve quality of life for individuals and families. This combination is a powerful impetus for developing a holistic model of health care. The book is likely to be helpful not only to medical practitioners but to practicing psychologists or psychiatrists in the medical centre and their students, other health professionals, and to hospital administrative colleagues.

It is anticipated that health-care facilities will benefit from the services provided by psychologists and psychiatrists in several ways. Firstly, they provide an opportunity to implement strategies derived from our biopsychosocial understanding of illness to improve the health of individuals. In 1997 the World Health Organization called for a new alliance between physical and social/psychological disciplines (Camic & Knight 1998), and the application of the knowledge emerging from this interface. Secondly, psychologists and psychiatrists will relieve medical practitioners of part of their demanding clinical commitments. As it has been estimated that about half the burden of illness has a psychological component, this relief can be substantial. Thirdly, medical practitioners will have available to them cognitive behavioural therapies for problems such as pain, sleep disorders and anxiety, as well as expert advice on appropriate psychotropic treatment, which can be helpful either alone or in combination with each other. Fourthly, health bills are likely to be cut drastically. Many of the problems which psychologists and psychiatrists can treat with non-physical methods are still taken to the physician, who has traditionally paid less attention to these problems. The problem is often not solved after consultation with the physician, the patient keeps coming back, and the bill keeps mounting. Furthermore, it has long been demonstrated that hospital attendances and length of stay can be reduced by helping this group of patients develop coping skills for situations where they currently do not function effectively (Milgrom et al 1994; Sank & Shapiro 1979; Kiesler et al 1979; Groth-Marnat & Edkins 1996; Vandenbos et al 1981).

Another source of cost reduction relates to the concept of preventive intervention. As early as 1974 the Canadian Minister of National Health and Welfare stated "vast sums are being spent on treating diseases that could have been prevented in the first place" (Lalonde 1974; Viney 1983). Today this is clearer than ever, as it is now recognized that ischaemic heart disease, lung cancer, respiratory diseases and suicide account for a sizeable proportion of morbidity and mortality rates, and that there are elements in the lifestyle of many people such as heavy smoking, high levels of anxiety, overeating, and alcohol addiction which contribute to the risk of death from these conditions, and which can be modified by psychological treatment. Preventive intervention does not result in immediately visible outcomes because the goals are long-term. However, funding for health promotion using psychological approaches to change maladaptive behaviours should be considered of at least equal importance to the funding of individual treatment in health-care systems (although Chapter 10 highlights the controversies in this area).

Finally, and perhaps most importantly, a psychological emphasis will help to restore part of the human interest that has been drained away by technological advances. Complex technology has been mastered but insufficient attention has been spent on integrating these procedures with the person's experience, as he or she is subjected to these "advances". It is hoped that the concept of care for the person will modify the current excessive concern with physical ailments found in many medical settings. The Australian Royal Commission on Human Relationships noted many years ago that: "heavily bureaucratized systems can have a generally dehumanizing influence on those who contact them" (Evatt 1977). Unfortunately, in the past, as today, governments have tended to focus on economic factors rather than human dignity in the area of health care. Growing pressure on the health dollar results in the risk of reverting back to treating only "visible" medical complaints, and ignoring the emotional experience of the patient.

Psychology and psychiatry have a major role to play in the health system to redress this balance. In this age of continued specialization and technological advances the relevance of human factors in health care increases rather than decreases. The emotional care of patients remains a neglected domain in medicine, and psychologists and psychiatrists have a lot to offer to maximize recovery from illness and maintain health.

An Overview of the Book

The following chapters begin with our theoretical understanding of mind–body relationships and take the reader carefully through a thorough exposition of the practice of psychology and psychiatry in the medical centre.

Chapter 2 provides a learned review of biopsychosocial influences on illness. It describes the mounting evidence for the effect of psychosocial factors such as socioeconomic status, stress, depression and anxiety on outcome, not only in terms of well-being but disease incidence and progression. Importantly, it highlights the lifestyle behaviours linked with major causes of mortality (e.g. cardiovascular disease and cancer). Effects of intervention are reviewed and cover both psychological treatment once illness has occurred and the critical role of prevention to maximize impact (this is further covered in Chapter 10). Psychological theories are presented, particularly those concerned with explaining health risk behaviour. This chapter includes a detailed account of biobehavioural mediators of disease, heralding a new era of collaborative research as we advance in our understanding of the underlying mechanisms linking psychological factors to illness.

Chapter 3 addresses methods of assessment, followed by consideration of the targets of assessment, and integration of the information. Goals can be directed towards prevention, treatment, or the promotion of coping. The focus of assessment is described as ideally based on assets and strengths of the patient and his/her environment, as well as the identification of problems. A two-way process occurs with the referring service, and where a medical cause of psychiatric illness is suspected, further tests are discussed with the referring team. The psychiatrist takes into account presenting symptoms in the context of an understanding of the physical illness and is careful to note medications being taken in order to avoid drug interactions. The psychologist can offer a range of psychometric methods which are relevant both to psychiatric populations and medico-surgical ones, and guidelines on their usage are provided. Common assessment approaches (e.g. interview methods) are covered and interventions including the pharmaceutical and psychological are dealt with in detail. Finally, the importance of the biopsychosocial model for integrative care is highlighted, as are unaddressed patient needs as suggested by the estimated prevalence of psychological disorder in medical populations, compared to low reported referral rates.

In the first part of Chapter 4, the consultation-liaison (C-L) psychiatrist describes the evolution of C-L psychiatry for managing medical and surgical patients with psychiatric symptoms, from the historical antecedents to recent developments. Their central role is substantiated by the epidemiology of psychiatric morbidity in medical populations reflecting high utilization of medical services by this population, financial burden, and profound resulting physical impairment. Next the stages of arriving at a diagnosis and the associated problems are covered. Several C-L models of mental health training to promote improvement in the pattern of health care provided by primary care professionals for the population under study are discussed.

An extensive information resource list of software applications is provided, giving the C-L psychiatrist access to data to help in decision-making. A comprehensive C-L psychiatry literature database is also available, together with software for providing access to it. Next are listed guidelines for C-L psychiatry sponsored by the United States Department of Health and Human Services, Public Health Service, Agency for Health Care Policy and Research (AHCPR), and the Cochrane database of systematic reviews, which should be useful in clinical decision-making by C-L personnel.

The psychologist's commentary in the second part of the chapter begins with issues of interest to psychologists practicing in a C-L setting, to their health colleagues and to the patients at the receiving end of their care. Problems of clinician–patient communication outlined in the previous section are discussed in greater detail. Psychology has much to teach about interpersonal skills in communication, and this is now an essential part of medical education in many countries. Factors in compliance and adherence to treatment are also considered. The psychologist has procedures for improving adherence as well as dealing with medical anxieties and phobias which can minimize stresses in both patients and clinicians and improve medical treatment. Lastly, preparing patients for invasive medical and surgical procedures can help achieve a favourable outcome, both in terms of well-being and use of medical resources.

A concluding section by both the psychiatrist and the psychologist covers the desirability of having both professionals on the treating team to conduct conjoint evaluation of the patient, implement treatment, and conduct conjoint research. A further list of available resources completes the chapter.

Pain is ubiquitous in medicine. Chapter 5 provides an important review of the application of psychological strategies of choice in overcoming clinical pain problems. Differences in the roles of clinical psychologists and psychiatrists in the assessment and management of these problems are outlined, with the implications for clinical practice.

Models of pain are described, together with their implications for treatment. Assessment will identify psychological factors, and target treatment goals, with special attention to comorbidity which may contribute to disability. Tests and questionnaires selected for use cover varied domains of interest, since pain is a multidimensional phenomenon. A list is given of appropriate instruments with established psychometric properties to cover these domains. Options for treatment are provided, followed by a brief discussion of the use of antidepressant medication in chronic pain management. Psychological treatments are covered at greater length, with evidence for their utility; this appears strongest for cognitive-behavioural techniques. The relationship between pain and depression is discussed, and the need for formulating causal hypotheses to aid in planning intervention. There is special reference to treatment of the severely depressed patient. As the treatment setting may be multidisciplinary or interdisciplinary, in a group setting or with individual patients, professional issues and the dynamics of teamwork are considered. In conclusion, a case history is used to illustrate methods used in the authors' pain clinic.

Cancer is a leading cause of death and is accompanied by significant suffering. Behavioral medicine has provided an important contribution to the role of psychology in evolving medical treatments in prevention, early detection, treatment, and palliative care in cancer patients and this is considered in Chapter 6. Psychological evaluation and treatment are discussed; early psychosocial intervention permits more effective coping with the stressful demands of surgery and/or adjuvant treatment that may be required and minimizes the likelihood of future psychiatric morbidity. The role of the psychologist in the oncology team includes patient care programs, consulting on treatment compliance issues and supporting staff, while the C-L psychiatrist addresses the interface of psychological and medical issues experienced by oncology patients. Treatments may include pharmacotherapy as well as psychotherapy, and management of psychiatric emergencies that may arise. A case history is presented to illustrate some of the complexities of mental health intervention with cancer patients. Although patients prefer to die at home, their medical care places a burden on the family. The palliative care model described in this chapter is an example of the benefits of integrated behavioral and medical care accomplished by interdisciplinary treatment teams.

An important final objective is primary prevention, tailored towards risk factors for disease. This includes educating medical practitioners about cancer risk factors and training health-care providers in cancer-prevention strategies.

Three areas have been chosen in Chapter 7 to illustrate psychological factors associated with adjustment, impact and treatment in a person who has become disabled. The first examines emotional issues and adjustment concerns associated with renal failure. The second section examines psychological aspects and psycho-social interventions in the management of traumatic spinal injury, and the third examines the emotional and psychiatric sequelae, treatment and interventions for people with traumatic brain injury. These themes were chosen because of the range and diversity of disabilities associated with the conditions, and the years of life affected by them. Each area has been considered under the headings of: physical impact and epidemiology; emotional issues and adjustment concerns; family and social issues; acute, rehabilitation and community needs; and approaches to assess-ment, treatment and interventions. This chapter provides a practical and compre-hensive coverage of psychological and psychiatric approaches to chronic illness and disability, an area where, once medical stabilization has occurred, psychological issues may be the paramount cause of concern.

Most patients with substance-related disorders seen by psychiatrists and psycholo-gists suffer not only from abuse or dependence, with one or more additional substance-related disorders, but also comorbid psychiatric conditions. Chapter 8 considers the definitions of these disorders, their epidemiology, comorbid conditions, and roles and responsibilities of clinicians working in this field. Details of diagnosis and assessment are given, together with information concerning assessment interviews, questionnaires and rating scales. Since a thorough physical examination of the substance abuser is mandatory, a list is given of the most important points to be sought in a physical examination.

While expectation of a total and permanent cure for substance-related disorders may be unrealistic, working in this area can be rewarding if one views treatment success as attenuation of the pattern of abuse with reduction in adverse social sequelae. Treatment methods are described, including detoxification programs, and details of psychosocial and pharmacological treatments, with information con-cerning the specific drugs involved. Special issues are considered, including vulner-able groups such as pregnant women, children, adolescents, and the elderly. Moreover, there are the situations of chronic pain patients who have become iatrogenically dependent on opioids, as well as physicians and other health profes-sionals impaired by substance abuse. In conclusion, cooperation between psycholo-gists and psychiatrists can enable substance-abusing patients to enjoy the full armamentarium of assessment and treatment practices, and improve their quality of life.

Coronary heart diseases are another major cause of premature death in Western countries, and the enormous social and psychological consequences of coronary heart disease are described. While many patients seem to adapt over time, anxiety and depression are prevalent at all stages of adaptation. There is growing evidence that vital exhaustion, hostility and anger, anxiety and especially depression may be associated with disease progression and/or cardiovascular mortality. Chapter 9 is concerned with psychological and psychiatric issues in the management of coronary heart disease.

This chapter concentrates on cardiac rehabilitation, with evidence of the beneficial effects of these programs on cardiovascular mortality, but surprisingly less evidence for their effects on morbidity or psychosocial recovery. The effects of health education and stress management programs are also discussed. These appear to have beneficial effects on cardiac mortality and morbidity, on risk factors for coronary heart disease and on health behaviours; effects on psychosocial outcomes are, however, inconsistent. The next section of the chapter discusses the psychological side-effects of cardiovascular drugs as well as cardiovascular effects of psychotropic drugs. The chapter concludes with recommendations concerning future research, and development and implementation of intervention programs.

The recognition that psychiatry and psychology can contribute to health promotion is now fairly well established: many areas, however, (most notably models of addictive behaviour) are relatively underdeveloped and hinder the progress of the field. Chapter 10 explores some of the problematic issues in current models of addiction and explores briefly the benefits to health promotion in developing new approaches to deal with the individual and social problems arising from substance use or abuse. The major area of concern in this chapter is cigarette smoking. Not only is tobacco the leading cause of preventable death in the modern world, but the status of its main psychoactive substance has recently been changed to addictive. The background to this decision and the social and legal ramifications of this change are outlined. Numerous efforts to reduce cigarette smoking have been tried, with mixed success. These have included the individually focused MRFIT study and the community-centred COMMIT program. The deficiencies in these approaches are discussed and suggestions made for a more effective approach to social change in substance use.

The final chapters in this volume address a number of issues of relevance to the future of psychology and psychiatry in the medical setting. Chapter 11 discusses teaching, training and research, both in their current form and with a view to improving integrated medical practice. The section "training psychiatrists and psychologists to function in medical settings" is concerned with incorporating the biopsychosocial perspective into the generic and specialist training of psychiatrists and psychologists.

Special attention is paid to the role that liaison psychiatry and health psychology can play in educating other health professionals in secondary and tertiary medical settings, not only medical practitioners (both GPs and specialists) but others such as social workers and physiotherapists. This section is followed by a description of the programs conducted by the University of Melbourne Department of Psychiatry for GPs in various fields (general psychiatry, child and family psychiatry, transcultural psychiatry, community psychiatry, hypnosis and cognitive behavioural psychiatry).

Finally, a section on "research into psychological, psychiatric and psychosomatic factors as they affect medical settings" gives an overview of opportunities for psychological research on medically ill populations and some of the practical and methodological issues which affect such research.

Chapter 12 draws together major issues raised in previous chapters, with an emphasis on the future, and on how to consolidate the role of psychiatry and psychology in the medical setting. Team-work is emphasized, including working with other specialties such as neuropsychology and when to refer to each other. The importance of the liaison function, as opposed to consultation, is discussed together with a suggested expansion of the role of the psychologist and psychiatrist to intervene within the organization (from trouble-shooting to bioethics to influencing policy-making). The context is understanding organizational structure, culture and the unwritten rules of conduct to best adapt mental health practice to the medical setting changes and the broader health care system. An overview, particularly in terms of implications for funding, the need for psychology and psychiatry to play the political game, is given. A thoughtful analysis of how to measure the value of mental health treatments is then provided. The chapter ends on a hopeful note, concluding that not only is there undeniable evidence of the relevance of psychological factors in health and illness but that mental health treatment may be justifiable on cost-effectiveness grounds. The future does indeed seem promising.

REFERENCES

Alexander F, French TM and Pollock GH: *Psychosomatic Specificity*. University of Chicago Press: Chicago and London, 1968.

APA (American Psychological Association): Committee on Training in Clinical Psychology: Recommended graduate training programs in clinical psychology. *American Psychologist*, **2**: 539–558, 1947.

APA (American Psychological Association): "Levels and Patterns of Professional Training in Psychology", Vail, Colorado, July 1973 (M Korman, Ed). APA: Washington, DC, 1976.

Bakal DA and Kaganov JA: Muscle contraction and migraine headache: psychophysiologic comparison. *Headache*, **17**: 208–215, 1977.

Baum A, Newman S, Weinman J, West R and McManus C (Eds) *Cambridge Handbook of Psychology, Health and Medicine*. Cambridge University Press: Cambridge, England, 1997.

Belar CD: Issues in training clinical health psychologists. *Psychology and Health*, **4**: 31–37, 1990.

Bellack AS and Hersen M (Eds): *Comprehensive Clinical Psychology*. Elsevier Science: Oxford, 1980.

Billings EG: Teaching psychiatry in the medical school general hospital: a practical plan. *JAMA*, **89**: 1949–1956, 1936.

Bishop GD: *Health Psychology. Integrating Mind and Body*. Allyn & Bacon: Boston, MA, 1994.

Bloom BL: *Health Psychology—A Psychosocial Perspective*. Prentice-Hall: Englewood Cliffs, NJ, 1988.

Boring EG: *A History of Experimental Psychology*. Prentice-Hall: Englewood Cliffs, NJ, 1950.

Breuer J and Freud S: *Studies on Hysteria. vol 2, The Standard Edition of Freud*, Ernest Jones (Ed), Hogarth Press: London, 1955, p 335.

Camic PM and Knight SJ (Eds): *Clinical Handbook of Health Psychology: A Practical Guide to Effective Interventions*. Hogrefe & Huber Publishers: Seattle, WA, 1998.

Cannon WB: *The Wisdom of the Body*. WW Norton & Co: New York, 1932.

Cassem NH and Hackett TP: Psychiatric consultation in a coronary care unit. *Annals of International Medicine*, **75**: 9–14, 1983.

Clark DM and Fairburn CG: *Science and Practice of Cognitive Behaviour Therapy*. Oxford Medical Publications: Oxford, 1997.

Engel GL: Medical education and the psychosomatic approach. A report on the Rochester experience 1946–1966. *Journal of Psychosomatic Research*, **11**: 77–85, 1967a.

Engel GL: Training in psychosomatic research. *Advances in Psychosomatic Medicine*, **5**: 16–24, 1967b.

Engel GL: The concept of psychosomatic disorder. *Journal of Psychosomatic Research*, **11**: 3–9, 1967c.

Engel GL: The need for a new medical model: a challenge for biomedicine. *Science*, **196**, 129–132, 1977.

Evatt E (Chair): The Australian Royal Commission on Human Relationships, Australian Government Printing Service: Canberra ACT, 1977.

Fiester AR: JACH standards for accreditation of community mental health service programs. *American Psychologist*, **33**: 1114–1121, 1978.

Flanders Dunbar H: Psychosomatic Diagnosis. Paul Hoeber Inc: New York and London, 1943.

Freud S: *Complete Psychological Works*, Standard Edition (J Strachey, Ed). Hogarth Press: London, 1953.

Groth-Marnat G and Edkins G: Professional psychologists in general health care settings: a review of the financial efficacy of direct treatment interventions. *Professional Psychological Research and Practice*, **27**: 161–174, 1996.

Harrison JA, Mullen PD and Green LW: A meta-analysis of studies of the health belief model with adults. *Health Education Research*, **7**: 107–116, 1992.

Henry GW: Some modern aspects of psychiatry in general hospital practice. *American Journal of Psychiatry*, **86**: 481–499, 1929.

Hersen S et al: *Adult Psychopathology and Diagnosis* (SM Turner and S Hersen, Eds). Wiley: New York, 1984.

Hutchinson S: Psycho-oncology: An overview and review of psychological interventions. Paper presented at the 20th National Conference, Australian Association for Cognitive Behavioural Therapy: Brisbane, Australia, 1997.

James W: *Principles of Psychology*. New York: Holt, 1890.

James W: *Varieties of Religious Experiencing: A Study in Human Nature*. Longmans Green: New York, 1902.

Judd FK and Brown DJ: Psychiatric consultation in a spinal injuries unit. *Australia and New Zealand Journal of Psychiatry*, **26**: 218–222, 1992.

Judd FK and Burrows GD: Liaison psychiatry in a spinal unit. *Paraplegia*, **24**: 6–19, 1986.

Kiesler CA, Cummings NA and Vandenbos GR (Eds): *Psychology and National Health Insurance: A Sourcebook*. APA: Washington, DC, 1979.

Lalonde M: A more positive approach to health promotion. *Canadian Nurse*, **70**: 19–20, 1974.

Leigh H and Reiser MF: *The Patient: Biological, Psychological and Social Dimensions of Medical Practice*, 3rd Edition. Plenum: New York, 1977.

Levitan SJ and Kornfeld DS: Clinical and cost benefits of liaison psychiatry. *American Journal of Psychiatry*, **138**: 790–793, 1981.

Lipowski ZJ: Review of consultation psychiatry and psychosomatic medicine. II. Clinical aspects. *Psychosomatic Medicine*, **29**: 201–224, 1967.

Lipowski ZJ: Psychiatric consultation: concepts and controversies. *American Journal of Psychiatry*, **134**: 523–528, 1977a.

Lipowski ZJ: Psychosomatic medicine in the seventies: an overview. *American Journal of Psychiatry*, **134**: 233–244, 1977b.

Lipowski ZJ: Consultation-liaison psychiatry: the first half century. *General Hospital Psychiatry*, **8**: 305–315, 1986.

Lipowski ZJ: Consultation-liaison psychiatry at century's end. *Psychosomatics*, **33**: 128–133, 1992.

Ludwigsen KR and Albright DG: *Professional Psychology. Research and Practice.* **25**: 241–246, 1994.

Marks D: EPPA task force on health psychology: recommendations on training (*Newsletter of the Special Group in Health Psychology*, Issue 17). The British Psychological Society: London, 1994.

Matarazzo JD: Behavioural health and behavioural medicine: Frontiers for a new health psychology. *American Psychologist*, **35**: 807–817, 1980.

Mendel WM: Psychiatric consultation education 1966. *American Journal of Psychiatry*, **123**: 150–155, 1966.

Milgrom J and Hardardottir D: Clinical health psychology: a specialty in its own right. *Bulletin of Australian Psychological Society*, **Oct**, 13–18, 1995.

Milgrom J, Nathan PR and Martin PR: Health psychology: Overview and practice in a general hospital setting. In Martin PR and Birnbrauer JS (Eds), *Clinical Psychology: Profession and Practice in Australia*, Ch 8, pp 191–235. MacMillan: Melbourne, 1996.

Milgrom J, Walter P and Green S: Cost savings following psychological intervention in a hospital setting: The need for Australian-based research. *Australian Psychologist*, **29**: 194–200, 1994.

Mosher JM: A consideration of the need of better provision for the treatment of mental disease in its early stage. *American Journal of Insanity*, **65**: 499–508, 1909.

Noyes R Jr, Wise TN and Hayes JR: Consultation liaison psychiatrists. How many are there and how are they funded? *Psychosomatics*, **33**: 123–127, 1992.

Olbrisch ME: Psychotherapeutic interventions in physical health. Effectiveness and economic efficiency. *American Psychologist*, **32**: 761–777, 1977.

Rachman S and Philips C: *Psychology and Medicine.* Temple Smith: London, 1975.

Rush B: *Sixteen Introductory Lectures to Courses of Lectures Upon the Institutes and Practice of Medicine, With a Syllabus of the Latter.* Bradford and Innskeep: Philadelphia, 1811. [Cited by Schwab (1989).]

Sachar E (Ed): *Hormones, Behavior and Psychopathology.* Raven Press: New York, American Psychological Association, 1976.

Sank LL and Shapiro JR: Case examples of the broadened role of psychology in health maintenance. *Professional Psychology, Research and Practice*, **10**: 402–408, 1979.

Sarafino EP: *Health Psychology: Biopsychosocial Interactions*, 2nd edn. Wiley: New York, 1994.

Saravay SM and Lavin M: Psychiatric comorbidity and length of stay in the general hospital. *Psychosomatics*, **35**: 233–252, 1994.

Schwab JJ: Consultation-liaison psychiatry: a historical overview. *Psychosomatics*, **30**: 245–254, 1989.

Selye H: General adaptation syndrome and diseases of adaptation. *Journal of Clinical Endocrinology and Metabolism*, **6**: 117–230, 1946.

Shakow D: Seventeen years later; clinical psychology in the light of the 1947 Committee on Training in Clinical Psychology Report. *American Psychologist*, **20**: 353–367, 1965.

Sheeran P and Abraham C: *The Health Belief Model.* In M Conner and P Norman (Eds), *Predicting Health Behaviour.* Open University Press: Buckingham, UK, 1998.

Sheridan CL and Radmacher SA: *Health Psychology: Challenging the Biomedical Model.* John Wiley: Singapore, 1992.

Stanley Hall G: *Adolescence: Its Psychology and its Relation to Physiology, Anthropology, Sociology, Sex, Crime, Religion and Education*. Appleton & Co: New York, 1911.

Stone GC, Cohen F, Adler NE et al: *Health Psychology, A Handbook. Theories and Applications*. Jossey Bass: San Francisco, CA, 1979.

Strain JJ: Needs for psychiatry in the general hospital. *Hospital and Community Psychiatry*, **33**: 996–1002, 1982.

Strain JJ, Lyons JS, Hammer JS et al: Cost offset from a psychiatric consultation-liaison intervention with elderly hip fracture patients. *American Journal of Psychiatry*, **148**: 1044–1049, 1991.

Strain JJ, Hammer JS and Fulop G: APM task force on psychosocial interventions in the general hospital inpatient setting. A review of cost-offset studies. *Psychosomatics*, **35**: 253–254, 1994.

Sweeney GH: Pioneering general hospital psychiatry (Pavilion F, 1902–1922). *Psychiatric Quarterly Supplement*, **36**: 217–219, 1962.

Taylor SE: *Health Psychology*. Random House: New York, 1986.

Taylor SE: *Health Psychology* (2nd edn). McGraw Hill: New York, 1990.

Taylor SE: *Health Psychology* (3rd edn). McGraw-Hill: New York, 1995.

Vandenbos GR, Stapp J and Kilburg RR: Health service providers in psychology. Results of the 1978 APA Human Resources survey. *American Psychologist*, **36**: 1395–1418, 1981.

Viney LL: *Images of Illness*. Krieger: Malabar, FL, 1983.

Watson RI: *The Clinical Method in Psychology*. Harper: New York, 1951.

Watson RI: A brief history of clinical psychology. *Psychology Bulletin*, **50**: 321–346, 1953.

Watson RI: *Psychology of the Child*. John Wiley: New York, 1965.

Weiner M and Walker JK: Utilization of basic and clinical health sciences personnel in a team approach for the achievement of competency in therapeutics. *Medical Education*, **11**: 114–118, 1977.

Weinman J, Petrie K, Moss-Morris R and Horne R: The illness perception questionnaire: A new method for assessing the cognitive representation of illness. *Psychology and Health*, **11**(3): 431–445, 1996.

2

Biopsychosocial Factors in Health
and Illness

David Copolov

The Mental Health Research Institute of Victoria and Departments of Psychiatry,
University of Melbourne and Monash University, Melbourne, Australia

Jack E. James

Department of Psychology, The National University of Ireland, Galway, Ireland

and

Jeannette Milgrom

Department of Psychology, University of Melbourne, and Austin & Repatriation Medical Centre,
Melbourne, Australia

SECTION A

BIOPSYCHOSOCIAL INFLUENCES ON ILLNESS: AN OVERVIEW

Substantial opportunities arise for psychologists and psychiatrists to influence the welfare of patients with non-psychiatric illnesses. These follow from the indubitable influences that psychological and behavioural factors impose on the predisposition to, course and outcome of, these illnesses, and the behavioural and psychological sequelae that result from them.

The pioneers of psychodynamically focused psychosomatic medicine emphasized particular constellations of intrapsychic conflict which led to specific disorders such as duodenal ulcer, asthma and hypertension (Alexander 1950). Replacing these overblown, theory-driven and eventually unsustainable claims, is a view that recognizes the bi-directionality of the relationship between behaviour and health and the breadth and richness of interactions between the two. This is a view which derives strength from the growing, but still quite underdeveloped, empirical bases which have accrued in the relevant areas of epidemiology, consultation-liaison psychiatry and health psychology. It is one which seeks not only to establish and modify causal

Psychology and Psychiatry: Integrating Medical Practice.
Edited by J. Milgrom and G. D. Burrows © 2001 John Wiley & Sons, Ltd.

relationships, but also to understand the mechanisms underlying those relationships by way of the investigational techniques which are used in disciplines such as neuroendocrinology and neuroimmunology, as reviewed later in this chapter.

That there is no separate and definable group of "psychosomatic disorders", but instead, that a broad raft of psychological states may affect physical disorders, was first given due recognition in the *Diagnostic and Statistical Manual of Mental Disorders* of the American Psychiatric Association in its third edition (DSM-III, APA 1980), with the introduction of the term "Psychological Factors Affecting Physical Conditions". The factors considered under this rubric have expanded in subsequent editions, so that in the most recent edition (DSM-IV, APA 1994) the factors include those which affect the course of general medical conditions, or heighten the risks or interfere with the treatment associated with such conditions. Also included under this heading in DSM-IV are stress-related physiological responses which precipitate or exacerbate the symptoms associated with general medical conditions. Examples of such responses are stress-induced cardiac arrhythmias or asthma.

The range of potential psychological influences on medical conditions and their treatment is recognized by DSM-IV to include not only psychiatric and personality disorders, but also psychological symptoms (e.g. anxiety), personality traits (e.g. suspiciousness and aloofness) and maladaptive behaviours (e.g. excessive alcohol and drug use, or unsafe sexual practices), which may be subthreshold for specific mental disorders.

This last group of behaviours, although not the obvious primary focus of the category in which it is subsumed, is the largest cause of preventable death in developed countries. Cigarette smoking, sedentary lifestyles, poor dietary habits and substance—especially alcohol—abuse contribute substantially to major causes of mortality in western countries (see Table 2.1) including cardiovascular disease, cancer, accidents and respiratory illnesses. The importance of population-based approaches to these problems is highlighted later in this section.

Although the vast majority of individuals who engage in such behaviours are not diagnosable as having a psychiatric disorder, such disorders may well lead to an

TABLE 2.1 Leading causes of death in Australia in 1994

Cause	Ranking
Malignant neoplasm (cancer)	1
Coronary heart disease (heart attack)	2
Cerebrovascular accidents (stroke)	3
Chronic obstructive pulmonary disease (includes asthma, emphysema and bronchitis)	4
Accidents, including motor vehicle	5
Diseases of arteries, including atherosclerosis and aortic aneurysm	6
Diabetes mellitus	7
Suicide	8

From: Australian Bureau of Statistics 1994

increase in these behaviours (for example, there is a high rate of smoking and alcohol abuse in people suffering from schizophrenia, estimated at 70% and greater; see Regier et al 1990; De Leon 1996). Even more importantly, when they occur in the "general population", these behaviours are amenable to psychological and public health promoting interventions, although this is not without controversy (see Chapter 10 of this book).

In addition to considering the manner in which psychological factors may influence non-psychiatric disorders, it is also very important to understand and be watchful for the obverse relationship. Medical or surgical conditions, as well as the treatment of these conditions, may give rise to distress, anxiety, depression, delirium, mood or personality changes or psychoses. In some cases, the relationship is a result of the individual's adaptation to their illness or injury (e.g. withdrawal, irritability and depression in a previously athletics-oriented man rendered a paraplegic after a diving accident), or aetiological in the sense that a plausible physiological explanation makes a significant contribution to the understanding of the consequential psychological symptoms. Post-stroke depression, which occurs in a major form in up to 25% of patients (Robinson 1997) provides a good example of the latter relationship. Although correlations have been noted between functional impairments following stroke and post-stroke depression, these have been of small magnitude (Robinson et al 1983; Eastwood et al 1989). Of greater apparent relevance is the location of the lesion. When major depression occurs after a stroke, the lesion is likely to be located in the left hemisphere, especially in anterior regions (Robinson et al 1984). When depression does occur after a right hemisphere lesion, it is usually minor depression (Robinson 1997) and is most likely to affect the parietal lobe (Starkstein et al 1989; Finset et al 1988). Emphasising the often inextricable interdependence of psychological and biomedical processes is the fact that patients with post-stroke depression are found to be more impaired than non-depressed stroke patients in activities of daily living two years after their strokes, despite similarities in many variables, including those relating to acute treatment and rehabilitation and to the size and location of the lesion (Parikh et al 1990).

Broadening our Approaches to Health and Illness

Throughout much of this century, health care in the western world has been virtually synonymous with biologically based medicine (Davis & George 1988; James 1994). However, some of the most widespread improvements in health and life expectancy that have occurred in this and previous centuries have not been due to biomedical advances. Infectious diseases (e.g. tuberculosis, cholera, typhoid, diphtheria, gastroenteritis) were the main causes of premature death in the pre-industrial societies of the past, and continue to be the main causes of premature death in the developing countries of today. Control of these diseases is achieved primarily by using technology of a non-medical kind. In particular, technological development has brought improvements in the supply and distribution of food, thereby raising levels of nutrition. Improved nutrition means greater host resistance to disease. Technological development has also brought improvements in the supply of uncontaminated water, thereby reducing exposure to waterborne diseases like cholera and typhoid. Similarly, developments in technology and enlightened social policies have fostered improved housing and the reduction of slums (where over-crowding and poor living conditions contribute to the spread of infectious diseases), improved education and raised standards of personal hygiene. Thus, the marked increases in health and life expectancy experienced in many countries over the past couple of centuries, are primarily attributable to engineering and social innovations (McKeown 1979).

A biopsychosocial approach to health and illness can benefit from taking a population-based approach to achieve greatest change. In countries where infectious diseases have declined markedly, illness patterns are characterized by chronic dis-eases that develop slowly, and persist or recur over long periods of time. Fairly consistently, in these countries, about four-fifths of deaths result from cardiovascular diseases, malignant neoplasms, diseases of the respiratory system, and accidents. These are the so-called "lifestyle" diseases, presumed to be caused in large part by the way people live. For patients who are acutely ill, medical care and individual psychological or psychiatric treatment can be strikingly effective in relieving suffer-ing and fostering recovery. However, the curative focus of biomedical practice is inadequate, and often irrelevant to the prevention of most of the major illnesses in contemporary developed societies. Diet, sedentary habits, cigarette smoking, exces-sive use of alcohol, and excessive life "stress" and/or poor adaptation to stress, are among the behavioural and social conditions that contribute to the development of major killers such as cardiovascular disease. There are also major behavioural and psychosocial causes of malignant neoplasms, including cigarette smoking (lung cancer), low intake of dietary fibre and/or high intake of animal fat (colon cancer), and excessive exposure to sunlight (skin cancer). Cigarette smoking, and to a lesser extent environmental pollution resulting from industrial processes and motor vehicle exhaust fumes, contributes to respiratory disease. Similarly, accidents are primarily caused by behavioural and social factors. Most accidental deaths involve motor vehicles, and most motor vehicle fatalities involve use of alcohol, excessive speed, and/or failure to use safety devices (e.g. seat belts). The fact that behavioural and social factors are profoundly implicated in the aetiology of most major health problems should not be interpreted as suggesting that biology is not important, only that biology alone is inadequate for promoting health and minimizing disease (Best & Proctor 1988; James 1994).

The Biopsychosocial Model

Increasingly, health and illness are being conceptualized from an ecological or systems perspective in which notions of univariate biological causality are being replaced by more complex explanations that take account of the multifactorial involvement in health of biological, behavioural, and social factors (Engel 1977, 1980). Indeed, the biopsychosocial model, as it has come to be known, is a central theme of this book. Each component of the model is essential, and each encompasses major subsystems. The biological component requires consideration of predisposing factors, including genetic and constitutional variability, and detailed study of physiological processes.

The psychological component is at the "crossroads of biological and social influences" (Rice 1998, p 69), and subsumes behavioural, cognitive, and emotional subsystems. Behaviour in turn subsumes the myriad actions collectively referred to as lifestyle, including variables that enhance health (e.g. physical exercise, adequate nutrition), increase vulnerability to illness (e.g. smoking, drug abuse, unsafe sex), and affect adherence to health-enhancing interventions (e.g. dietary restriction, medication use). Emotions are the subjective experiences and physiological variations that accompany changes in affective tone, especially anxiety, depression, and hostility. The cognitive subsystem includes beliefs about susceptibility to disease, attributions of causation, perceived control or social support, and the complex decision processes that underpin health-affecting life choices (e.g. whether to smoke, take exercise, to use safe-sex practices).

The social component includes a complex array of socioeconomic factors. In general, lower socioeconomic status is associated with increased levels of health-risk behaviour and decreased health-protective behaviour (Anderson & Armstead 1995). In particular, persons of lower socioeconomic status are more likely to smoke, consume higher levels of dietary fat, are less physically active, and are less knowledgeable about health. The complexity of the relationship between social factors and health cannot be overstated. No one factor, whether it be income, education, occupational status, geography (e.g. urban versus rural residence), cultural and ethnic background, or access to medical services, provides a satisfactory explanation of the disparities in longevity and health between higher and lower socioeconomic groups. Moreover, differences in health status between socioeconomic groups do not appear to be due entirely to material inequalities. Much of the effect of socioeconomic status on health appears to be due to perceptions of difference and other psychological processes (Carroll et al 1993).

Considering the extreme complexity of the subject of health, Rice (1998) has suggested that it may be a matter of evolutionary necessity that disciplines that have worked independently amassing knowledge would now be well served to combine this information as the foundation for integrative, multidisciplinary, biopsychosocial explanations of human health and illness. This chapter will begin with a review of psychological factors found to have a role in illness and then follow with the emerging evidence for biobehavioural mediators of disease. The last section of the chapter will consider implications for intervention, both the efficacy of psychological interventions and current concepts in preventive health behaviour.

SECTION B

BEHAVIOURAL AND PSYCHOLOGICAL FACTORS IN ILLNESS

Prediction of Health-Related Outcomes

Evidence for the influence of psychological factors on health-related outcomes is growing (Rozanski et al 1999). In general, five psychosocial domains are found to be predictive of a range of health outcomes. These comprise: (1) anxiety/acute stress; (2) depression; (3) personality factors and character traits; (4) social isolation and support; (5) chronic life stress. Health outcomes under study are broad and include a range of disease entities as well as health-threatening behaviours and health services usage (Martin, Prior & Milgrom 2001).

Table 2.2 summarizes a small number of articles, reviews and meta-analyses which provide examples of the diversity of health outcomes under study, and the impact of psychological factors.

Three psychological factors that repeatedly emerge from these studies as key constructs are stress, depression and social support, and these are discussed below. In general, these factors exert their influence on health in two ways: by a direct effect on the body's ability to remain healthy or via their impact on health-impairing behaviours (Baum & Posluszny 1999).

Stress and Health

Stress is a major psychosocial construct that has been proposed to influence health and illness (Chrousos 1998). In general terms, stress occurs when people face demands which threaten their ability to adapt. Although psychosocial stress is widely believed by both lay people and professionals to be causally related to illness, the true nature of the relationship is complex and remains poorly understood. Stress may refer to situational variables (e.g. "stressful" work), a physical or mental reaction (feeling "stressed"), or the person–environment interaction (the "transaction" between the person and the situation).

Stress may affect health by producing changes in behaviour and/or physiology. There is evidence that under high levels of stress, health-enhancing behaviour declines and health-threatening behaviour increases (i.e. people are more likely to engage in behaviour that increases the risk of illness and injury). For example, during periods of high stress, consumption of nicotine, alcohol, and other drugs may increase, diet may deteriorate, physical exercise may decline, and risk of accidents may increase (Rozanski et al 1999). Direct stress-induced physiological changes may also promote the onset of illness and affect its progression. In particular, physiological stress responses can affect the function of major organ systems, including the cardiovascular system, the gastrointestinal system, the endocrine

TABLE 2.2 Psychological factors predicting health-related outcomes

Study	Type	Psychological factor	Health outcome predicted
Holden (1991)	Meta-analysis of 56 studies	Self-efficacy	Smoking cessation; pain tolerance; weight loss; adherence to exercise; tolerance of dental procedures.
Booth-Kewley & Friedman (1987)	Meta-analytical study	Depression; anger; anxiety	Heart disease outcome including angina, atherosclerosis, myocardial infarct, cardiac death; asthma; ulcer; arthritis; headache.
(Although the magnitude of relationship between psychological factors and heart disease outcome was small ($r = 0.15$) these psychological variables were as important as cholesterol and smoking.)			
Cohen & Williamson (1991)	Review	Negative emotional states or social introversion	Complaints of illness; susceptibility to herpes and viral infection; immune functioning; utilization of medical services.
Allison et al (1995)	Follow-up	Psychological distress	Re-hospitalization and further coronary events; 6-month hospital charges were $9504 or $2146 for distressed compared to non-distressed population.
Shapiro et al (1995)	Follow-up	Personality	Survival in organ transplant cases.
Everson et al (1996)	Follow-up of 2428 Finnish middle-aged men	Hopelessness	Men high on hopelessness were four times more likely to have died of heart disease at 6-year follow-up and twice as likely to have died of cancer.
Watson et al (1998)	100 breast cancer patients	Anxiety; previous experience of symptoms	Anticipatory nausea in patients on chemotherapy.

system, and the kidneys. Most importantly, stress can affect functions of the immune system possibly through the hypothalamus–pituitary–adrenal (HPA) axis. These underlying biological mechanisms will be covered in the next section. It is important to note, however, that humans appear well able to cope with acute stress. Impairment of immune function and other adverse effects on health are likely to occur mainly when stress is prolonged (Singer & Ryff 1999). For instance, Lundberg (1999) suggested that longstanding stress is induced by psychosocial conditions such as low-status jobs, which involve a person in constant tension and results in an inability to recover from high states of arousal and may be linked with neck, shoulder, and back problems. Moreover, illness itself is stressful, having the potential to undermine further preventive health behaviour. An important pathway of influence of the stress of illness itself is the patient's perception of their illness and treatment. It has been suggested that this is more important than illness severity in predicting adherence to treatment, delay in health-seeking behaviour and rehabilitation attendance factors, which in turn have a significant effect on illness and recovery. Illness perception involves factors such as beliefs about the identity or cause of illness, perceived consequences, perception of control and timeline beliefs (Weinman et al 1996; Petrie & Weinman 1997). Horne Weinman (1999), in a study of 324 patients from four illness groups, found that medication beliefs were powerful predictors of reported adherence and more important than clinical and sociodemographic factors. Patients appeared to engage in a cost–benefit analysis in which beliefs about the necessity of their medication was weighed against concerns about the potential adverse effects.

As described previously the influence of stress on illness may occur through either behaviour or physiology, and this appears to be a factor in many medical conditions. For example, 84% of diabetes mellitus patients report increased levels of glucose when stressed. A possible explanation is that stress-related neurohormonal activity may directly increase blood glucose via sympathetic nervous system activation, which inhibits insulin production and action. Alternatively, it is possible that when stressed, eating habits are changed (Surwit et al 1992). Similarly, chronic life stress has been found to explain 79% of the variance of symptom intensity over 16 months in patients with irritable bowel syndrome (Bennett et al 1998).

The effect of stressors is further mediated by individual differences such as cognitive appraisals. For instance, in a recent study the effect of acute stress on immune functioning was found to be buffered by an optimistic perspective (Cohen et al 1999). Some individuals may therefore be more vulnerable to stress and again this may occur via behaviour (e.g. having a more optimistic framework) or via individual differences in physiology. Krantz et al (1999) compared patients who demonstrated ischaemia in response to mental stress to those who did not. Survival analysis over 3.5 years indicated that those with mental stress ischaemia experienced cardiac events more frequently.

This concept of individual differences adds a further complexity to the proposed effect of stress on health. Baum Posluszny (1999) provide an excellent coverage of how to include this concept in our understanding of biobehavioural contributions to the disease process. Individual differences in coping and cognitive style moderate the amount of stress experienced. A stress and coping perspective postulates that stress arises as a result of imbalance between perceived demands, both personal and social and perceived resources (Lazarus Folkman 1984). The stress experience of emotional arousal is usually associated with discomfort/tension accompanied by non-specific biological and behavioural changes which can be thought of as a stress response. For instance, the individual engages his or her resources to minimize, deflect or manage this distress. Coping strategies can therefore be conceptualized as a specific stress response which moderates the influence of stress. The arousal that motivates and supports these actions is thought to be one mechanism by which stress affects health, increasing the "wear and tear" and affecting particular systems. Coping may be protective (e.g. exercise) or negative (engaging in potentially harmful behaviour such as drinking). It may also mediate the direct physiological effects of stress. For instance, Olff (1999) reviewed 78 articles and suggested that individual variability in immune responses to stress is largely determined by the way a subject copes with stress, and in turn this may be mediated by changes in the HPA axis. Gender, age and other personal resources were also identified as influencing this process.

Whilst further interdisciplinary research is therefore necessary to continue to elucidate more clearly the mechanisms whereby stress may affect disease onset and progression, the next major task is to develop interventions that improve coping responses to stress, and evaluate their effectiveness on health outcome.

Depression

Depression has been found to be co-morbidly associated with a number of medical conditions. There is growing interest in the debate of whether depression is a consequence or an aetiological factor in conditions such as coronary heart disease (Dwight & Stoudemire 1997). Major depression has been estimated to affect about one in five patients with myocardial infarct. It appears that depressive illness (perhaps together with anxiety or stress) may trigger cardiovascular events and possibly contribute to processes such as atherosclerosis (Esler et al 1999). Whilst studies linking depression to early death are poorly controlled and do not take into account mediating factors, they suggest that depression substantially increases the risk of death, especially death by unnatural causes and cardiovascular disease. For instance, Frasure-Smith et al (1999) found that cardiac mortality was related to Beck Depression Inventory Scores reflecting moderate to severe depression. The odds ratio for depressed versus non-depressed women was 3.29 and for men 3.05. Suicide accounts for fewer than 1% of deaths in medical samples, suggesting this is not the mechanism. Depression is also associated with new coronary heart disease events. Penninx et al (1998a), in a prospective cohort of 3701 men and women older than 70 years, found that newly depressed older men, but not women, were twice as likely to have a cardiovascular disease event than those who were never depressed. Interestingly, despite preliminary evidence that co-morbidity of depression and ischaemic heart disease is associated with increased morbidity and mortality (Musselman & Nemeroff 2000; Carney et al 1995), there is a paucity of treatment research and randomized trials designed to evaluate whether improving diagnosis and treatment of depression might have an impact on disease progression and quality of life (Musselman et al 1997).

Depression has been linked not only with cardiovascular disease but also with other medical conditions. For instance, in diabetes mellitus (DM) major depression is five times more likely and is linked with prior history, poor illness control and increased reporting of symptoms. Once again, it is unclear whether depression is a reaction to the stressors introduced by DM, the poor correlation between self-care and health outcome resulting in feelings of helplessness (a construct which predicts depression) or neurophysiological changes associated with DM (Lustman et al 1986). Whilst there is less evidence that depression and cancer outcome are linked, Buccheni (1998) reported a significantly lowered survival rate in depressed lung cancer patients followed longitudinally, and Penninx et al (1999) reported in a prospective study of 4825 persons, that when present for at least six years, depression was associated with a generally increased risk of cancer. Finally, Ormel et al (1998) surveyed 5279 middle-aged and older persons, some with medical conditions and some without, and found that persons with symptoms of depression displayed greater dysfunction, health perception and well-being. This study underscored the importance of detection and management of depression in older people.

Depression has been predicted by the World Health Organization to become the leading cause of disability, accounting for 10.7% of the global burden of disability (Murray & Lopez 1996). Therefore, the relevance of depression both as a co-morbid or aetiological factor in disease assumes major public health significance. Future well controlled studies of high-risk groups, such as those with myocardial infarct, may guide efforts to develop treatments that reduce the burden of the disease and possibly the mortality risk of depression (Wulsin et al 1999).

Social Factors

Psychosocial stress is believed to be influenced by a variety of demographic variables, including age, gender, ethnicity and socioeconomic status (Chrousos 1998). Pickering (1999) reviewed the consistent finding that the prevalence of cardiovascular disease is higher in those of lower socioeconomic status (SES). This could be related to the higher rates of health-impairing behaviours such as smoking, obesity and physical inactivity found in lower SES populations. However, as the relationship between hypertension, cholesterol and SES was weak, Pickering suggested that the other pathways of influence could be chronic stress, differences in lifestyle, behaviour patterns and access to health care. Baum et al (1999) further reviewed the relationship between stress and low SES, highlighting yet other factors that may be relevant as stressors, such as crowding, crime, noise pollution and discrimination. In addition, the impact of stress may vary according to the pre-existing physical and psychological well-being of the individual, which in turn is a function of preventive health practice. For example, regular physical exercise is believed to promote resistance to the potentially adverse effects of stress (Kaplan et al 1996; Blumenthal et al 1997).

Another important variable, and one that is receiving increased attention from researchers, is social support (i.e. the relationships that exist between the individual and family, friends, work colleagues, social groups, and the wider community) (e.g. Gorkin et al 1994; Kaplan & Keil 1993; Kaplan & Lynch 1999). Although definitions vary, a distinction is often made between structural and functional features of social support. The former refers to such features as the breadth of the social network, the number of people in the network who are supportive, and the frequency of supportive social contacts. Functional features are the qualitative aspects of the support that is received, and include instrumental support (money, useful material objects, time), informational support (relevant information, advice, guidance), appraisal support (approval, affirmation), and emotional support (affection, reassurance, sympathy, friendship, concern). Robinson et al (1999) for instance, reported an association between an impaired relationship with the patient's "closest other" prior to stroke and post-stroke depression and recovery. Knox et al (1998) once again highlighted the complexity of the relationship in a study of 2300 high-risk people with a familial predisposition for cardiovascular disease. They found an interaction between hostility and low social support on cardiovascular disease after controlling for exercise, smoking and body mass.

Although there is much evidence showing an association between levels of perceived social support and health, the findings are largely correlational (Thorsteinsson et al 1998; Uchino et al 1996). As such, the existence of a causal relationship for both social support and SES still has to be confirmed, and the biopsychosocial mechanisms for the causal link (if one exists) have still to be explicated.

SECTION C

BIOBEHAVIOURAL MEDIATORS OF DISEASE

The burgeoning study of the psychological influences on neuroendocrine, immunological and cardiovascular processes is complementary to the epidemiological and clinical investigation of the reciprocal relationship between behaviour and health. The delineation of the physiology and pathophysiology of these processes in response to internal and external stressors is an important element in modern psychosomatic research because it provides buttressing validity to the relationship by characterizing biologically plausible mechanisms which might explain how psychological factors might give rise to medical disorders and how these disorders might result in psychological dysfunction. The study of biobehavioural mediators is also important because it might lead to the discovery of processes which prove to be therapeutically susceptible.

Neuroendocrine Mediators

Although the neuroendocrine response to stress in humans is extremely complex (Stratakis & Chrousos 1995), varies from individual to individual (Meikle et al 1988), and is still far from being fully understood (Vingerhoets & Assies 1991), there is no doubt that the hypothalamo–pituitary–adrenal (HPA) axis represents its most important component. Stress causes neurons in the paraventricular nucleus of the hypothalamus to release corticotrophin-releasing hormone (CRH) and arginine vasopressin (AVP) which, in turn, results in the secretion of adrenocorticotrophic hormone (ACTH) from the anterior pituitary gland and, consequently, glucocorticoids—predominantly cortisol—from the adrenal gland. Cortisol binds to high-affinity intracytosolic glucocorticoid receptors. The hormone–receptor complex binds to specific sequences of DNA called glucocorticoid recognition elements which are found on numerous genes in the nuclei of cells throughout the body, thereby affecting the expression of a large variety of genes (Herman 1993). The net result of cortisol's effect on genetic transcription, and therefore of HPA activation, has been conceptualized as resulting in the mobilization of energy, via the generation of glucose, amino acids and free fatty acids (Sapolsky 1992), the switching off of non-essential body systems (Munck et al 1984) and the counter-regulation of inflammatory processes (Maier et al 1994) in response to immediate or chronic stresses.

The mechanisms by which stress might result in a dysfunction of the body's two major stress-responding systems, the HPA and the sympathetic nervous system, have recently been categorized (McEwen 1998) into those in which: (a) normal physiological responses must cope with repetitive stressors of the type which do not lead to adaptation; (b) the physiological response to repetitive stress would normally lead to adaptation but fails to do so; (c) there is an unusually prolonged physiological response to a limited number of stressors; and (d) an inadequate physiological response is mounted in response to a stressor—with, for example, underactivity of the HPA resulting in the abnormal release of cytokines normally under counter-regulatory control by glucocorticoids.

This classification is a useful addition to the conceptualization of the physiological response to stress because it highlights the fact that when considering the HPA axis, for example, dysfunction cannot be simply understood in terms of "overactivity". Furthermore, it gives due attention to the fact that when heightened activity does occur in the HPA, this may be due to the nature and frequency of various stressors or to different types of impairment of the negative and positive regulatory circuits, which control HPA function, circuits which normally enable the HPA to be in a state of optimal readiness to respond rapidly and efficiently to stress, but which also ensure that it is adequately dampened in the absence of it.

An interesting distinction has been suggested with regard to different types of stressors by Herman and colleagues (Herman et al 1996; Herman & Cullinan 1997). They propose that systemic stressors of immediate survival value such as haemorrhage, hypoglycaemia or hypoxia trigger HPA responses as a result of direct effects on ACTH-controlling neuropeptides in the paraventricular nucleus—probably via brainstem catecholaminergic neurons, whereas stressors that require interpretation by higher brain structures, such as fear-conditioned stimuli or exposure to novel environments, influence paraventricular nucleus activity more indirectly via limbic circuitry including the frontal cortex, hippocampus and amygdala. This hypothesized distinction between "limbic insensitive" and "limbic sensitive" stressors has received some support from lesion studies (Herman et al 1996).

The most comprehensive investigation of HPA dysfunction in humans has taken place in relation to major depressive disorder. Hypercortisolaemia is found in more than 50% of patients with the disorder (Rubin et al 1996), and is frequently associated with non-suppression in the dexamethasone suppression test (DST) (Arana et al 1985). This non-suppression, which indicates impaired negative feed-back within the HPA axis, is not specific to major depression and is also found in several other psychiatric conditions including schizophrenia, mania, bulimia nervosa and alcoholism (Godwin 1984; APA Task Force 1987; Joyce et al 1987; O'Brien et al 1988; Copolov et al 1989; Yeragani 1990).

Associated with HPA axis overactivity in DST non-suppressors with major depression, have been reports of elevations in CRH in the cerebrospinal fluid (Roy et al 1987; Pitts et al 1990) and blunted ACTH responses to exogenously administered CRH (Gold et al 1984; Kathol et al 1989)—both suggestive that hypersecretion of CRH may play an important role in the HPA axis hyperactivity in the disorder. In addition, there have been reports from magnetic resonance imaging (MRI) studies of both pituitary gland (Krishnan et al 1991) and adrenal gland (Rubin et al 1996) enlargement in depression.

The identification of the likely consequences of HPA axis dysfunction in major depression, in other psychiatric disorders and following threatening life events (Willis et al 1987; Calloway & Dolan 1989) is currently the subject of intense research interest. One possibility is that in initially non-depressed individuals HPA axis hyperactivity may predispose to the development of depression, whereas in depressed individuals it may contribute to the perpetuation of the mood disturbance. Supporting this proposition is the fact that the hypercortisolaemia which characterizes Cushing's syndrome is associated with depression in approximately 50% of patients (Checkley 1996).

There is also great interest in the possibility that HPA axis overactivity may contribute to the impairment of cognitive function which is a feature of both Cushing's syndrome (Starkman et al 1992; Newcomer et al 1994) and major depression (McAllister 1981). This interest arises from convincing animal studies which have shown that several weeks' administration of the glucocorticoid cortico-sterone (Sapolsky 1985) or application of restraint stress (Watanabe et al 1992) causes atrophy of neurons in the CA3 region of the hippocampus. The hippocampus possesses the highest concentrations of receptors for both glucocorticoid receptors (GRs) and related mineralocorticoid receptors (MRs) in the brain, inhibits the HPA axis' response to stress (Reul & de Kloet 1985; Jacobson & Sapolsky 1991; Herman et al 1989; Herman 1993; Albeck et al 1994) and is important in cognitive function—especially in verbal and contextual memory (Eichenbaum & Otto 1992). (Contextual memory involves remembering the time and place of events which possess emotional valence.)

The morphological change results from the atrophy of apical dendrites (Woolley et al 1990) by mechanisms in which both glucocorticoids and excitatory amino acids are implicated (McEwen et al 1995). The permanence of the stress-related structural change in the hippocampus is determined by the duration of the stress—varying from reversible with short-term stress, to permanent with long-term stress (McEwen & Magarinos 1997). The extent to which the MRI-determined hippocampal volume reductions which have been noted in some studies of patients with recurrent depressive illnesses, Cushing's disease, post-traumatic stress disorder and schizophrenia (McEwen & Magarinos 1997; Velakoulis et al 1998) relate to alterations in HPA axis dysfunction is currently unknown.

In addition to the frank and overt physical and psychological consequences occurring as a result of Cushing's syndrome, HPA axis hyperfunction or dysfunction occurring in response to stress or illness may play an important role in the development of certain deleterious sequelae, including abnormalities of immune function (see the next section), osteoporosis (Michelson et al 1996), poor metabolic control in diabetes (Stratakis & Chrousos 1995) and hypofunction of the hypothalamo–pituitary–gonadal axis (Beitins & Dufan 1986; Brooks-Gunn 1985). It must be emphasized, however, that knowledge in this field is incomplete and that the HPA axis is just one of several highly complex and interrelated physiological systems which the body activates in response to stress (Stratakis & Chrousos 1995).

Neuroimmunological Mediators

Even the pioneers in the study of psychoneuroimmunology, such as Robert Ader, Nicholas Cohen and David Felten (1995), acknowledge that while a great deal has been learnt about the mechanisms and molecules involved in the transfer of information from the nervous system to the immune system and back again, and although there is strong evidence of the effect of stress and depression on disease, there is still a lack of compelling and cohesive evidence in favour of the hypothesis that changes in immune function are mediating variables by which stress and depression affect disease onset and progression in humans.

Over the recent two decades the strongest empirical base in the field of psychoimmunology has been developed as a result of animal studies which have shown that behaviour can have a significant influence on immune function. One of the most interesting streams of research in this field commenced with the work of Ader and colleagues in 1975 (Ader & Cohen 1975) which showed that in rats immunosuppression induced by the drug cyclophosphamide could be conditioned by pairing the drug with an unconditioned stimulus—namely, saccharin-flavoured drinking water—so that the subsequent exposure of the animals to the flavoured drinking water, in the absence of cyclophosphamide, could suppress antibody responses to foreign antigens. Subsequent research has demonstrated that unconditioned stimuli other than immunosuppressant drugs (electric shocks, for example) can be paired with conditioned stimuli to alter immune function (e.g. Sato et al 1984; Zalcman et al 1989); that changes in cell-induced as well as humoral immunity can occur in response to conditioned stimuli (e.g. Bovberg et al 1982); and that conditioned enhancement, as well as conditioned suppression, can be elicited (Bovberg et al 1987).

Although the immunological response to conditioned stimuli has uncertain clinical significance, is sometimes modest or undemonstrable, and when present is not specific to any particular component(s) of the immune system, the discovery of conditioned immunosuppression and immunoenhancement as general reproducible phenomena has been one of the major catalysts in the development of psychoneuroimmunological research because it seriously challenged the previously held view of the immune system as functionally autonomous by demonstrating that the central nervous system is able to influence its activity.

Many studies in laboratory animals have demonstrated that the application of a wide range of stressors can suppress one or more components of the immune response (summarized by Maier et al 1994), but in order to understand how such effects might arise, it is important to determine whether the stressors have their effects via local or non-specific mechanisms (for example, soft tissue damage or altered vascular reactivity following exposure to electric shocks or immersion in cold water), or whether processing by the central nervous system is likely to be involved. A good example of one of many strategies to tease out such issues is provided by the work of Fleshner et al (1989). They demonstrated that the suppression of antibody response to antigen administration which follows upon a newcomer male rat enduring social defeat when placed in a well established colony of male rat peers, correlated with the amount of time the newcomer engaged in submissive behaviours rather than the amount of physical damage he sustained.

Some of the most interesting findings in the literature on the effect of psychological factors on immune function in humans involve studies in depression, infectious diseases and cancer. According to a meta-analysis of well designed studies conducted by Herbert and Cohen in 1993, depressed patients, particularly those who are older and hospitalized, demonstrate a number of alterations in immune function, including lowered lymphocyte proliferative responses to mitogens, lowered natural killer cell activity, decreased numbers of natural killer (NK), T and B lymphocytes and increased numbers of neutrophils and monocytes. Data from a few studies which have carefully controlled confounding variables such as weight loss, or cigarette or alcohol use (Irwin et al 1987, 1990) suggest that these factors cannot explain the identified immunological changes.

Interestingly, the conclusions from influential studies that pointed to depression as a predisposing risk factor for the development of cancer (Shekelle et al 1981; Persky et al 1987) have not been supported by two large and more recent epidemiological studies (Zonderman et al 1989; Vogt et al 1994). Some of the psychosocial factors which do appear to have an impact upon cancer progression—such as the protective effects of being married (Goodwin et al 1987) or having good social supports in a more general sense (Reynolds & Kaplan 1990; Hislop et al 1987), and possessing a "fighting spirit" (Greer et al 1979; Greer 1991)—may exert their influences by means of general health-promoting activities such as better sleep, better diet, more exercise and greater adherence to treatment regimens (Spiegel & Kato 1996).

Neuroimmunological processes may, however, also be affected either directly or indirectly (Herbert & Cohen 1993; Anderson et al 1994) by such factors, and may, in part, play a mediating role in determining how and why the cancer patient's clinical course proceeds as it does. One of the most interesting studies on this topic (Fawzy et al 1990) involved an investigation of the effect on patients with recently treated stage I and II melanomas of a randomly allocated six-week structured group intervention or no intervention. The patients in the intervention group showed increases in natural killer (NK) cell numbers and interferon-alpha in NK activity in comparison to controls and also reduced mortality (9% vs 29%) at six-year follow-up (Fawzy et al 1993). Although the biological relevance of the immunological changes noted in this study is still to be determined, its findings are worthy of exploration and its design calls out for emulation, since there is a troubling paucity of cancer intervention studies which track psychosocial, immunological, morbidity and mortality data.

A similar need exists in the field of psychoneuroimmunology of infectious diseases. For example, although there are reasonably strong data linking mood (Longo & Clum 1989) and coping skills (Cassidy et al 1997) to recurrences of genital herpes simplex (HSV-2), there are few studies in this area which incorporate immunological measures, together with psychological and disease-related data. One notable exception is the study by Kemeny et al (1989) which showed that a negative mood state correlated to a significant degree with both an increased number of recurrences and a decrease in $CD8^+$ lymphocytes, which are important effector cells in the body's immune response against HSV-2 (Posavad et al 1996).

Although the extent to which neuroimmunological processes mediate the relationship between behaviour and health has yet to be properly understood, there has been considerable progress in understanding the nature of the reciprocal relationships between the immune and nervous systems—thereby providing an increasingly solid base from which to propose that functional relationships between the two systems may be relevant to psychosomatic medicine and health psychology.

Immunocompetent cells process binding sites for a wide range of neurotransmitters, neuropeptides and hormones, including opioid, corticotropin-releasing hormone, insulin, oestradiol, testosterone and β-adrenergic binding sites (for reviews on this and related matters see Reichlin 1993, and Besedovsky & del Rey 1996). The nervous system can release neuromodulators which bind to these sites either via the direct and rich noradrenergic sympathetic innervation of primary and secondary lymphoid organs, including bone marrow, thymus, spleen, lymph nodes and intestinal Peyer's patches (Bellinger et al 1992), or as a result of anatomically imprecise neuroendocrine mechanisms.

Because of its role in stress, particular interest has focused on the hypothalamo–pituitary–adrenal axis and its effect on immunomodulation. HPA axis activation, largely as a result of the actions of glucocorticoids, tends to dampen cellular immunity (McEwen et al 1998) perhaps as a mechanism by which to check overexuberant responses (Reichlin 1993). The effect of such activation is not simple, however. Glucocorticoids also contribute to shoring up local immunological defences by "marginating" immunocompetent cells such as lymphocytes and macrophages along blood vessel walls and within relevant compartments in order to ready the host for immunological challenges (McEwen et al 1998).

Just as the central nervous and neuroendocrine systems can affect the immune system, so too can the immune system affect these systems. For example, the brain possesses receptors for many cytokines (or immune-derived chemicals) including interleukin (IL)-1, IL-6, tumour necrosis factor (TNF) and granulocyte colony stimulating factor (GCSF) (Besedovsky & del Rey 1996). Occupancy of these receptors is thought to transduce the effects of infection on thermoregulation, sleep, behaviour and neuroendrocrine responses (Sternberg 1997). As an example of the last effect, cytokines produced from only one million lymphocytes can result in a several-fold increase in ACTH and glucocorticoid levels when injected into normal animals (Besedovsky et al 1981, 1985).

Neuropeptides

The investigation of the behavioural effects of neuropeptides has flourished since the 1970s and has held out much as yet unrealized therapeutic promise. Dozens of neuropeptides, including cholecystokinin, substance P, somatostatin, insulin and vasopressin, have been localized in the brain (Nicholls 1994). These cleavage products of precursor proteins are present in widespread locations throughout the brain in very low concentrations and are often stored in the same nerve terminals as classical neurotransmitters such as acetylcholine and serotonin. In contrast to these classical neurotransmitters, which are stored in small synaptic vesicles and are released into synapses, neuropeptides are segregated by being stored in large dense core vesicles and are usually released at non-synaptic sites. Many of these features together with their electrophysiological effects, suggest that neuropeptides act as neuromodulators, that is, that they affect the responsiveness of neurons to other neurochemical mediators.

Peptides of special relevance to the relationship of behaviour to disease include CRH and the opioid peptides. The intracerebroventricular administration of CRH to experimental animals results in a range of physiological and behavioural responses which resemble the behavioural response to a number of stressors, including activation of the sympathetic nervous system, with resultant increases in heart rate and blood pressure, inhibition of the parasympathetic nervous system, increases in general arousal and agitation, as well as thermogenesis and hypophagia in unfamiliar settings (Herbert 1993; De Souza 1995). Thus in addition to playing a key role in the orchestration of the neuroendocrine responses to stress, CRH may play an important role in integrating these responses with autonomic and behavioural ones—either by means of direct effects on the CNS or indirectly, by HPA-mediated mechanisms.

Consistent with a significant non-endocrine neuromodulatory role for CRH is its distribution in the brain. Not only is it present in the paraventricular nucleus of the hypothalamus, it is also found in the cerebral cortex, hippocampus, amygdala, olfactory tubercle, lateral septal nuclei, caudate-putamen and locus coeruleus (De Souza 1995; Hartline et al 1996).

Opioid peptides are also distributed in both hypothalamic and extra-hypothalamic sites. These peptides have been grouped into three families on the basis of their precursors—the Pro-opiomelanocortin (POMC) family, which includes β, γ and α endorphin; the Pro-enkephalin family, which includes met- and leu-enkephalin; and the Prodynorphin family, which includes dynorphin A and B, and α and β neo-endorphin (Simon & Hiller 1994). The opioid peptides bind to a number of receptors, namely the mu (μ) receptor, for which β endorphin has been considered the classical peptide ligand, the delta (δ) receptor for which the enkephalins show preferential affinity and the kappa (κ) receptor for which dynorphin peptides show selectivity (Terenius 1992).

Significant progress has been made in recent years in elaborating the complexity of opioid peptides and their receptors. For example, the cloning of the three major receptors (Evans et al 1992; Chen et al 1993; Fukuda et al 1993; Meng et al 1993) has enabled all of them to be identified as members of the same super-family of G-protein coupled receptors, with high sequence homologies (Akil et al 1997).

Of the more than 20 opioid peptides that have been characterized (Akil et al 1997), two recently identified ones—endomorphins 1 and 2 (Zadina et al 1997)—are of particular interest. It has been known for a long time that although β endorphin has been characterized as the classical peptide ligand for the mu receptor (the opioid receptor which is most important in analgesia), it has poor selectivity for the receptor—displaying nearly equipotent affinities for mu and delta receptors (Chang & Chang 1983; Hewlett & Barchas 1983). In contrast, the endomorphins show selectivity for the mu receptor over the delta receptor which is thousands of times greater than that demonstrated by β endorphin (Zadina et al 1997). It is possible that the endomorphins may be the natural ligands for mu receptors and that endomorphin-like drugs might possess an ability to induce analgesia with a relative sparing of such side-effects of morphine-like drugs as nausea, respiratory depression and addiction (Julius 1997).

The involvement of opioid peptides in the control of pain is one of the most studied aspects of opioid biology—as would be expected of an arena of research which arose in large part from the discovery of stereochemically selective receptors for morphine and related drugs in the brain (Pert & Snyder 1973).

Although opioid agonists produce analgesic effects at peripheral receptors (Ferreira & Nakamura 1979) and at the level of the spinal cord, where its administration results in inhibition of the firing of dorsal horn neurons (Yaksh 1993), greatest attention has been focused on the manner by which opioids act on the brain stem to exert their pain-modulating properties. The injection of opioids into the periaqueductal grey matter of the mid-brain or the rostral ventral medulla gives rise to analgesia which is reversed by the mu receptor antagonist, naloxone (Fields et al 1988; Yaksh et al 1988), and is mimicked by electrical stimulation (stimulation-produced analgesia) of the same regions (Hosobuchi et al 1977; Oliveras et al 1975; Llewelyn et al 1986).

Although opioid analgesia at the brain stem level is thought to arise as a result of descending inhibitory influences on the dorsal horn of the spinal cord (Basbaum & Fields 1984), other mechanisms of action may include the direct inhibition of noxious throughput at the level of the brain stem and direct cortical or thalamic inhibition (Jensen 1997). It is a notable fact, however, that the role of the thalamus and of many other subcortical and cortical regions of the forebrain in opioid analgesia is quite unclear (Kanjhan 1995). This partly explains why it has been difficult to properly understand the role that opioids might play in modulating the effects that psychosocial factors play on the perception of and response to pain (Von Korff & Simon 1996), even though these influences have been well documented, as have been the relationship between stress and opioids (Olson et al 1997) and the fact that stress can induce naloxone-reversible analgesia (Terman et al 1986).

Recent studies relying on advances in gene knockout technology have highlighted the importance of the mu receptor and β endorphin in analgesia. Mice lacking mu receptors as a result of homologous recombination demonstrated no analgesic effect when treated with morphine (Matthes et al 1996), thereby demonstrating that the mu receptor is mandatory for the action of this drug and calling into question the role played by δ and κ receptors in morphine-induced analgesia (there were no observable alterations in δ or κ receptors in the transgenic animals). Gene knockout technology has also been useful in showing that mice lacking β endorphin as a result of targeted mutagenesis do not display stress-induced analgesia (SIA) (Rubinstein et al 1996), therefore suggesting that β endorphin plays an essential role in this form of analgesia.

As well as being involved in stress-induced analgesia, opioids such as β endorphin have also been implicated in placebo-induced analgesia. A key study pointing towards such an involvement was conducted by Levine and colleagues (1978), who reported that naloxone reduced placebo-induced analgesia following wisdom tooth extraction. This finding has had less experimental follow-up than might have been expected, with two studies of experimental ischaemic pain (Grevert et al 1983) supporting Levine et al's conclusions and two other studies, one also involving experimental ischaemic pain (Posner & Burke 1985) and another involving post-surgical pain (Gracely et al 1983), challenging them.

Of recent note has been the study of nocebos—inert substances which produce negative effects—an important matter, given the common occurrence of adverse events in patients taking pharmacologically inactive tablets in double-blind control trials and the prevalence of sometimes severe side-effects in patients who have negative expectations about treatment—such as patients experiencing anticipatory nausea and emesis while undergoing cancer chemotherapy (Straus & Cavanaugh 1996). Benedetti and Amanzio (1997) have proposed that the neuropeptide cholecystokinin may be involved in mediating the nocebo effect on the basis of the fact that the cholecystokinin antagonist proglumide enhances placebo analgesia— thereby suggesting that cholecystokinin may inhibit placebo analgesia.

The understanding of the mechanisms by which placebos work is at a very early stage of development (Harrington 1997). Very little, if anything, is known about the manner in which neurobiological mediators vary with and subsequently affect various psychological and physiological outcomes in response to subject expectations, clinician–patient relationships, prior experience and conditioning, and various treatment variables, including the size, type, number and colour of tablets (Straus & Cavanaugh 1996).

Furthermore, although the discussion above has primarily addressed placebo-induced analgesia, a full understanding of the neurobiology of placebos must provide explanations for the mechanisms by which non-specific treatment factors can substantially influence symptoms in conditions as diverse as the common cold, asthma, hypertension, depression, duodenal ulcers, anxiety disorders and schizophrenia (Beecher 1955; Benson & Epstein 1975; Dobrilla & Scarpignato 1994).

BIOLOGICAL FACTORS CONTRIBUTING TO CORONARY ARTERY DISEASE AND SUDDEN CARDIAC DEATH

There are many vascular, neural and metabolic processes which may be affected by the psychosocial and lifestyle factors which are considered risk factors either for coronary artery disease (CAD) or sudden cardiac death. These factors include cigarette smoking, sedentary activity, poor diet, hostility, depressive symptoms, hopelessness, life stress, low socioeconomic status, and social isolation (Kamarck & Jennings 1991; Goldstein & Niaura 1992; Wilson 1994; Everson et al 1996; Chesney 1996; Williams & Barefoot 1988).

For the purposes of this brief overview, attention will be drawn to the processes by which psychosocial factors might affect the development of atherosclerosis, influence the pathogenesis of the events leading to coronary artery thrombosis, and finally play a contributing role in the generation of serious cardiac arrhythmias.

The development of coronary atherosclerosis, which takes place over decades, involves endothelial injury (which is particularly affected by local haemodynamic factors), lipid entry and macrophage recruitment into the arterial wall, followed by connective tissue production (which involves smooth muscle cell proliferation) and increasing extracellular lipid accumulation (McLaughlin & Fuster 1995). There are several steps in the progression of the lesion which might be accelerated by neuro-humoral factors responsive to psychological stressors such as adrenaline and nor-adrenaline. For example, these vasoactive amines may lead to chronic endothelial injury in a manner which predisposes to lipid entry into the arterial wall (Fuster et al 1992a). The possible synergistic effect of high plasma catecholamines and high cholesterol on atherogenesis lesions is suggested by Mikat et al's 1991 findings that Egyptian sand rats provided with a high cholesterol diet and infused with noradrenaline took only two months to develop atherosclerostic lesions of the same severity that developed in sand rats over six to eight months when they were fed on a high cholesterol diet but were not infused with noradrenaline.

Relevant to this observation is the fact that in subjects with high hostility scores there was a positive association between the release of plasma catecholamines and fasting plasma cholesterol, whereas in subjects with low hostility scores there was a trend towards a negative relationship between these two measures (Suarez et al 1991). Williams (1994) speculates that in hostile individuals the combination of elevated cholesterol and catecholamines leads to altered plaque-enhancing macrophage activation as a result of increased intracellular cyclic AMP levels. He also suggests ways in which this hypothesis might be tested using circulatory macrophage precursors (monocytes) in human subjects. This suggestion highlights the difficulty of studying the biobehaviour mediators of atherogenesis in human subjects. The changes in the activation patterns of circulatory monocytes may or may not be relevant to the processes occurring in the walls of the coronary arteries. It is, clearly, very difficult if not impossible to study the development of coronary atherosclerosis in asymptomatic individuals over the many years necessary for such a study because of the time course involved and, more importantly, the intrusiveness of the techniques currently available to determine coronary artery pathology.

It is for this reason that the studies of atherosclerosis in Old World monkeys—cynomolgus macaques—are so germane. Kaplan and colleagues have performed an interesting series of experiments which showed that dominant male cynomolgus monkeys fed an atherogenic diet and housed in an unstable social environment, developed approximately twice the amount of coronary atherosclerosis of animals raised in stable social environments (Kaplan et al 1982). This effect, which was unrelated to blood pressure or serum lipid concentrations, was able to be prevented by the use of the beta-adrenoreceptor antagonist propranolol (Kaplan et al 1987, 1989), suggesting that activation of the sympathetic nervous system may play a role in accelerating atherogenesis. In this regard, it is interesting to note that during social reorganization the heart rate of dominant monkeys in the unmedicated condition was significantly higher than that of subordinates during certain behavioural states. This heightened cardiac reactivity was ameliorated by propranolol (Manuck et al 1991).

These experiments raise the issue of responsivity of both heart rate and blood pressure as intervening variables in the psychosocial predisposition to atherosclerosis in humans. Although there have been reports of a relationship between cardiac responsivity to mental stressors and ischaemia and arrhythmia in coronary artery disease patients (Krantz et al 1991; Zotti et al 1991) and of higher cognitively induced cardiac responsivity in males with type-A behaviour (summarized in Harbin 1989), the value of this psychophysiological factor as a predictor of CHD onset is yet to be appropriately tested (Schneiderman & Orth-Gomer 1996). Furthermore, although the use of beta-blockers has been shown to have an advantageous effect over thiazide diuretics in the prevention of coronary events in hypertensive patients (Wikstrand et al 1991), no controlled trials have been reported on the usefulness of beta-blockers in the primary prevention of coronary artery disease in normotensive subjects (Hansson 1991).

Many factors contribute to the formation of thrombosis on unstable or vulnerable atherosclerotic plaques. These factors include plaque fissuring and rupture, platelet activation and aggregation, clotting cascade activation, the extent to which previous residual thrombi are present, and coronary vasoconstriction (which enhances thrombogenicity) (McLaughlin & Fuster 1995; Markovitz & Matthews 1991).

There is great interest in understanding the mechanisms whereby emotional stress might promote thrombus formation and other processes which lead to reduction or cessation of coronary blood flow and to clinically apparent coronary artery disease—as reflected by, for example, the increased rate of heart attacks in Israeli citizens following the threat of Iraqi missile attack (Meisel et al 1991) and amongst the populace of Athens following their 1981 earthquake (Trichopoulos et al 1983; Muller & Verrier 1996).

Platelet aggregation is a central process in the thrombus formation which may be affected not only by vessel wall factors such as the degree of plaque disruption, but also by systemic features such as plasma catecholamine concentrations. Adrenaline and, to a lesser extent, noradrenaline cause the aggregation of platelets—possibly, but not necessarily—as a result of occupancy of alpha-2-adrenergic receptors on their cell walls (Markovitz & Matthews 1991). The release of these catecholamines is likely to explain the enhancement of platelet aggregation which has been shown to occur in the coronary arteries of rats exposed to environmental stressors (e.g. Haft & Fani 1973a,b). Interestingly, plasma catecholamines, as well as causing in vitro platelet responsivity, have been shown to increase during the early hours of the morning in human subjects (Tofler et al 1987)—a time during which the risk for myocardial infarction and sudden coronary death is highest (Muller et al 1989).

While these findings are suggestive of a role for the sympathetic nervous system as a mediator of stress-related coronary artery events, there is inconsistent and sparse evidence in the human experimental literature that mental stress or psychological factors putatively linked to coronary artery disease is associated with increased platelet activity (Kamarck & Jennings 1991; Markovitz & Matthews 1991). The exception to this conclusion is the recent finding by Markovitz et al that hostility is associated with greater platelet reactivity—using plasma beta thromboglobulin as a marker of such activation (Markovitz et al 1996).

Another mechanism by which psychological factors might result in symptomatic coronary artery disease is by the induction of coronary artery spasm. In dogs with experimentally produced coronary artery stenoses, it has been shown that coronary artery vasoconstriction leading to myocardial infarction can be induced by the provocation of intense anger (Verrier et al 1987). Extreme emotion in humans, in the form of panic attacks, has also been shown to be associated with documented cardiac ischaemia, presumably due to coronary spasm, in a report on three patients (Mansour et al 1998), all of whom showed no evidence of atherosclerosis on coronary angiography. This finding is congruent with epidemiological data that patients with panic disorder are at higher risk of sudden cardiac death than patients with other forms of psychiatric disorder (Coryell et al 1982). That stress may alter coronary vascular tone under less emotionally charged circumstances is evidenced by the finding that mental arithmetic can reduce the cross-sectional area in the coronary arteries of patients with stable angina, as determined by angiography

(Rebecca et al 1986). The results from similar studies have not been consistent, however (Kamarck & Jennings 1991).

While it might be assumed that psychological factors may reduce coronary blood flow primarily by means of activation of the sympathetic nervous system, this is not a ready explanation because although coronary arteries possess alpha-1-adrenergic receptors and these are associated with vasoconstriction (Kamarck & Jennings 1991), the infusion of adrenaline or sympathetic nervous system stimulation usually produces vasodilation as a result of the occupancy of beta-adrenergic receptors (Hjemdahl 1990).

The role of sympathetic nervous system activation in the genesis of serious cardiac arrhythmias is more compelling. In approximately 70–85% of patients who experience sudden cardiac death in non-hospital settings, but who are monitored during the event, ventricular arrhythmias are noted (Cobb et al. 1980; and Liberthson et al 1974; Bayes de Luna et al 1989). Because sudden cardiac death is usually associated with severe coronary artery stenosis (but is not, interestingly, in 40% of cases—Liberthson et al 1974), many of the cardiovascular processes discussed above must be considered as acting in concert with the factors contributing to lethal cardiac arrhythmias.

That these latter factors include sympathetic nervous system arousal is suggested by both animal and human studies. For example, stimulation of the left stellate ganglion which provides sympathetic nervous innervation to posterior walls of the ventricles results in ventricular tachycardia (Randall 1977), whereas ablation of this ganglion reduced cardiac arrhythmias and deaths following myocardial ischaemia (Schwartz & Stone 1980). In humans, an association has been noted between increased resting heart rate—a measure which may reflect increased sympathetic drive—and fatal cardiac events (Coumel et al 1987). Related to this finding are the observations that in the hour prior to the onset of ventricular arrhythmias there is an increase in heart rate (Adgey et al 1982; Kempf & Josephson 1984). Of even greater salience to the relationship between sympathetic nervous system activation and ventricular arrhythmias is the ability of beta-adrenergic blocking drugs to reduce the mortality in post-infarct patients due to sudden cardiac death (May et al 1982; Zipes 1992).

Major depression (Lesperance et al 1996) and anxiety (Moser & Dracup 1996) have both been identified as increasing the risk of mortality or arrhythmias after myocardial infarction. It is postulated that increased sympathetic drive might contribute to these associations (Cameron 1996).

Although attention has been focused on the role of the sympathetic nervous system on the induction of ventricular arrhythmias, it is important to point out that there are many relevant complexities relating to the sympathetic innervation to the heart (some are discussed in Schwartz 1984) which cannot be addressed in this brief review. Furthermore, many other factors, including the parasympathetic nervous system, specific brain regions, cardiac muscle cell structure and function, and intracardiac electrical signalling mechanisms need to be considered as possible sites of dysfunction in this often fatal condition (Kamarck & Jennings 1991; Zipes 1992), sites which might be influenced by psychosocial variables.

SUMMARY

The scientific evidence presented in this section provides some support for biobehavioural processes in mediating the effect of psychological states on disease onset and progression. In reviewing the role of neuroendocrine, immunological, neuropeptide and cardiovascular system responses, the complexity of a causal model for disease involves input at multiple levels.

When confronted with a stressor, it seems that a number of adaptive processes may occur within the neuroendocrine system to maintain homeostasis. Chronic stress or situations in which effective adaptation is compromised may lead to dysfunction in the two main systems that are activated in response to stress: the HPA axis and sympathetic nervous system. These dysfunctional responses have been associated with stressful life events, various psychiatric disorders, and cognitive deficit.

The field of psychoneuroimmunology has attempted to uncover the mechanisms by which immune function mediates the effects of psychological factors on disease. Animal studies have demonstrated the influence of behaviour on immune function via the process of classical conditioning and have shown the effects of stress on the immune response. In humans, studies have focused on the effects of depression and the incidence of infectious disease and cancer; however, many studies are beset with methodological shortcomings. Despite strong evidence for the influence of stress and depression on disease, many questions remain regarding the role of the immune system and the central nervous system in mediating these effects.

Neuropeptides, such as CRH and the opioid peptides, can be considered as neuromodulators, which have particular relevance to the relationship of behaviour to disease. Evidence suggests that CRH plays a role in the orchestration of the neuroendocrine responses to stress and in integrating these with autonomic and behavioural responses. The identification and delineation of the mechanisms of opioid peptides and receptors is also a progressive field of research. It is well established that opioid peptides are involved in the control of pain via production of analgesic effects; however, the mechanisms underlying the phenomena of stress- and placebo-induced analgesia and the nocebo effect are still unclear. A better understanding of these phenomena will have significant implications for the pharmacological and clinical treatment of pain.

Subjective states and lifestyle factors act as biobehavioural mediators of coronary artery disease and sudden cardiac death. In particular, psychological stressors and hostility exert their influence via the production of catecholamines, which in turn are associated with pathological changes, such as atherosclerosis and thrombosis, and consequently with the pathophysiology of the cardiovascular system.

This section has reviewed the accumulating knowledge that may explain the relationship between behavioural and psychological factors and health outcomes. The following section will discuss implications for intervention, both from a micro-perspective (i.e. the individual) and importantly move the discussion back to a macroview of intervention. Preventive population-based approaches are necessary for maximum impact in changing the health outcome of the population and intrinsic to a full consideration of a biopsychosocial perspective of disease. Psychologists and psychiatrists have important roles to play in such approaches, since one important way to influence the population is through our understanding of individual differences that influence preventive health behaviours.

SECTION D

IMPLICATIONS FOR INTERVENTION

Evidence-based Intervention

In light of reports that many common medical practices are without empirical validation (e.g. Ferguson 1999), the need to ensure the use of interventions that are evidence-based has become an issue of debate within medicine. Objective verification of outcomes is increasingly being expected of practitioners, thereby increasing the demand for interventions that have been, or have the potential to be, validated empirically. Although the prospects for the increased uptake and future development of the practice of psychology and psychiatry in medical settings appear to be good, there are several potentially serious limiting factors (James 1997). First, it is not enough simply to establish empirical validity. In medicine, attempts have also been made to gauge the extent to which medical practitioners in actual clinical settings employ empirically validated interventions effectively and appropriately. The latter considerations relate to the notion of "quality of care" (Kassirer 1993). One aspect of quality of care is "appropriateness" (e.g. Phelps 1993), which refers to treatment not being applied when it is not needed (i.e. the avoidance of over-servicing). For instance, the wide variation in caesarean delivery rates among regions within the United States has been the focus of considerable attention because of increased maternal morbidity associated with the procedure without apparent impact on infant mortality (Menard 1999; Socol & Peaceman 1999). Another aspect of quality of care is the concept of "necessity" (Kahan et al 1994), which refers to accessibility to care by persons in need of treatment (i.e. avoidance of under-servicing). Among the reasons for concern about levels of appropriateness of medical care is that medical over-servicing contributes to the costs of health care. The measurement of necessity of treatment is equally important, because of humanitarian and equity concerns. Indeed, of the two concerns, appropriateness (avoidance of over-servicing) and necessity (avoidance of under-servicing), the latter would appear to be the more serious problem, when it comes to the application of psychology and psychiatry in medical settings.

   With these cautionary words in mind, it is interesting to review current progress in psychological intervention. Evidence for the effectiveness of psychological interventions in reducing biopsychosocial risk factors is inconclusive. There are preliminary studies suggesting that psychological intervention may improve a number of health outcomes, although the number of high-quality studies is limited. The rationale for these interventions, which generally aim to provide support, coping skills and psychoeducation, is based on studies such as those of Faller et al (1997), who found that the best psychological predictor of survival in cancer patients was "active" coping. Spiegel et al (1989) and similarly Fawzy et al (1993) reported that group intervention providing psychological support improves survival in cancer patients. Being male and having poorer coping skills (particularly minimization) predicted poorer survival. Others have warned that a broader sociological perspective is required, as social support and isolation are important intervening variables on health outcome (Edelman & Kidman 1997) and the relationship between survival and coping style requires further investigation (Faller et al 1999). Inconsistent results in intervention studies have been attributed to the many confounding variables not adequately controlled for, including compliance, age, socioeconomic factors, self-care, diet and health status and stage of disease at entry (Cwikel et al 1997). Hutchinson (1997) reviewed the broad outcomes that have been targeted. There are a number of psychosocial intervention trials (e.g. Spiegel 1999), suggesting improvements in adjustment in five main areas:

1. Emotional adjustment—fear, anxiety, depression, denial, self-esteem, satisfaction.
2. Functional adjustment—social behaviour, return to work.
3. Treatment and disease-related symptoms—nausea, vomiting, pain, cough, nutrition, weight.
4. Medical measures—disease progression, immune functioning.
5. Survival.

Further randomized trials are required to substantiate studies supporting the effectiveness of psychological interventions although meta-analyses are beginning to suggest which factors are most amenable to intervention. For instance, Sheard and Maguire (1999) reported the results of two meta-analyses of studies with cancer patients which suggested that preventive psychological interventions may have a moderate effect on anxiety, but not on depression. Furthermore, interventions targeted at those with existing psychological distress were particularly effective.

Biopsychosocial Outcomes

To date, interest in the psychosocial aspects of physical health has focused on illness causation. Notwithstanding the strength of the evidence implicating behaviour and social conditions as causes of illness, Kaplan (1990) has called for a change in focus from psychosocial causes of physical outcomes (i.e. illness) to behavioural health outcomes. For Kaplan (1990), it is not enough to assume that illness is caused by biological and psychosocial factors. For him, the real interest lies in the behavioural effects of these causal processes. He identified two general classes of behavioural outcomes: length of life and health-related quality of life. Kaplan has argued that all illness, ranging from the common cold to terminal cancer, can be characterized in terms of behavioural outcomes. For example, although arthritis can be described with reference to the physical pathology thought to be involved, it is also characterized by its disabling behavioural effects, including limping, difficulty manipulating objects, crippling pain, disrupted activity patterns, decreased work capacity, and so on. From this perspective, the biological knowledge central to curative medicine, and the more recent accumulation of knowledge about psycho-social causes, can be used to predict behavioural outcomes. For example, asymptomatic disease (e.g. hypertension, early HIV infection) arouse concern, because the observed biological indicators are predictive of important behavioural outcomes. These behavioural outcomes, particularly health-related quality of life, have become important measures of the success of intervention and form a central argument in justifying the use of psychological interventions (see Chapter 12 for further discussion of this issue).

Preventive Health Behaviour and the Influences of Cognitions

Although behaviour has major influences on health, changing behaviour after a major health problem has developed is of limited benefit. Undertaking health-enhancing behaviour after an illness event is typically much less effective in promoting health and longevity than engaging in behaviour that protects against the development of disease in the first place. For example, undertaking regular exercise may assist rehabilitation following a myocardial infarction, but as the heart is often already damaged, the benefits, whilst important, are limited by the existing pathology. Thus, life-long regular exercise, as a "primary" preventive health behaviour, is likely to be even more effective in avoiding premature death from coronary heart disease than taking up exercise once the disease process has begun.

In essence, primary prevention as it pertains to health behaviour involves:

1. The adoption of health-enhancing behaviour patterns that positively promote good health (e.g. a low-fat, low-salt, balanced diet; abundant sleep; regular exercise).
2. Changing potentially health-damaging habits before the damage is done (e.g. stopping smoking; desisting from consuming more than the recommended maximum weekly intake of alcohol; effective management of stressful life demands).

Changing behaviour, such as reducing salt intake, lowering lipids and increasing exercise, may therefore be a particularly useful strategy for population-based approaches to tackle problems such as hypertension. However, whilst the straight-forward assumption that changing risk factors known to contribute to risk for disease will reduce the incidence of the disease is reasonable, substantial further research is required. To date, most support for behavioural interventions comes from cross-sectional studies. The Cochrane Review of multiple risk factor interventions for primary prevention of coronary disease (Ebrahim & Davey Smith 2000) suggests that we still have to refine our health promotion methods, as changing the prevalence of risk factors in the community is not easily achieved. Disappointingly, current studies targeting risk factors such as blood cholesterol, blood pressure and smoking in general and workplace populations of middle-aged persons are subject to substantial hetero-geneity. The authors conclude that current approaches are in general ineffective in achieving reductions in both risk factors and cardiovascular disease mortality. However, factors such as method of intervention may have contributed to these poor results. For instance, smoking rates fell more substantially when individual smoking advice was given by a physician. There was also strong associations between baseline levels of risk factors and net falls in cholesterol and blood pressure experienced, suggesting that interventions may be more effective in populations with high risk profiles. This suggests that an important factor may be that participants are more likely to change their behaviours once they have had a myocardial infarct.

Owing to its massive public health importance, further research is needed to determine which population-based methods are most effective. For instance, pro-spective randomized trials are needed to evaluate the effectiveness of behavioural (non-pharmacological) interventions and the additive/interactive effects of using a range of techniques to reduce multiple behavioural risk factors with and without the use of drugs. Most importantly, psychologists and psychiatrists are in an important position to contribute their knowledge of how to change behaviour since primary prevention to promote behavioural change in health-risk behaviours (diet, smoking cessation) remains the most likely method to produce large changes in the commu-nity. As it is clear there is a need to improve our public campaigns, we need to review our theories of factors that may enhance or retard behaviour change in order to target our campaigns more appropriately, and the next section tackles the question of why people often continue to engage in health-risk behaviours.

Secondary prevention, involving early detection through preventive health behaviours such as skin or breast self-examination, is another important avenue for enhancing health. There is also scope for improving the percentage of the population that participate in these procedures by further understanding psycho-logical or social mechanisms that moderate individual differences in health behaviours, e.g. ruminative worry, family history or socioeconomic factors may make some individuals more likely to self-examine.

Tertiary prevention is concerned with reducing morbidity by shortening the delay to seek a diagnosis once a physical symptom is discovered and improving adherence to treatment. Psychological research in this area has investigated symptom inter-pretation and delayed help-seeking (Petrie & Weinman 1997). Factors facilitating compliance and appropriate self-care are also relevant.

The adoption of preventive health behaviour is obstructed by a number of barriers. First, people tend to underestimate their vulnerability to illness, are often inclined to ignore potential health threats despite clear warnings, and continue to expose themselves to preventable threats (e.g. continue to smoke, drink to excess, take unnecessary risks when driving). Such risk-taking may be due to a lack of direct experience with the threatened consequences. For example, the experience of coronary heart disease or lung cancer sometimes provides belated strong and effective encouragement to quit smoking. In addition, people generally assess themselves to be less likely to become ill (across a wide range of illnesses) than others of their own age and gender. Since the extent of such beliefs exceeds the statistical levels of risk attached to various illnesses, such beliefs have been described as indicating unrealistic optimism (Weinstein 1989).

The adoption of preventive health behaviour involves choices. The question arises of why, when health is valued, people frequently forsake preventive health behaviour and engage in actions that threaten health. An answer is suggested by behavioural conceptions of self-control and impulsivity (e.g. Logue 1988). Self-control involves choosing a larger, more delayed reinforcer in preference to a smaller, less delayed reinforcer, and impulsivity is the exact reverse. In general, behavioural choices are a function of the relative strength of competing reinforcers and the length of delay in receiving reinforcement. All other things being equal, behaviour leading to a larger reinforcer will be chosen in preference to behaviour leading to a smaller reinforcer. Also, other things being equal, an immediate reinforcer will be chosen in preference to a delayed one. Thus, although avoiding lung cancer is a bigger reinforcer than the pleasure derived from smoking, smoking (in persons who are aware of the hazards) occurs partly because the pleasure of smoking is immediate whereas lung cancer and other smoking-induced disease develop only after a long period of time (if at all).

Cognition and Health

The self-control evidenced by engagement in preventive health behaviour varies as a function of age, gender, socioeconomic status and cultural factors (Bennett & Murphy 1997). This variability, as well as the variation evident between people who share common demographic characteristics, may be due in part to differences in cognitive variables, especially health-related attitudes, beliefs and expectations.

Considerable cognitive (and social-cognitive) theorizing has gone into trying to explain and predict individual differences in the adoption of preventive health behaviour. Much of this theorizing assumes that people perceive their world, more or less, in terms of attributable causes and effects. Attribution theory holds that perceptions of causality vary between individuals along a number of continua (e.g. Abramson et al 1978). Individuals may differ in the extent to which they attribute causes of illness to being external versus internal, the belief that causes are stable versus changeable, that particular health behaviours are instances of global traits versus specific dispositions, and that causes of illness are subject to their control versus being uncontrollable. For example, one person might attribute a recently diagnosed heart condition to their history of continuing to smoke despite warnings about the hazards (internal attribution) whereas another person might attribute the same condition to stress at work (external attribution). In turn, perceived causes of illness, such as smoking and stress at work, may be seen as being stable (e.g. in the past the person has tried and failed to quit smoking or to lessen work stress) or changeable (e.g. under the threat of declining health, the person feels that the changed circumstances will allow them to effect behavioural changes where they have tried and failed in the past). Furthermore, a health-risk behaviour such as smoking may be perceived as being an instance of a global disposition towards an unhealthy lifestyle versus a specific behaviour which should not prevent them from adopting other health-enhancing behaviours. Finally, once illness occurs, individuals differ in the extent to which they perceive themselves as being able to control the course of the disease as against believing that progression of the disease is beyond their control.

Controllability has received specific attention, especially in relation to the construct of internality versus externality. In particular, Rotter's (1966) general concept of locus of control (which refers to general beliefs about personal control) has been adapted for the purpose of assessing individual health locus of control (Wallston et al 1987). Persons who have an internal locus of control believe that their health is controllable by them. Conversely, health may be regarded as not being under personal control, but as being a matter of luck or fate, or as being under the control of powerful others (e.g. one's physician). While the concept has intuitive appeal, it is not without limitations. For example, consulting a health professional could be indicative of an external locus in that the health professional is perceived as a powerful other who can cure illness. Conversely, consulting health professionals could be indicative of an internal locus in that it represents an active search for appropriate assistance. Moreover, the empirical findings generally indicate that health locus of control is at best a weak predictor of health behaviour. This is hardly surprising, considering the simplicity of the construct and the complex nature of the psychosocial determinants of health and illness.

Attempts to predict preventive health behaviour using social-cognitive theory have taken more elaborate forms. One such theory is the Health Belief Model, which proposes that health behaviour is a function of the perceived level of threat of disease, and the perceived relative costs and benefits of preventive action (Rosenstock et al 1988). There are several variants of the theory, all of which give a central role to individual perceptions of susceptibility to disease (i.e. risk of becoming ill or succumbing to a particular illness), and the perception of the severity (i.e. seriousness) of the illness were the individual to succumb. Whether action is taken to lessen the risk depends on the perceived balance of costs (e.g. time and effort involved in taking preventive action) and benefits (perceived reductions in risk), and the occurrence of cues to action which may be internal (as in the case of illness symptoms) or external (e.g. overt illness signs observed by a health professional). Health-promotion programmes based on the Health Belief Model make explicit use of external cues. For example, a programme designed to encourage smoking cessation might include informational input, including fear-arousing warnings (e.g. "smoking causes lung cancer and heart disease") and advice on how to quit that is intended to strengthen perceived personal benefits and reduce perceived costs, and thereby increase the likelihood of preventive action.

Another prominent theory of health behaviour is the Theory of Reasoned Action (Fishbein & Ajzen 1975), which emphasizes the role of intentions as determinants of behaviour. Intentions are seen as being primarily influenced by two factors. First, intentions are linked to the individual's attitude towards the particular action, and attitudes are in turn a function of expected outcomes and the value associated with these outcomes. Secondly, intentions are influenced by subjective norms about the appropriateness of the action, taking account of the normative beliefs of the individual's peers and the importance the individual attaches to these beliefs. There is some evidence to suggest that the Theory of Reasoned Action, which was subsequently extended and renamed the Theory of Planned Behaviour (Ajzen & Madden 1986), has slightly better predictive value than the Health Belief Model. Overall, however, social-cognitive theories have had limited success in predicting preventive health behaviour. One criticism of these theories is that they may exaggerate the extent to which behaviour results from a process in which individuals consider their options, evaluate multiple hypothetical consequences, and act rationally in ways designed to maximize future personal benefits. These theories invest the individual with considerable powers of deliberation and control. In reality, everyday life circumstances may often discourage people from behaving in ways that are strictly rational.

Despite the burgeoning number of alternative models proposed to explain health behaviour, empirical evidence strongly supporting these models remains sparse. For instance, Harrison et al (1992) conducted one of the most comprehensive meta-analytic reviews of the Health Belief Model. They identified 234 published tests of the predictive reliability of the model. The range of application of the Health Belief Model were impressive and included studies of preventive behaviours, such as screening of cervical cancer, risk behaviours such as smoking and alcohol, health behaviours such as cholera prevention, influenza vaccination, breast self-examination, contraceptive use, dental behaviour and adherence to antihypertensive, diabetic and renal regimens. Whilst susceptibility, severity, benefits and barriers were often predictors of behaviours, their effects were very small in substantive terms. In addition, poor operationalization of the model and failure to check reliability and validity of constructs imply that significant ongoing research is necessary to elucidate important components predictive of health behaviours.

Because of the complexity and multidetermined nature of health behaviour, it is likely that models such as Health Belief Model and concepts of locus of control are too simplistic, and current evidence does not support them as key explanatory concepts. For instance, the importance individuals place on their health, disease-specific issues, age, gender, socioeconomic and cultural factors have been suggested as critical factors moderating not only causal beliefs but the relationship between behaviour and health. Thus development of refined models is likely to become increasingly complex as they include socio-cultural factors and interactions between variables. Such models are necessary as they have heuristic value in guiding health promotion approaches to target key elements influencing health behaviours, and despite the problems described significant advances in health promotion planning and modification of health behaviour have been made (e.g. Green & Kreuter 1991; Glanz et al 1997). Further research is necessary, however, to combine variables from the numerous theoretical approaches that exist (van der Velde & van der Pligt 1991) and to combine cognitive approaches with behavioural interventions (e.g. reinforcement) derived from learning theory (Greenberg & Silverstein 1983). It may also be important to consider method of delivery; and a combination of approaches using individual face-to-face, telephone and community interventions may be necessary.

CONCLUDING REMARKS

This chapter has reviewed current understanding of the complex relationship between psychological factors and health, and the possible mechanisms underlying these effects. It has also challenged us to consider interventions not just within the hospital but outside its walls and targeting individuals who are not yet symptomatic. As such, psychology and psychiatry have a challenging role to play in examining the evidence to date and applying their skills at diagnosis and behaviour change to best influence these processes. The following chapters describe the ways in which the psychologist and psychiatrist are increasingly becoming integrated in medical practice, with a focus on particular medical conditions and also a consideration of the health-promotion approaches and professional issues that arise.

ACKNOWLEDGEMENTS

Eliza Sims provided invaluable assistance in the preparation of this chapter.

REFERENCES

Abramson LY, Seligman MEP and Teasdale JD: Learned helplessness in humans: critique and reformation. *J Abnorm Psychol* **87**(1): 49–74, 1978.

Ader R and Cohen N: Behaviorally conditioned immunosuppression. *Psychosom Med* **37**: 333–340, 1975.

Ader R, Cohen N and Felten D: Psychoneuroimmunology: conditioning and stress. *Annu Rev Psychol* **44**: 53–85, 1995.

Adgey AA, Devlin JE, Webb SW and Mulholland HC: Initiation of ventricular fibrillation outside hospital in patients with acute ischemic heart disease. *Br Heart J* **47**: 55–61, 1982.

Ajzen I and Madden TJ: Prediction of goal-directed behavior attitudes, intentions and perceived behavioral control. *J Exp Soc Psychol* **22**: 453–474, 1986.

Akil H, Meng F, Devine DP and Watson SJ: Molecular and neuroanatomical properties of the endogenous opioid system: implications for treatment of opioid addiction. *Semin Neurosci* **9**: 70–83, 1997.

Albeck DS, Hastings NB and McEwen BS: Effects of adrenalectomy and Type I or Type II glucocorticoid receptor action on AVP and CRH mRNA in the rat hypothalamus. *Mol Brain Res* **26**: 129–134, 1994.

Alexander F: *Psychosomatic Medicine: Its Principles and Applications.* WW Norton: New York, 1950.

Allison TG, Williams DE, Miller TD, Patten CA, Bailey KR, Squires RW and Gau GT: Medical and economic costs of psychologic distress in patients with coronary artery disease. *Mayo Clin Proc* **70**: 734–742, 1995.

Anderson BL, Kiecolt-Glaser JK and Glaser R: A biobehavioral model of cancer stress and disease course. *Am Psychologist* **49**: 389–404, 1994.

Anderson NB and Armstead CA: Toward understanding the association of socioeconomic status and health—a new challenge for the biopsychosocial approach. *Psychosom Med* **57**: 213–225, 1995.

APA (American Psychiatric Association): *Diagnostic and Statistical Manual of Mental Disorders* (3rd edition; DSM-III). APA: Washington, DC, 1980.

APA (American Psychiatric Association): *Diagnostic and Statistical Manual of Mental Disorders* (4th edition; DSM-IV). APA: Washington, DC, 1994.

APA Task Force on Laboratory Tests in Psychiatry: The dexamethasone suppression test: an overview of its current status in psychiatry. *Am J Psychiatry* **144**: 1253–1262, 1987.

Arana GW, Baldessarini RJ and Ornsteen M: The dexamethasone suppression test for diagnosis and prognosis in psychiatry. *Arch Gen Psychiatry* **42**: 1193–1204, 1985.

Australian Bureau of Statistics: *Causes of death: Australia. ABS Cat No 3303.0.* Australian Government Publishing Service: Canberra, 1994.

Basbaum AI and Fields HM: Endogenous pain control systems: brainstem spinal pathways and endorphin circuitry. *Annu Rev Neurosci* **7**: 309–338, 1984.

Baum A and Posluszny DM: Health psychology: mapping biobehavioural contributions to health and illness. *Annu Rev Psychol* **50**: 137–163, 1999.

Baum A, Garofalo JP and Yali AM: Socioeconomic status and chronic stress. Does stress account for SES effects on health? *Ann NY Acad Sci* **896**: 131–144, 1999.

Bayes de Luna A, Coumel P and Leclerq JR: Ambulatory sudden cardiac death: mechanisms of production of fatal arrhythmia on the basis of data from 157 cases. *Am Heart J* **117**: 151–159, 1989.

Beecher HK: The powerful placebo. *JAMA* **159**: 1602–1606, 1955.

Beitins IZ and Dufau ML: Pulsatile secretions of progesterone from the human corpus luteum and poor correlation with bioactive LH pulses. *Acta Endocrinol* **111**: 553–557, 1986.

Bellinger D, Lorton D, Felten SY and Felten DL: Innervation of lymphoid organs and implications in development, aging and autoimmunity. *Int J Immunopharmacol* **14**: 329–344, 1992.

Benedetti F and Amanzio M: The neurobiology of placebo analgesia—from endogenous opioids to cholecystokinin. *Prog Neurobiol* **52**: 109–125, 1997.

Bennett EJ, Tennant CC, Piesse C, Badcock CA and Kellow JE: Level of chronic life stress predicts clinical outcome in irritable bowel syndrome. *Gut* **43**(2): 256–261, 1998.

Bennett P and Murphy S: *Psychology and Health Promotion.* Open University Press: Buckingham, 1997.

Benson H and Epstein MD: The placebo effect: a neglected asset in the care of patients. *JAMA* **232**: 1225–1227, 1975.

Besedovsky HO and del Rey A: Immune-neuro-endocrine interactions: facts and hypotheses. *Endocrine Rev* **17**: 64–102, 1996.

Besedovsky HO, del Rey A and Sorkin E: Lymphokine containing supernatants from Con A-stimulated cells increase corticosterone blood levels. *J Immunol* **126**: 385–387, 1981.

Besedovsky HO, del Rey A, Sorkin E, Lotz W and Schwulera U: Lymphoid cells produce an immunoregulatory glucocorticoid increasing factor (GIF) acting through the pituitary gland. *Clin Exp Immunol* **59**: 622–628, 1985.

Best JA and Proctor S: Behavioral medicine training from a public health perspective. *Ann Behav Med* **10**: 19–22, 1988.

Blumenthal JA, Wei J, Babyak M et al: Stress management and exercise training in cardiac patients with myocardial ischemia: effects on prognosis and on markers of myocardial ischemia. *Arch Intern Med* **157**: 2213–2223, 1997.

Booth-Kewley S and Friedman HS: Psychological predictors of heart disease: a quantitative review. *Psychol Bull* **101**: 343–362, 1987.

Bovberg DH, Ader R and Cohen N: Behaviorally conditioned suppression of a graft versus host response. *Proc Natl Acad Sci USA* **79**: 583–585, 1982.

Bovberg DH, Cohen N and Ader R: Behaviorally conditioned enhancement of delayed hypersensitivity response in the mouse. *Brain Behav Immun* **1**: 64–71, 1987.

Brooks-Gunn J: The salience and timing of the menstrual flow. *Psychosom Med* **47**: 363–371, 1985.

Buccheri G: Depressive reactions to lung cancer are common and often followed by a poor outcome. *Eur Resp J* **11**(1): 173–178, 1998.

Calloway P and Dolan R: Endocrine changes and clinical profiles in depression. In GW Brown and TO Harris (Eds), *Life Events and Illness*, pp 139–160. Unwin Hyman: London, 1989.

Cameron O: Depression increases post-MI mortality: how? *Psychosom Med* **58**: 111–112, 1996.

Carney RM, Freedland KE, Rich MW et al: Depression as a risk factor for cardiac events in established coronary heart disease: a review of possible mechanisms. *Ann Behav Med* **17**: 142–149, 1995.

Carroll D, Bennett P and Smith GD: Socio-economic health inequalities: their origins and implications. *Psychol Health* **8**: 295–316, 1993.

Cassidy L, Meadows J, Catalan J and Barton S: Are reported stress and coping style associated with frequent recurrence of genital herpes? *Genitourin Med* **73**: 263–266, 1997.

Chang JK and Chang KJ: The role of amino-terminal sequence of beta-endorphin and dynorphin in the determination of opiate receptor type selectivity. *Life Sci* **33**: 267–269, 1983.

Checkley S: The neuroendocrinology of depression and chronic stress. *Br Med Bull* **52**: 597–617, 1996.

Chen Y, Mestek A, Liu J, Hurley JA and Yu L: Molecular cloning and functional expression of a m-opioid receptor from rat brain. *Mol Pharmacol* **44**: 8–12, 1993.

Chesney MA: New behavioral risk factors for coronary heart disease: implications for intervention. In K Orth-Gomer and N Schneiderman (Eds), *Behavioral Medicine Approaches to Cardiovascular Disease Prevention*. Lawrence Erlbaum Associates Inc: New Jersey, 1996.

Chrousos GP: Stressors, stress, and neuroendocrine integration of the adaptive response. The 1997 Hans Selye Memorial Lecture. *Ann NY Acad Sci* [Lectures]: **851**: 311–335, 1998.

Cobb LA, Werner JA and Trobaugh GB: Sudden cardiac death: I. A decade's experience with out-of-hospital resuscitation. *Modern Concepts Cardiovasc Dis* **49**: 31–36, 1980.

Cohen F, Kearney KA, Zegans LS, Kemeny ME, Neuhaus JM and Stites DP: Persistent stress as a prediction of genital herpes recurrence. *Brain, Behavior & Immunity* **13**(2): 155–174, 1999.

Cohen S and Williamson EA: Stress and infectious disease in humans. *Psychol Bull* **109**(1): 5–24, 1991.

Copolov DL, Rubin RT, Stuart GW, Poland RE, Mander AJ, Sashidharan SP, Whitehouse AM, Blackburn IM Freeman CP and Blackwood DH: Specificity of the salivary cortisol dexamethasone suppression test across psychiatric diagnoses. *Biol Psychiatry* **25**: 879–893, 1989.

Coryell W, Noyes R and Clancy J: Excess mortality in panic disorder. A comparison with primary unipolar depression. *Arch Gen Psychiatry* **39**: 701–703, 1982.

Coumel P, Leclerq J and Leenhardt AV: Arrhythmias as predictors of sudden death. *Am Heart J* **114**: 929–937, 1987.

Cwikel JG, Behar LC & Zabora Jr: Psychosocial factors that affect the survival of adult cancer patients: a review of research. *J Psychosocial Oncol* **15**: 1–34, 1997.

Davis A and George J: *States of Health: Health and Illness in Australia.* Harper & Row: Sydney, 1988.

De Leon J: Smoking and vulnerability for schizophrenia. *Schiz Bull* **22**: 405–409, 1996.

De Souza EB: Corticotropin-releasing factor receptors: physiology, pharmacology, biochemistry and role in central nervous system and immune disorders. *Psychoneuroendocrinology* **20**: 789–819, 1995.

Dobrilla G and Scarpignato C: Placebo and placebo effect. Their impact on the evaluation of drug response in patients. *Dig Dis* **12**: 368–377, 1994.

Dwight MM and Stoudemire A: Effects of depressive disorders on coronary artery disease: a review. *Harvard Rev of Psychiatry* **5**(3): 115–122, 1997.

Eastwood MR, Rifat SL, Nobbs H and Ruderman J: Mood disorder following cerebrovascular accident. *Br J Psychiatry* **154**: 195–200, 1989.

Ebrahim S and Davey Smith G: Multiple risk factor interventions for primary prevention of coronary heart disease (Cochrane Review). In: *The Cochrane Library.* Update Software: Oxford, 2000, Issue 4.

Edelman S and Kidman AD: Mind and cancer: is there a relationship? A review of evidence. *Aust Psychologist* **32**: 79–85, 1997.

Eichenbaum H and Otto T: The hippocampus: what does it do? *Behav Neural Biol* **57**: 2–36, 1992.

Engel GL: The need for a new medical model: a challenge for biomedicine. *Science* **196**: 129–136, 1977.

Engel GL: The clinical application of the biopsychosocial model. *Am J Psychiatry* **137**: 535–544, 1980.

Esler M, Lambert G and Kaye D: Neurobiology of psychosomatic heart disease. *Personal communication,* 1999.

Evans CJ, Keith DE Jr, Morrison H, Magendzo K and Edwards RH: Cloning of a delta opioid receptor by functional expression. *Science* **258**: 1952–1955, 1992.

Everson SA, Goldberg DE, Kaplan GA, Cohen RD, Pukkala E, Tuomilehto J and Salonen JT: Hopelessness and risk of mortality and incidence of myocardial infarction and cancer. *Psychosom Med* **58**: 113–121, 1996.

Faller H, Buelzebruck H, Schilling S, Drings P and Lang H: Do psychological factors influence survival in cancer patients. Findings of an empirical study with lung cancer patients. *Psychother Psychosom Med Psychol* **47**: 206–218, 1997.

Faller H, Bulzebruck H, Drings P and Lang H: Coping, distress, and survival among patients with lung cancer. *Arch Gen Psychiatry* **56**(8): 756–762, 1999.

Fawzy FI, Kemeny ME, Fawzy NW, Elashoff R, Morton D, Cousins N and Fahey L: A structured psychiatric intervention for cancer patients II. Changes over time in immunological measures. *Arch Gen Psychiatry* **47**: 729–735, 1990.

Fawzy FI, Fawzy N, Hyun CS, Elashoff R, Guthrie D, Fahey L and Morton D: Malignant melanoma: effects of an early structured intervention, coping and affective state on recurrence and survival 6 years later. *Arch Gen Psychiatry* **50**: 681–689, 1993.

Ferguson JH: Curative and population medicine: bridging the great divide. *Neuroepidemiology* **18**: 111–119, 1999.

Ferreira SH and Nakamura M: Prostaglandin hyperalgesia: the peripheral analgesic activity of morphine, enkephalins and opioid antagonists. *Prostaglandins* **18**: 191–200, 1979.

Fields HL, Barbaro NM and Heinricher MM: Brain stem neuronal circuitry underlying the antinociceptive action of opiates. *Prog Brain Res* **77**: 245–257, 1988.

Finset A, Sundet K and Haakonsen M: Neuropsychological syndromes in right hemisphere stroke patients. *Scand J Psychol* **29**: 9–20, 1988.

Fishbein M and Ajzen I: *Belief, Attitude and Behavior: An Introduction to Theory and Research.* Addison-Wesley: Reading, MA, 1975.

Fleshner M, Landenslager ML, Simons L and Maier SF: Reduced serum antibodies associated with social defeat in rats. *Physiol Behav* **45**: 1183–1187, 1989.

Frasure-Smith N, Lesperance F, Juneau M, Talajic M and Bourassa MG: Gender, depression, and one-year prognosis after myocardial infarction. *Psychosom Med* **61**(1): 26–37, 1999.

Fukuda K, Kato S, Mori K, Nishi M and Takeshima H: Primary structures and expression from cDNAs of rat opioid receptor d- and m-subtypes. *FEBS Lett* **327**: 311–314, 1993.

Fuster V, Badimon L, Badimon JJ and Chesebro JH: The pathogenesis of coronary artery disease and the acute coronary artery syndromes (1). *N Engl J Med* **326**: 242–250, 1992a.

Fuster V, Badimon L, Badimon JJ and Chesebro JH: The pathogenesis of coronary artery disease and the acute coronary artery syndromes (2). *N Engl J Med* **326**: 310–318, 1992b.

Glanz K, Lewis FM and Rimer BK (Eds): *Health Behavior and Health Education: Theory, Research, and Practice*, 2nd edn. Jossey-Bass: San Francisco, 1997.

Godwin CD: The dexamethasone suppression test in acute mania. *J Affect Dis* **7**: 281–286, 1984.

Gold PW, Chrousos G, Kellner C, Post R, Roy A, Augerinos P, Schulte H, Oldfield E and Loriaux DL: Psychiatric implications of basic and clinical studies with corticotropin-releasing factor. *Am J Psychiatry* **141**: 619–627, 1984.

Goldstein M and Niaura R: Psychological factors affecting physical condition. Cardiovascular disease literature review. Part I: Coronary artery disease and sudden death. *Psychosomatics* **33**: 134–145, 1992.

Goodwin JS, Hunt WC, Key CR and Samet JM: The effect of marital status on stage, treatment and survival of cancer patients. *JAMA* **258**: 3125–3130, 1987.

Gorkin L, Follick MJ, Wilkin DL and Niaura R: Social support and the progression and treatment of cardiovascular disease. In SA Shumaker and SM Czajkowski (Eds), *Social Support and Cardiovascular Disease*, pp 281–299. Plenum Press: New York, NY, 1994.

Gracely RH, Dubner R, Wolskee PJ and Deeter WR: Placebo and naloxone can alter post-surgical pain by separate mechanisms. *Nature* **306**: 264–265, 1983.

Green LW and Kreuter M: Health promotion planning: an educational and environmental approach. Mayfield Publishing Company: Mountain View, 1991.

Greenberg MS and Silverstein ML: Cognitive and behavioral treatments of depressive disorders: interventions with adults. In Morrison HL (Ed.), *Children of Depressed Parents: Risk, Identification, and Intervention*, pp 189–220. Grune & Stratton: New York, 1983.

Greer S: Psychological response to cancer and survival. *Psychol Med* **21**: 43–49, 1991.

Greer S, Morris T and Pettingale KW: Psychological response to breast cancer: effect on outcome. *Lancet* **ii**: 785–787, 1979.

Grevert P, Albert LH and Goldstein A: Partial antagonism of placebo analgesia by naloxone. *Pain* **16**: 129–143, 1983.

Haft JL and Fani K: Intravascular platelet aggregation in the heart induced by stress. *Circulation* **47**: 353–358, 1973a.

Haft JL and Fani K: Stress and the induction of intravascular platelet aggregation. *Circulation* **48**: 164–169, 1973b.

Hansson L: Shortcomings of current antihypertensive therapy. *Am J Hypertens* **4**(2): 308–311, 1991.

Harbin TJ: The relationship between the type A behavior pattern and physiological responsivity: a quantitative review. *Psychophysiology* **28**: 110–119, 1989.

Harrington A: *The Placebo Effect: An Interdisciplinary Exploration.* Cambridge University Press: Cambridge, MA, 1997.

Harrison JA, Mullen PD and Green LW: A meta-analysis of studies of the health belief model with adults. *Health Educ Res* **7**: 107–116, 1992.

Hartline KM, Owens MJ and Nemeroff CB: Postmortem and cerebrospinal fluid studies of corticotropin-releasing factor in humans. *Ann NY Acad Sci* **780**: 96–105, 1996.

Herbert J: Peptides in the limbic system: neurochemical codes for co-ordinated adaptive responses to behavioural and physiological demand. *Progr Neurobiol* **41**: 723–791, 1993.

Herbert TB and Cohen S: Depression and immunity: a meta-analytic review. *Psychol Bull* **113**: 472–486, 1993.

Herman JP: Regulation of adrenocorticosteroid receptor mRNA expression in the central nervous system. *Cell Mol Neurobiol* **13**: 349–372, 1993.

Herman JP and Cullinan WE: Neurocircuitry of stress: central control of the hypothalamo–pituitary–adrenocortical axis. *TINS* **20**: 78–84, 1997.

Herman JP, Patel PD, Akil H and Watson SJ: Localization and regulation of glucocorticoid and mineralocorticoid receptor messenger RNAs in the hippocampal formation of the rat. *Endocrinology* **3**: 1886–1894, 1989.

Herman JP, Prewitt CMF and Cullinan WE: Neuronal circuit regulation of the hypothalamo–pituitary–adrenocortical stress axis. *Crit Rev Neurobiol* **10**: 371–394, 1996.

Hewlett WA and Barchas JD: Regional interactions of opioid peptides at mu and delta sites in rat brain. *Peptides* **4**: 853–858, 1983.

Hislop TG, Waxler NE, Coldman AJ, Elwood JM and Kan L: The prognostic significance of psychosocial relationships in women with breast cancer. *J Chronic Dis* **40**: 729–735, 1987.

Hjemdahl P, Larsson K, Johansson MC, Zetterlund A and Eklund A: Beta-adrenoceptors in human alveolar macrophages isolated by elutriation. *Br J Clin Pharmacol* **30**: 673–682, 1990.

Holden G: The relationship of self-efficacy appraisals to subsequent health related outcomes: a meta-analysis. *Soc Work Health Care* **16**: 53–93, 1991.

Horne R and Weinman J: Patient's beliefs about prescribed medicines and their role in adherence to treatment in chronic physical illness. *J Psychosom Res* **47**(6): 555–567, 1999.

Hosobuchi Y, Adams JE and Linchitz R: Pain relief by electrical stimulation of the central gray matter in humans and its reversal by naloxone. *Science* **197**: 183–186, 1977.

Hutchinson S: Psycho-oncology: an overview and review of psychological interventions. Paper presented at the 20th National Conference, Australian Association for Cognitive Behavioural Therapy, Brisbane, Australia, 1997.

Irwin M, Daniels M, Smith T, Bloom E and Weiner H: Impaired natural killer cell activity during bereavement. *Brain, Behav Immun* **1**: 98–104, 1987.

Irwin M, Hauger RL, Jones L, Provincio M and Britton KT: Sympathetic nervous system mediates central corticotropin-releasing factor induced suppression of natural killer cytotoxicity. *J Pharmacol Exp Ther* **255**: 101–107, 1990.

Jacobson L and Sapolsky R: The role of the hippocampus in feedback regulation of the hypothalamic–pituitary–adrenocortical axis. *Endocr Rev* **12**: 118–134, 1991.

James JE: Health care, psychology, and the scientist-practitioner model. *Aust Psychologist* **29**: 511, 1994.

James JE: Empirically validated treatments: health psychology interventions. *Behav Change* **14**: 6–8, 1997.

Jensen TS: Opioids in the brain: supraspinal mechanisms in pain control. *Acta Anaesthesiol Scand Suppl* **41**: 123–132, 1997.

Joyce PR, Brinded PJ, Sellman D, Donald RA and Elder PA: The dexamethasone suppression test in psychiatry. *NZ Med J* **100**: 173–175, 1987.

Julius D: Another opiate for the masses? *Nature* **386**: 442, 1997.

Kahan JP, Bernstein SJ, Leape LL, Hilborne LH, Park RE, Parker L, Kornberg CJ and Brook RH: Measuring the necessity of medical procedures. *Med Care* **32**: 357–365, 1994.

Kamarck T and Jennings JR: Biobehavioral factors in sudden cardiac death. *Psychol Bull* **109**: 42–75, 1991.

Kanjhan R: Opioids and pain. *Clin Exp Pharmacol Physiol* **22**: 397–403, 1995.

Kaplan AS, Garfinkel PE and Brown GM: The DST and TRH test in bulimia nervosa. *Br J Psychiatry* **154**: 86–92, 1989.

Kaplan GA and Keil JE: Socioeconomic factors and cardiovascular disease: a review of the literature. *Circulation* **88**: 1973–1998, 1993.

Kaplan GA and Lynch JW: Socioeconomic considerations in the primordial prevention of cardiovascular disease [Review]. *Prev Med* **29**(6 Pt 2): S30–35, 1999.

Kaplan GA, Strawbridge WJ, Cohen RD and Hungerford LR: Natural history of leisure-time physical activity and its correlates: associations with mortality from all causes and cardiovascular disease over 28 years. *Am J Epidemiol* **144**(8): 793–797, 1996.

Kaplan JR, Manuck SB, Clarkson TB, Lusso FM and Taub DM: Social status, environment and atherosclerosis in cynomolgus monkeys. *Arteriosclerosis* **2**: 359–368, 1982.

Kaplan JR, Manuck SB, Adams MR, Weingand KW and Clarkson TB: Inhibition of coronary atherosclerosis by propranolol in behaviorally predisposed monkeys fed an atherogenic diet. *Circulation* **76**: 1364–1372, 1987.

Kaplan RM: Behavior as the central outcome in health care. *Am Psychologist* **45**: 1211–1220, 1990.

Kassirer J: The quality of care and the quality of measuring it. *N Engl J Med* **329**: 1263–1265, 1993.

Kathol RG, Jaeckle RS, Lopez JR and Meller WH: Consistent reduction of ACTH responses to stimulation with CRH, vasopressin and hypoglycaemia in patients with depression. *Br J Psychiatry* **155**: 468–478, 1989.

Kemeny ME, Cohen F, Zegans LS and Conant MA: Psychological and immunological predictors of genital herpes recurrence. *Psychosom Med* **51**: 195–208, 1989.

Kempf FC and Josephson ME: Cardiac arrest recorded on ambulatory electrocardiograms. *Am J Cardiol* **53**: 1577–1582, 1984.

Knox SS, Siegmund KD, Weidner G, Ellison RC, Adelman A and Paton C: Hostility, social support, and coronary heart disease in the National Heart, Lung and Blood Institution Family Health Study. *Am J Cardiol* **82**(10): 1192–1196, 1998.

Krantz DS, Helmers KF, Bairey CN, Nebel LE, Hedges SM and Rozanski A: Cardiovascular reactivity and mental-stress induced myocardial ischemia in patients with coronary artery disease. *Psychosom Med* **53**: 1–12, 1991.

Krantz DS, Santiago HT, Kop WJ, Bairey Merz CN, Rozanski A and Gottdiener JS: Prognostic value of mental stress testing in coronary artery disease. *Am J Cardiol* **84**(1): 1292–1297, 1999.

Krishnan KRR, Doraiswamy PM, Lurie SN, Figiel GS, Husain MM, Boyko OB, Ellinwood EH Jr and Nemeroff CB: Pituitary size in depression. *J Clin Endocrinol Metab* **72**: 256–259, 1991.

Lazarus RS and Folkman S: *Stress, Appraisal and Coping.* Springer: New York, 1984.

Lesperance F, Frasure-Smith N and Talajic M: Major depression before and after myocardial infarction: its nature and consequences. *Psychosom Med* **58**: 99–110, 1996.

Levine JD, Gordon NC and Fields HL: The mechanism of placebo analgesia. *Lancet* **ii**: 654–657, 1978.

Liberthson RR, Nagel EL, Hirschman JC, Nussenfeld SR, Blackbourne BD and Davis JH: Pathophysiologic observations in prehospital ventricular fibrillation and sudden cardiac death. *Circulation* **49**: 790–798, 1974.

Llewelyn MB, Azami J and Roberts MH: Brainstem mechanisms of antinociception. Effects of electrical stimulation and injection of morphine into the nucleus raphe magnus. *Neuropharmacology* **25**: 727–735, 1986.

Logue AW: Research on self-control: an integrating framework. *Behav Brain Sci* **11**: 665–709, 1988.

Longo DJ and Clum GA: Psychosocial factors affecting genital herpes recurrences: linear vs mediating models. *J Psychosom Res* **33**: 161–166, 1989.

Lundberg U: Stress responses in low-status jobs and their relationship to health risks: musculoskeletal disorders. *Ann NY Acad Sci* **896**: 162–172, 1999.

Lustman PJ, Griffith LS, Clouse RE and Gryer RE: Psychiatric illness in diabetes mellitus: relationship to symptoms and illness control. *J Nerv Ment Dis* **174**: 736–742, 1986.

Maier SF, Watkins LR and Fleshner M: Psychoneuroimmunology. The interface between behavior, brain and immunity. *Am Psychologist* **49**: 1004–1017, 1994.

Mansour VM, Wilkinson DJ, Jennings GL, Schwarz RG, Thompson JM and Esler MD: Panic disorder: coronary spasm as a basis for cardiac risk? *Med J Aust* **168**: 390–392, 1998.

Manuck SB, Kaplan JR, Muldoon MF et al: The behavioral exacerbation of atherosclerosis and its inhibition by propranolol. In PM McCabe, N Schneiderman, TM Field et al (Eds), *Stress, Coping and Disease*, pp 51–72. Lawrence Erlbaum and Associates: Hillsdale, NJ, 1991.

Markovitz JH and Matthews KA: Platelets and coronary heart disease: potential psychophysiological mechanisms. *Psychosom Med* **53**: 643–668, 1991.

Markovitz JH, Matthews KA, Kiss J and Smitherman TC: Effects of hostility on platelet reactivity to psychological stress in coronary heart disease patients and in healthy controls. *Psychosom Med* **58**: 143–149, 1996.

Martin PR, Prior M and Milgrom J (Eds): Psychological factors in illness. In *Health and Medical Research: Contribution of the Social and Behavioural Sciences*. Academy of the Social Sciences in Australia: Canberra, 2001.

Matthes HWD, Maldonado R, Simonin F, Valverde O, Slowe S, Kitchen I, Befort K, Dierich A, Le Meur M, Dolle P, Tzavara E, Hanoune J, Roques BP and Kieffer BL: Loss of morphine-induced analgesia, reward effect and withdrawal symptoms in mice lacking the m-opioid-receptor gene. *Nature* **383**: 819–823, 1996.

May GS, Eberlein KA, Furberg CD, Passamani ER and DeMetz DC: Secondary primary prevention after myocardial infarction: a review of long-term trials. *Prog Cardiovasc Dis* **24**: 331–352, 1982.

McAllister TW: Cognitive functioning in the affective disorders. *Comprehens Psychiatry* **22**: 572–586, 1981.

McEwen BS: Protective and damaging effects of stress mediators. *N Engl J Med* **338**(3): 171–179, 1998.

McEwen BS and Magarinos AM: Stress effects on morphology and function of the hippocampus. *Ann NY Acad Sci* **821**: 271–284, 1997.

McEwen BS, Albeck D, Cameron H, Chao HM, Gould E, Hastings N, Kuroda Y, Luine V, Magarinos AM, McKittrick CR, Orchinik M, Pavlides C, Vaher P, Watanabe Y and Weiland N: Stress and the brain: a paradoxical role for adrenal steroids. In GD Litwack (Ed), *Vitamins and Hormones*, pp 371–402, 1995.

McKeown T: *The Role of Medicine: Dream, Mirage or Nemesis?* Basil Blackwell: Oxford, 1979.

McLaughlin and Fuster V: The three mechanisms for coronary artery disease progression: insights into future management. *Mt Sinai J Med* **62**: 265–274, 1995.

Meikle AW, Stringham JD, Woodward MG and Bishop DT: Heritability of variation of plasma cortisol levels. *Metabolism* **37**: 514–517, 1988.

Meisel SR, Kutz I, Dayan KI, Pauzner H, Chetboun I, Arbel Y and David D: Effect of Iraqi missile war on incidence of acute myocardial infarction and sudden death in Israeli civilians. *Lancet* **338**: 660–661, 1991.

Menard MK: Cesarean delivery rates in the United States. The 1990s. *Obst Gynecol Clin Am* **26**(2): 275–286, 1999.

Meng F, Xie GX, Thompson RC, Mansour A, Goldstein A, Watson SJ and Akil H: Cloning and pharmacological characterization of a rat kappa opiod receptor. *Proc Natl Acad Sci USA* **90**: 9954–9958, 1993.

Michelson D, Stratakis C, Hill L, Reynolds J, Galliven E, Chrousos G and Gold P: Bone mineral density in women with depression. *N Engl J Med* **335**: 1176–1181, 1996.

Mikat EM, Bartolome JV, Weiss JM, Schanberg SN, Kuhn CM and Williams RB: Chronic norepinephrine infusion accelerates atherosclerotic lesion development in sand rats maintained on a high cholesterol diet. [Abstract] *Psychosom Med* **53**: 212–213, 1991.

Moser DK and Dracup K: Is anxiety after myocardial infarction associated with subsequent ischemic and arrhythmic events? *Psychosom Med* **58**: 395–401, 1996.

Muller JE and Verrier RL: Triggering of sudden death Lessons from an earthquake. *N Engl J Med* **334**: 460–461, 1996.

Muller JE, Tofler GH and Stone PH: Circadian variation and triggers of onset of acute cardiovascular disease. *Circulation* **79**: 733–743, 1989.

Munck A, Guyre PM and Holbrook NJ: Physiological functions of glucocorticoids in stress and their relations to pharmacological actions. *Endocrine Rev* **5**: 25–44, 1984.

Murray CJL and Lopez AD (Eds): *The Global Burden of Disease*. The Harvard School of Public Health: Boston, 1996.

Musselman DL and Nemeroff CB: Depression really does hurt your heart: stress, depression, and cardiovascular disease. *Prog Brain Res* **122**: 43–59, 2000.

Musselman DL, Evans DL and Nemeroff CB: The relationship of depression to cardiovascular disease. *Ann Behav Med* **19**: 264–270, 1997.

Newcomer JW, Craft S, Hershey T, Askins K and Bardgett ME: Glucocorticoid-induced impairment in declarative memory performance in adult humans. *J Neurosci* **14**: 2047–2053, 1994.

Nicholls D: *Proteins, Transmitters and Synapses*. Blackwell: Oxford, 1994.

O'Brien G, Hassanyeh F, Leake A, Schapira K, White M and Ferrier IN: The dexamethasone suppression test in bulimia nervosa. *Br J Psychiatry* **152**: 654–656, 1988.

Olff M: Stress, depression and immunity: the role of defense and coping styles. *Psychol Res* **85**(1): 7–15, 1999.

Oliveras JL, Redjemi F, Guilbaud G and Besson JM: Analgesia produced by electrical stimulation of the inferior centralis nucleus of the raphe in the cat. *Pain* **1**: 139–145, 1975.

Olson GA, Olson RD and Kastin AJ: Endogenous opiates: 1996. *Peptides* **18**: 1651–1688, 1997.

Ormel J, Kempen GI, Deeg DJ, Brilman EI, van Sonderen E and Relyveld J: Functioning, well-being, and health perception in late middle-aged and older people: comparing the effects of depressive symptoms and chronic medical conditions. *J Am Geriar Soc* **46**(1): 39–48, 1998.

Parikh RM, Robinson RG, Lipsey JR, Starkstein SE, Fedoroff JP and Price TR: The impact of post stroke depression on recovery in activities of daily living over two year follow-up. *Arch Neurol* **47**: 785–789, 1990.

Penninx BW, Guralnik JM, Mendes de Leon CF, Pahor M, Visser M, Corti MC and Wallace RB: Cardiovascular events and mortality in newly and chronically depressed persons >70 years of age. *Am J Cardiol* **81**(8): 988–994, 1998a.

Penninx BW, Guralnik JM, Pahor M, Ferrucci L, Cerhan JR, Wallace RB and Havlik RJ: Chronically depressed mood and cancer risk in older persons. *J Natl Cancer Inst* **90**(24): 1888–1893, 1998b.

Persky VH, Kempthorne-Rawson J and Shekelle RB: Personality and risk of cancer: 20-year follow-up of Western Electric Study. *Psychosom Med* **49**: 435–449, 1987.

Pert CB and Snyder SH: Opiate receptors: demonstration in nervous tissue. *Science* **179**: 1011–1014, 1973.

Petrie K and Weinman J (Eds): *Perceptions of Health and Illness: Current Research and Applications*. Harwood Academic Publishers: Singapore, 1997.

Phelps CE: The methodologic foundations of studies of appropriateness of medical care. *N Engl J Med* **329**: 1242–1245, 1993.

Pickering T: Cardiovascular pathways: socioeconomic status and stress effects on hypertension and cardiovascular function. *Ann NY Acad Sci* **896**: 262–277, 1999.

Pitts AF, Kathol RG, Gehris TL et al: Elevated cerebrospinal fluid corticotropin-releasing hormone and arginine vasopressin in depressed patients with dexamethasone nonsuppression. *Soc Neurosci Abs* **16**: 454, 1990.

Posavad CM, Koelle DM and Corey L: High frequency of CD8+ cytotoxic T-lymphocyte precursors specific for Herpes Simplex viruses in persons with genital herpes. *J Virol* **70**: 8165–8168, 1996.

Posner J and Burke CA: The effects of naloxone on opiate and placebo analgesia in healthy volunteers. *Psychopharmacology* **87**: 468–472, 1985.

Randall WC (Ed): *Neural Regulation of the Heart*. Oxford University Press: New York, 1977.

Rebecca G, Wayne R, Zebede J, D'Adamo A, Hanlon B, Sandor T, Ganz P and Selwyn A: Pathogenic mechanisms causing transient myocardial ischemia with mental arousal in patients with coronary artery disease. *Clin Res* **34**: 338A, 1986.

Regier DA, Farmer ME, Rae DS, Locke BZ, Keith SJ, Judd LL and Goodwin FK: Comorbidity of mental disorders with alcohol and other drug abuse. *JAMA* **264**: 2511–2518, 1990.

Reichlin S: Mechanisms of disease. Neuroendocrine-immune interactions. *N Engl J Med* **329**: 1246–1253, 1993.

Reul JMHM and de Kloet ER: Two receptor systems for corticosterone in rat brain: microdistribution and differential occupation. *Endocrinology* **117**: 2505–2511, 1985.

Reynolds P and Kaplan GA: Social connections and risk for cancer: prospective evidence from the Alameda County Study. *Behav Med* **16**: 101–110, 1990.

Rice PL: *Health Psychology*. Brooks/Cole: Pacific Grove, 1998.

Robinson RG: Neuropsychiatric consequences of stroke. *Annu Rev Med* **48**: 217–229, 1997.

Robinson RG, Starr LB, Kubos KL and Price TR: A two year longitudinal study of post-stroke mood disorders: findings during the initial evaluation. *Stroke* **14**: 736–744, 1983.

Robinson RG, Kubos KL, Starr LB, Rao K and Price TR: Mood disorders in stroke patients: importance of location of lesion. *Brain* **107**: 81–93, 1984.

Robinson RG, Murata Y and Shimoda K: Dimensions of social impairment and their effect on depression and recovery following stroke. *Inter Psychogeriatrics* **11**(4): 375–384, 1999.

Rosenstock IM, Strecher VJ and Becker MH: Social learning theory and the health belief model. *Health Educ Q* **15**: 175–183, 1988.

Rotter JB: Generalized expectancies for internal versus external control of reinforcement. *Psychol Monogr* **80**: 1–28, 1966.

Roy A, Pickar D, Paul S, Doran A, Chrousos GP and Gold PW: CSF corticotropin-releasing hormone in depressed patients and normal control subjects. *Am J Psychiatry* **144**: 641–645, 1987.

Rozanski A, Blumenthal JA and Kaplan J: Impact of psychological factors on the pathogenesis of cardiovascular disease and implications for therapy. *Circulation* **99**: 2192–2217, 1999.

Rubin RT, Phillips JJ, McCracken JT and Sadow TF: Adrenal gland volume in major depression: relationship to basal and stimulated pituitary–adrenal cortical axis function. *Biol Psychiatry* **40**: 89–97, 1996.

Rubinstein M, Mogil JS, Japon M, Chan EV, Allen RG and Low MJ: Absence of opioid stress-induced analgesia in mice lacking β-endorphin by site-directed mutagenesis. *Proc Natl Acad Sci USA* **93**: 3995–4000, 1996.

Sapolsky RM: Glucocorticoids potentiate ischemic injury to neurons: therapeutic implications. *Science* **229**: 1397–1400, 1985.

Sapolsky RM: *Stress: The Aging Brain and the Mechanisms of Neuron Death*. MIT Press: Cambridge, MA, 1992.

Sato K, Flood JF and Makinodan T: Influence of conditioned psychological stress on immunological recovery in mice exposed to low-dose X-irradiation. *Radiat Res* **98**: 381–388, 1984.

Schneiderman N and Orth-Gomer K: Blending traditions: a concluding perspective on behavioral medicine approaches to coronary heart disease prevention. In K Orth-Gomer and N Schneiderman (Eds), *Behavioral Medicine Approaches to Cardiovascular Disease Prevention*, pp 279–299. Lawrence Erlbaum Associates Inc: New Jersey, 1996.

Schwartz PJ: Sympathetic imbalance and cardiac arrhthymias. In W Randall (Ed), *Nervous Control of Cardiovascular Function*, pp 225–252. Oxford University Press: New York, 1984.

Schwartz PJ and Stone HL: Left stellectomy in the prevention of ventricular fibrillation caused by acute myocardial ischemia in conscious dogs with anterior myocardial infarction. *Circulation* **62**: 1256–1265, 1980.

Shapiro PA, Williams DL, Foray AT, Gelman IS, Wukich N and Sciacca R: Psychosocial evaluation and prediction of compliance problems and morbidity after heart transplantation. *Transplantation* **60**: 1462–1466, 1995.

Sheard T and Maguire P: The effect of psychological interventions on anxiety and depression in cancer patients: results of two meta-analyses. *Br J Cancer* **80**(11): 1770–1780, 1999.

Shekelle RB, Raynor WJ Jr, Ostfeld AM, Garron DC, Bieliauskaus LA, Liu SC, Maliza C and Paul O: Psychological depression and 17-year risk of death from cancer. *Psychosom Med* **43**: 117–125, 1981.

Simon EJ and Hiller JM: Opioid peptides and opioid receptors. In G Siegel, B Agranoff, R Albers and P Molinoff (Eds), *Basic Neurochemistry, 5th Edition*. Raven Press: New York, 1994.

Singer B and Ryff CD: Life histories and associated health risks. *Ann NY Acad Sci* **896**: 96–115, 1999.

Socol ML and Peaceman AM: Active management of labor. *Obst & Gynecol Clin N Am* **26**(2): 287–294, 1999.

Spiegel D: Embodying the mind in psychooncology research. *Adv Mind Body Med* **15**: 267–273, 1999.

Spiegel D and Kato PM: Psychosocial influences on cancer incidence and progression. *Harvard Rev Psychiatry* **4**: 10–26, 1996.

Spiegel DS, Bloom JR, Kraemer HC and Gottheil E: Effect of a psychosocial treatment on survival of patients with metastatic breast cancer. *Lancet* **ii**: 888–891, 1989.

Starkman M, Gebarski S, Berent S and Schteingart D: Hippocampal formation volume, memory dysfunction, and cortisol levels in patients with Cushing's syndrome. *Biol Psychiatry* **32**: 756–765, 1992.

Starkstein SE, Robinson RG, Honig MA, Parikh RM, Joselyn J and Price TR: Mood changes after right hemisphere lesion. *Br J Psychiatry* **155**: 79–85, 1989.

Sternberg EM: Emotions and disease. From balance of humors to balance of molecules. *Nature Medicine* **3**: 264–267, 1997.

Stratakis CA and Chrousos GP: Neuroendocrinology and pathophysiology of the stress system. *Ann NY Acad Sci* **771**: 1–18, 1995.

Straus JL and Cavanaugh S: Placebo effects: issues for clinical practice in psychiatry and medicine. *Psychosomatics* **37**: 315–326, 1996.

Suarez EC, Williams RB, Kuhn CM, Zimmerman EH and Schanberg SM: Biobehavioral basis of coronary-prone behavior in middle-aged men. Part II. Serum cholesterol, the Type A behavior pattern, and hostility as interactive modulators of physiological reactivity. *Psychosom Med* **53**: 528–537, 1991.

Surwit RS, Schneider MS and Feinglos MN: Stress and diabetes mellitus. *Diabetes Care* **15**: 1413–1422, 1992.

Terenius L: Opioid peptides, pain and stress. *Progr Brain Res* **92**: 375–383, 1992.

Terman GW, Morgan MJ and Liebeskind JC: Opioid and non-opioid stress analgesia from cold water swim: importance of stress severity. *Brain Res* **372**: 167–171, 1986.

Thorsteinsson EB, James JE and Gregg ME: Effects of video-played social support on hemodynamic reactivity and salivary cortisol during laboratory-based behavioral challenge. *Health Psychol* **17**: 436–444, 1998.

Tofler GH, Brezinski D, Schafer AI, Czeisler CA, Rutherford JD, Willich SN, Gleason RE, Williams GH and Muller JE: Concurrent morning increase in platelet aggregability and the risk of myocardial infarction and sudden cardiac death. *N Engl J Med* **316**: 1514–1518, 1987.

Trichopoulos D, Katsouyanni K, Zavitsanos X, Tzonou A and Dalla-Vorgia P: Psychological stress and fatal heart attack: the Athens (1981) earthquake natural experiment. *Lancet* **i**: 441–443, 1983.

Uchino BN, Cacioppo JT and Kiecolt-Glaser: The relationship between social support and physiological processes on underlying mechanisms and implications for health. *Psychol Bull* **119**: 488–531, 1996.

van der Velde FW and van der Pligt J: AIDS-related health behaviour: Coping, protection motivation and previous behaviour. *J Behav Med* **14**: 429–451, 1991.

Velakoulis D, Pantelis C, McGorry PD, Dudgeon P, Brewer W, Cook M, Desmond P, Bridle N, Tierney P, Murrie V, Singh B and Copolov D: Hippocampal volume in first episode psychoses and chronic schizophrenia: a high resolution magnetic resonance imaging study. *Arch Gen Psychiatry* **56**: 133–141, 1998.

Verrier RL, Hagestad EL and Lown B: Delayed myocardial infarction induced by anger. *Circulation* **75**: 249–254, 1987.

Vingerhoets AJJM and Assies J: Psychoneuroendocrinology of stress and emotions: Issues for future research. *Psychother Psychosom* **55**: 69–75, 1991.

Vogt T, Pope C, Mullooly J and Hollis J: Mental health status as a predictor of morbidity and mortality: a 15-year follow-up of members of a health maintenance organization. *Am J Public Health* **84**: 227–231, 1994.

Von Korff M and Simon G: The relationship between pain and depression. *Br J Psychiatry* **168** (suppl 30): 101–108, 1996.

Wallston KA, Wallston BS, Smith S and Dobbins CJ: Perceived control and health. *Curr Psychol Res & Rev* **6**: 5–25, 1987.

Watanabe Y, Gould E, Cameron HA, Daniels DC and McEwen BS: Phenytoin prevents stress- and corticosterone-induced atrophy of CA3 pyramidal neurons. *Hippocampus* **2**: 431–436, 1992.

Watson M, Meyer L, Thomson A and Osofsky S: Psychological factors predicting nausea and vomiting in breast cancer patients on chemotherapy. *Eur J Cancer* **34**(6): 831–837, 1998.

Weinman J, Petrie KJ, Moss-Morris R and Horne R: The illness perception questionnaire: a new method for assessing the cognitive representation of illness. *Psychol Health* **11**(3): 431–445, 1996.

Wikstrand J, Berglund G and Tuomilehto J: Beta blockade in the primary prevention of coronary heart disease in hypertensive patients. Review of present evidence. *Circulation* **84** (Suppl 6): VI 93–100, 1991.

Williams RB: Basic biological mechanisms. In AW Siegman and TW Smith (Eds), *Anger, Hostility and the Heart*, pp 117–125. Lawrence Erlbaum: Hillsdale, NJ, 1994.

Williams RB and Barefoot JC: Coronary-prone behavior: the emerging role of the hostility complex. In BK Houston and CR Snyder (Eds), *Type A Behavior Pattern: Research, Theory, and Intervention*, pp 189–211. Wiley: New York, 1988.

Willis L, Thomas P, Garry PJ and Goodwin J: A prospective study of response to stressful life events in initially healthy elders. *J Gerontol* **42**: 627–630, 1987.

Wilson PW: Established risk factors and coronary heart disease. The Framingham Study. *Am J Hypertens* **7**: 7S–12S, 1994.

Woolley CS, Gould E and McEwen BS: Exposure to excess glucocorticoids alters dendritic morphology of adult hippocampal pyramidal neurons. *Brain Res* **531**: 225–231, 1990.

Wulsin LR, Vaillant GE and Wells VE: A systematic review of the mortality of depression. *Psychosom Med* **61**: 6–17, 1999.

Yaksh TL: The spinal action of opioids. In A Herz (Ed), *Opioids II*, pp 53–90. Springer Verlag: Berlin, 1993.

Yaksh TL, Al-Rodhan NRF and Jensen TS: Sites of action of opiates in production of analgesia. *Prog Brain Res* **77**: 371–394, 1988.

Yeragani VK: The incidence of abnormal dexamethasone suppression in schizophrenia: a review and a meta-analytic comparison with the incidence in normal controls. *Can J Psychiatry* **35**: 128–132, 1990.

Zadina JE, Hackler L, Ge LJ and Kastin AJ: A potent and selective agonist for the mu opiate receptor. *Nature* **386**: 449–502, 1997.

Zalcman S, Richter M and Anisman H: Alterations of immune functioning following exposure to stress-related cues. *Brain Behav Immun* **3**: 99–109, 1989.

Zipes DP: Sudden cardiac death. Future approaches. *Circulation* **85**: 1160–1166, 1992.

Zonderman AB, Costa P and McCrae RR: Depression as a risk for cancer morbidity and mortality in a nationally representative sample. *JAMA* **262**: 1191–1195, 1989.

Zotti AM, Bettinardi O, Soffiantino F, Tavazzi L and Steptoe A: Psychophysiological stress testing in postinfarct patients: psychological correlates of cardiovascular arousal and abnormal cardiac responses. *Circulation* **83** (Suppl 4): 1125–1135, 1991.

3

Assessment and Intervention in a Medical Environment

Cynthia D. Belar
University of Florida, USA
Nick Paoletti
*Department of Psychiatry, University of Melbourne and
Austin & Repatriation Medical Centre, Melbourne, Australia*

and

Caren Jordan
University of Florida, USA

INTRODUCTION

Research on the psychological and behavioral aspects of health and illness is based on using a variety of different models, each having emphases on different components. For example, researchers who adopt frameworks that are primarily biobehavioral, biomedical, intrapsychic, social-ecological, psychosocial or biopsychosocial may choose very different variables for intensive study and model-building. Indeed, knowledge obtained from each approach contributes important information for the entire field. However, the practicing clinician who wishes to understand a particular patient must use the model most likely to provide a comprehensive understanding of the individual case. Thus, for decades, both psychologists and psychiatrists have advocated the use of the biopsychosocial model in clinical endeavors (e.g. Engel 1977; Lipowski 1967; Belar 1980; Millon 1982). In this chapter the biopsychosocial model in assessment and intervention is articulated as basic to practice for all clinicians working with medical patients. Although an individual discipline may have more expertise in one or more aspects of this model, it is our belief that all practitioners must have some knowledge in all areas, and that an integrative approach to practice has the potential to serve the patient best.

The kinds of problems addressed in the medical environment are varied. Lipowski (1967) described reasons for referrals to psychiatric consultation and

Psychology and Psychiatry: Integrating Medical Practice.
Edited by J. Milgrom and G. D. Burrows © 2001 John Wiley & Sons, Ltd.

liaison (C-L) teams as related to: (a) psychological presentations of medical illness, (b) psychological complications of illness, (c) emotional reactions to illness, (d) somatic effects of emotional distress, and (e) somatic presentations of psychiatric illness. A review of recent data from a variety of C-L services supports Lipowski's report, but also demonstrates considerable variability across settings in reasons for referral (Collins et al 1992; Freyne et al 1992; Levenson et al 1992; Neehall & Beharry 1993; Ormont et al 1997). In these reports, the most common referrals were for patients who had (a) attempted suicide (19–68% of referrals), (b) presented management or behavioral problems on the unit (6–34%) or (c) required differential diagnosis, including a determination regarding competency (6–29%). Variability in diagnosis was also apparent, the most common being adjustment reaction (2–41%), affective disorder (5–24%), substance abuse (7–29%), personality disorder (1–20%), and organic cognitive impairment (6–19%). The variability across settings may be accounted for by such factors as cultural differences and hospital policies affecting referral patterns, or professional preferences of consultants along with the availability of particular areas of expertise (e.g. pain management, neuropsychology). Historically, many health professionals entering independent practice have developed practices consistent with their preferences rather than documented community needs.

Despite the estimated 25% prevalence rate of actual psychological disorder in medical populations (Kamerow et al 1986), in the research cited above, the reported referral rates varied from 1.3% to 3% of hospitalized patients, suggesting that many patient needs may be going unaddressed. In ambulatory care settings it has been stated that up to 80% of medical patients have evidence of significant psychological distress (Barsky 1981), thus many psychologists and psychiatrists are paying increased attention to practice in primary care settings in an effort to improve the delivery of mental health services. However, as scientific knowledge in behavioral medicine has advanced over the past two decades, it has also been argued that "100% of all medical visits are psychological and that Cartesian mind–body dualism simply does not belong in any conceptualization or implementation of the health-care system. Behavior and health are inextricably intertwined . . . " (Belar 1996, p.78).

With the growth of behavioral medicine, and the increasing numbers of psychologists in medical settings, problems addressed in the health-care system have increasingly included those related to (a) treatment of psychophysiological disorders (e.g. headache, irritable bowel syndrome), (b) prediction of response to medical-surgical treatments (e.g. back surgery, oocyte donation, organ transplantation), (c) adherence to medical regimens (e.g. medication and dietary management), (d) reduction of destructive health behavior (e.g. smoking, excessive eating), (e) promotion of healthy behavior (e.g. exercise), (f) treatment of side-effects of medical treatments (e.g. anticipatory nausea), (g) anxiety management and preparation for stressful medical procedures, (h) use of preventive health behaviors (e.g. sunscreen and seatbelt usage), (i) physician–patient communication, (j) health care staff burnout, and (k) health care systems design with special attention to quality of life issues.

It is difficult to determine from the literature which types of problems are seen primarily by psychologists or psychiatrists, or both, since many C-L teams are multidisciplinary in nature. However, from a review of records of a C-L team responsible for inpatient services in a large capitated care system, approximately 50% of all referrals involved services of the psychiatrist, with psychiatric resources tending to be utilized for medication management and psychiatric admissions (Belar 1995). The other 50% were managed by psychologists and psychiatric nurse specialists. More subjectively, in comparing experiences obtained from two multidisciplinary C-L teams, directing a medical psychology service at an academic health science center, and developing a behavioral medicine outpatient team in a capitated care system, the first author has hypothesized that psychiatrists tend to receive more consultations regarding suicidal and combative behavior, psychotropic medications and mental status changes, while psychologists receive relatively more requests concerning coping with illness, compliance, preparation for surgery, pre-treatment screenings, pain management, and psychometric assessment (Belar et al 1987). Many of these problems are referred directly to clinical health psychologists who do not serve on traditional psychiatric C-L teams, but work independently in health center-based departments of psychology or in a variety of medical-surgical units throughout the health-care system (e.g. neurology, pediatrics, pain centers, burn units). In fact in the United States, only one-half of all psychologists employed in academic health science centers are in a department of psychiatry (Clayson & Mensh 1987).

Clearly there are large areas of overlap in the practice of psychology and psychiatry, and within each profession there is considerable heterogeneity with respect to specific areas of expertise. But there are distinctive background features as well. For example, psychiatrists possess a firm grounding in biomedical sciences with skills in the management of psychotropic medications. Psychologists possess a firm grounding in the behavioral sciences with skills in the measurement of behavior and research methods (e.g. diagnostic and outcomes assessment). However, as noted above, both psychologists and psychiatrists must be well-grounded in the foundations of the biopsychosocial model, in order to practice effectively with medical patients. The model for assessment and intervention is equally applicable to both disciplines, even if particular skills in implementation are more specific to one discipline.

ASSESSMENT

Historically, psychological and psychiatric assessment followed a medical model approach which tended to focus on the identification and treatment of mental health disorders. The primary focus was the patient's mind, while medical-surgical personnel focused on the treatment of bodily disease (often without consideration of emotional and behavioral factors). For integrative care, a blending of these models is extremely important.

Assessment is critical because it is the initial step in understanding a particular patient and in developing an appropriate intervention program. In working with medical patients, assessment and consultation activities are usually intertwined, as information obtained must be communicated in a meaningful manner to both the patient and the referral source. The type of referral question determines the type of assessment conducted, but all assessment must address interactions among the patient's medical and psychological state and his/her environment.

Based on work by Engel (1977) and Leigh & Reiser (1980), a model for assessment has been proposed that facilitates organization of information and thus decision-making about choice of assessment strategies and interventions (Belar et al 1987). The model is described as a series of building blocks of information, which unfortunately can convey a compartmentalized, reductionistic view of very complex inter-related processes. This is not our intention, but seems to be an artifact of inadequate schemata to represent the biopsychosocial model. Our model is briefly summarized below, but more fully described in Belar & Deardorff (1995). The implementation of aspects of this model is detailed with respect to selected patient problems in other chapters throughout this volume.

Targets of Assessment

Table 3.1 describes the targets for clinical assessment by domain of information (biological/physical, affective, cognitive, behavioral) and unit of assessment (patient or environment, including health-care providers, family and sociocultural context). Each block lists examples of the kinds of information that should be gathered during assessment. Also to be considered in each block is the associated developmental or historical perspective. The patient's current status, changes since onset of illness, and past history should be understood in each area as well. Finally, the focus of assessment should be on assets and strengths of the patient and his/her environment, and not only on the identification of problems.

Patient Targets

Although there are exceptions (e.g. comatose patients, children), the individual patient is usually the starting point in the assessment process, although this is often after a brief discussion of the referral with ward staff.

Biological/Physical Targets

The main physical assessment would already have been carried out by the medical/surgical team. However, especially where a psychiatric assessment is required, physical concomitants of psychiatric illness, such as the psychomotor retardation of depression and the reduced sensorium of delirium, would always be noted. An assessment of somatizing as an idiom of distress presenting as physical illness or, more usually in medical wards, superimposed on the symptoms expectable of the physical illness, needs to be made. A full history of the development of symptoms, as well as of past patterns of symptom expression, would be useful guides. It is critical to understand the specifics of the disease or injury involved, especially how the latter might affect presentation in other areas of assessment (e.g. effect of liver failure on cognitive functioning). Where a medical cause of psychiatric illness is suspected (e.g. brain tumor, hypothyroidism), further tests will need to be discussed with the referring team. Although this is relatively rare, a medical diagnosis may have been missed in the initial medical assessment (Antonowicz 1998), thus all C-L clinicians must be vigilant of such an eventuality. Finally, an understanding of the physical illness and a note of medications being taken or potentially to be taken is a crucial part of the assessment, especially if the use of psychotropic medication is contemplated, in order to avoid drug interactions. The clinician also must not forget to note over-the-counter medications and herbal supplements the patient could be using.

McDaniel et al (1995) herald the future possibility that biological markers, such as neuroendocrine, neurochemical, and neuroanatomical alterations associated with depression, may aid in the diagnosis of depression in medically ill patients.

Affective Targets

Assessment should provide an understanding of the patient's current mood and affect, their contextual elements and historical features, and the patient's feelings about self, future, social support, illness, treatment, and health-care providers. Special care needs to be taken with somatization, as patients with this type of presentation often do not see themselves as having psychological problems, thus affective components may be more obscured. When somatizing occurs as an affective manifestation in medically ill patients, matters become even more complicated.

Cognitive Targets

The clinician needs to understand the patient's content and pattern of thinking, knowledge, attitudes, perceptions, general cognitive style, cognitive capacity and philosophy of life. Particularly important is the patient's health belief model, including his or her knowledge and attitudes about the illness, treatment, and health-care providers; perceptions about costs and benefits of treatment; perceived threat of illness and control over symptoms; expectations regarding outcome; and perceived meaning of the illness.

Behavioral Targets

Patients' patterns of behavior in the areas of interpersonal, recreational and occupational functioning require attention. Of special importance is self-care behavior

TABLE 3.1 Targets for Clinical Assessment

Domain of information	Patient	Environment			
		Family	Health-care system	Sociocultural context
Biological or physical	Age, sex, race	Characteristics of home setting	Characteristics of the treatment setting	Social services
	Physical appearance	Economic resources	Characteristics of medical procedures and treatment regimens	Financial resources
	Symptoms, health status	Size of the family		Social networks
	Physical examination	Familial patterning (e.g. headache history)	Availability of prosthetic aids	Occupational setting
	Vital signs, lab data	Other illness in family		Physical job requirements
	Medications			Health hazards
	Psychophysiological data			
	Constitutional factors			
	Genetics			
	History of injury, disease, and surgery			
Affective	Mood	Members' feelings about patient, illness, and treatment	Providers' feelings about patient, illness, and treatment	Sentiments of culture regarding patient, illness, and treatment
	Affect			
	Feelings about illness, treatment, health-care providers, self, family, job, and social network			
	History of affective disturbance			

Cognitive	Cognitive style Thought content Intelligence Education Knowledge about disease Health beliefs Attitudes and expectations regarding illness, treatment, health care, and providers Perceived meaning of the illness Philosophy of life Religious beliefs	Knowledge about illness and treatment Attitudes and expectations about patient, illness, and treatment Intellectual resources	Providers' knowledge Providers' attitude toward patient, illness, and treatment	Current state of knowledge Cultural attitudes toward patient and illness
Behavioral	Activity level Interactions with family, friends, and coworkers Health habits Health-care utilization (previous medications and psychological treatment) Compliance Ability to control physical symptoms	Participation in patient care Reinforcement contingencies for health and illness	Providers' skills in education and training patients Reinforcement contingencies for health and illness	Employment policies Laws regulating health-care practice, disability, provision of care, health habits Handicapped access Customs in symptom-reporting and help-seeking

From Belar & Deardorff, 1995
Copyright © 1995 by the American Psychological Association. Adapted with permission.

(including health habits such as smoking and substance use), interaction patterns with health-care providers, and past and current health-care utilization patterns. It is particularly crucial to consider the patient's history with respect to adherence to previous treatment regimens.

Environmental Targets

The biopsychosocial model requires attention to the patient's environment, including the family, health-care system, and sociocultural context.

Family Environment

It is important to be aware of available economic resources and, in some cases, the physical features of the home environment. The clinician also needs to consider the family's developmental history, size, and experience of recent changes, and history of illness in other family members. In the affective domain, important aspects are the family's feelings about the patient and his or her illness and treatments. In the cognitive domain, the clinician should assess family members' expectations, perceptions, and attitudes about the patient, his or her illness and treatment, and future. In the behavioral domain, family interaction patterns plus any changes within the family since the onset of the illness are important to understand, especially with respect to contingencies for health or illness behavior.

Health-Care System

Clinicians must pay attention to the physical characteristics of the setting in which the patient is being assessed, and the nature of the environment in which treatment is to occur. In the affective domain, it is helpful to understand how health-care providers feel about the patient and about his or her illness. In the cognitive domain, there needs to be some understanding of the knowledge base held by the health-care providers regarding the patient's problem, as well as their attitudes and expectations regarding outcome. Skills in communication and patient education are also important. For the overall health-care system, one needs to be aware of rules, policies, and regulations that will affect the patient and treatment.

Sociocultural Environment

Included in the patient's sociocultural environment are the physical and psychological requirements of the patient's occupation and the availability of social services. It is important to gain an understanding of occupational health hazards. In the cognitive and affective domains, one should understand cultural expectations, attitudes and sentiments in relation to specific aspects of the patient such as age, gender, ethnicity (e.g. migrant groups, particularly if living in "enclaves", may have "calcification" of traditional attitudes and behaviors, that may reflect neither the current prevalent position in the country of origin, nor that in the host country—Paoletti 1990), religion, sexual orientation, particular illness and nature of treatment. Knowledge of laws regulating health-care practice and employment will also facilitate an understanding of resources available, and the behavior of others toward the patient.

METHODS OF ASSESSMENT

The choice of particular assessment methods depends on the target being assessed, the purpose of assessment and the clinician's competence. Although only briefly summarized below, there is a considerable body of clinical and research literature on each method. Other chapters in this volume will detail methods relevant to particular clinical problems.

Archival Methods

Since understanding illness components that can affect clinical presentation and course is critical to the biopsychosocial model, a review of medical records is always necessary in working with medical patients. It is mandatory in hospital consultations, and must be formally acknowledged in the written report.

Clinicians must understand manifestations of organic disease processes, as well as the effects of medications and other medical treatments on behavior. Clinicians must also be aware of which physical illnesses can present as behavioral, emotional or cognitive problems. For psychiatrists, medical education comprises a substantial portion of training. For psychologists without specialty training in the area, interpreting medical information could be problematic. However, information is easily accessible in texts, on-line, and from referring physicians. With the development of specialty training in health psychology, future clinicians are likely to be well-informed in this area.

One particularly difficult issue, already raised above, is the determination of when previous medical work-ups have been sufficient. This is relatively easy for psychiatrists and psychologists working within a consultation-liaison psychiatry team. Clinical health psychologists working in independent departments solve this problem by developing close working relationships with physicians in a variety of specialty areas who provide ongoing consultation regarding standards of care relevant to particular problems; in fact these psychologists are often members of multispecialty medical-surgical teams that contain multiple areas of expertise (e.g. organ transplantation teams). The interactions that occur across specialties and disciplines are mutually beneficial, and provide for more integrative care for all patients.

In addition to information about illness, medical record data often reveal patterns in the patient's help-seeking and adherence, as well as providers' responses to patients. Archival data are also used when clinicians research current literature on the presenting problem.

Interview

A cornerstone method of assessment is the clinical interview, since it can provide both historical and current data across all domains of information, and it allows for collection of self-report and observational data from patients, family members, health-care providers and significant others. Interviews can also help establish rapport with the patient. The content and style of interviews vary depending on the assessment question. Some are structured approaches to assess particular issues, e.g., Psychosocial Adjustment to Illness Scale (PAIS—Derogatis 1986).

A problem that both psychiatrists and psychologists face on interview is the mind–body dualism extant in the culture. Patients often perceive that referral means that their doctor thinks their problem is "all in the head", with subsequent defensiveness if not outright hostility. This issue always needs to be addressed early in the interview. Special ethical problems arise when there is a lack of confidentiality due to site of service (e.g. burn unit, semi-private room), and a team approach to care. Limits to confidentiality must be carefully discussed in order to obtain informed consent prior to evaluation.

Mental State Examination

It is not the purpose here to set out how to assess the mental state and for that the reader is referred to the standard textbooks (e.g. Sadock & Sadock 2000). Whilst the psychiatrist has particular expertise in mental state examination, the emphasis here will be on those issues that may be different or highlighted in the general medical patient by any mental health professional.

Beginning with observation, the presence of clouding of consciousness is vital to the diagnosis of delirium. While the patient who has a moderately severe impairment may be recognizable instantly, it is the mildly impaired patient who presents a challenge. Irritability may be an indicator, but is certainly not diagnostic. Distractibility may be observed during the course of the interview and, while the patient may not be floridly incoherent, s/he may have difficulty with maintaining attention. The more floridly impaired patient may be picking at the bedclothes, for example, to remove hallucinatory spiders. As the level of delirium deepens, the patient may become verbally or physically aggressive or pull at intravenous lines. However, subsequent settling and quietness may not represent an improvement, but may represent a deepening of the delirium.

With more subtle cases of delirium, returning in the evening may clinch the diagnosis, as these patients typically are worse in the evening and at night.

Just as delirium may represent a challenge, so do anxiety and, in particular, depression, in the medical setting. The patient may not recognize its presence or, seeing it as "logical" to the situation, may not volunteer it. Anhedonia may be present as a clue. Other indicators, like anorexia, psychomotor retardation and somatization, may be helpful, but need to be interpreted in the context of medical co-pathology that may produce or mimic them. The presence of guilt, to even frank delusional level in the more severe cases, would also generally be an indicator of depression.

Auditory and visual hallucinations, especially if mood-congruent, may indicate severe depression, but, again, co-existence of delirium may need to be excluded. It must be remembered that, with a rapidly changing medical state, the exclusion of delirium yesterday may not apply to today!

The assessment of cognition, in a patient who may be mildly demented, mildly delirious, moderately anxious and not depressed, may present a further challenge. Serial administration of the Mini-Mental State Examination (Folstein et al 1975) may be helpful.

Finally, any comments on "insight", a much abused term, must be assuaged by such factors as understanding of personality and culture. A middle-aged business-woman who is irascible because she is not coping with a new-found dependence, or a depressed, somatizing elderly migrant man may be both unjustly labelled as "lacking insight".

Observation

Another fundamental method of assessment is observation. Observations can be made by health-care providers and family members as well as the clinician. They can occur during the interview or in naturalistic settings (e.g. during burn debride-ment). Sometimes rating methods are used to quantify observations, e.g. the Hamil-ton Anxiety Scale (Hamilton 1959). And with the development of new technologies, "observation" through ambulatory monitoring is increasingly possible (e.g. amount of exercise in back pain patients). In interpreting data from observations it is important to consider the influence of the measurement process itself. Both inter-view and observation methods have considerable reactive components.

Since a substantial part of graduate education of psychologists is devoted to the measurement of behavior, psychologists often use a variety of well-researched behavioral observation methods that have developed within the discipline and that have demonstrated reliability and ecological validity (e.g. to assess parent–child interactions, or self-administration of insulin in people with diabetes).

Observations relating to sick role and abnormal illness behavior (e.g. changes of behavior when different people are present; changes in behavior over the course of the day and night, as in delirium) may be crucial in evaluation and management.

Questionnaires and Diaries

Also useful in the assessment process are problem-focused, clinician-developed questionnaires. Both psychologists and psychiatrists have found these methods to be timesavers on interview; these methods can provide a systematic recording of data that is later helpful in treatment as well.

A variety of diary methods are available to record both overt and covert behaviors (e.g. eating behavior, fears about cancer). Diaries serve as baseline measures and measures of treatment effectiveness; they can also be interventions to foster self-awareness.

Psychometrics

With an education and training background that emphasizes the measurement of behavior, psychologists often use psychometric methods in the assessment process. Psychological tests can be broadband in nature, such as measures of intelligence and personality, e.g. Minnesota Multiphasic Personality Inventory (Hathaway & Mc-Kinley 1967), or more narrowly focused measures of particular symptoms or syndromes, e.g. Beck Depression Inventory (Beck 1972), Mini-Mental State Exam (Folstein et al 1975). Measures can be illness-oriented in general, e.g. Millon Behavioral Health Inventory (Millon et al 1982), McGill Pain Questionnaire (Melzack 1975), or disease-specific, e.g. Arthritis Impact Measurement Scale (Meenan et al 1982). Although most often used to obtain information about the individual patient, tests can also be used to assess aspects of family, work, and sociocultural features, e.g. Family Environment Scale (Moos & Moos 1981), Work Environment Scale (Moos 1981), as well as measures of cultural values and ethnic identification. Choice of measures is guided by the question to be addressed and the knowledge of scientific data concerning a measure's validity for that particular usage. No test is "valid" in and of itself. The use of tests in the diagnostic process is recommended as part of a multiple measurement, convergent–divergent hypothesis testing approach to assessment, a core component of training of psychologists. A useful text describing methods and measures for psychological assessment in medical settings is that by Rozensky et al (1997).

A significant ethical (and malpractice) issue can arise when tests normed on psychiatric populations are applied to medical-surgical ones. Knowledge of the appropriate research literature is critical, as well as an awareness of relevant norms, some of which are often gathered locally. The use of computerized testing can increase risks in psychological testing, as practitioners unaware of scoring algorithms and the validity of interpretations may be misled by rather slick computer reports. To help guide professional behavior, the American Psychological Association has published *Guidelines for Computer-Based Tests and Interpretations* (APA 1986).

Psychophysiological Measures

Psychophysiological measures are commonly used by psychologists and psychiatrists, especially in disorders with stress-related components. Examples of frequently used methods are electromyographic recording in tension headache, polysomnography in sleep disorders, peripheral temperature in Raynaud's Disease, plethysmography in sexual dysfunction and blood pressure in hypertension. Autonomic nervous system stress-profiling is used for many psychophysiological disorders, and measurements of bodily functions are integral to the design of many intervention programs (e.g. anal sphincter activity for biofeedback training of fecal incontinence). Psychologists and psychiatrists who use these methods have expertise not only in the measurement of behavior, but in psychophysiological processes, bioelectric recordings and instrumentation, signal-processing methods and potential artifacts.

INTEGRATING ASSESSMENT INFORMATION

Information from the assessment process must be integrated in case conceptualization. However, case conceptualization is not a linear process, as information obtained in one of the building blocks of assessment will influence the interpretation of results in another. For example, age may mediate psychological response to loss of reproductive capacity, gender can influence help-seeking behavior, ammonia levels will affect cognitive functioning, social prejudices might influence patient report of symptoms, physician skills in listening will influence the report of pertinent medical information, organic disease can produce affective changes, family response to illness will influence patient self-management, belief in personal control influences perception of pain, knowledge of disease affects adherence to medical regimens, attitudes towards death and dying influence emotional reactions to terminal illness, psychiatric illness can affect compliance with medical regimens, social support can determine caretaker availability, employment policies will affect return to work, insurance coverage will affect access to care, current medications may affect performance on cognitive tasks, ethnicity may affect health belief models, preferred coping strategies may relate to success in dealing with stressful medical procedures. These are only a few examples of how findings must be interpreted in light of information obtained in the various building blocks of assessment. The list of possible interactions is extensive, as the body of knowledge concerning relationships between health and behavior has mushroomed over the past two decades. Thus to accurately assess psychological issues in medical patients, the clinician must have a firm grounding in the scientific knowledge base.

At the end of the assessment process, the clinician should have a clear understanding of the nature of the disease and its treatment, as well as the patient's cognitive, affective, and behavioral components. Patient psychopathology as well as coping resources must be understood. The clinician must also identify relevant contextual issues, especially those related to family issues, the health-care system, and the work environment.

INTERVENTION

In choosing an intervention, clinicians consider the scientific bases of specific interventions, the appropriateness of treatment goals, the impact of interventions on other domains, the feasibility of treatment delivery, the potential for staff cooperation (if needed), an analysis of cost–benefit issues, and professional competence in carrying out the intervention. To obtain informed consent and to assess treatment effectiveness, treatment goals must be clearly articulated and operationalized (e.g. "take medications with meals three times a day" versus "improve compliance"). It is especially important to distinguish whether goals are for prevention, cure or the promotion of coping.

Although, as with assessment, there are multiple targets for intervention, rarely can clinicians focus on a single target, since interventions in one domain have effects in others, some of which may impact on treatment: for example, as low back pain patients increase activity levels, family overprotectiveness might increase; patients who learn control of physiological processes can experience an increased sense of mastery and decreased anxiety; patients with increased assertion skills can disrupt stable marital dynamics; and intensive relaxation training can cause changes in insulin needs that must be carefully monitored in people with diabetes. Lack of knowledge and/or inattention to the potential effects of interventions across domains can result in treatment failure and unintended negative side-effects.

Targets of Intervention

Interventions can be targeted at the individual patient level, the family, the health-care system, the sociocultural context or any combination of these.

Patient Targets

At the individual patient level, the clinician can intervene in the biological, affective, cognitive, and behavioral domains.

Biological Targets

The sine qua non of treatment strategies targeted to biologic factors are the medical interventions carried out by physicians. Moreover, symptoms in other domains (e.g. affective) are often treated biologically through the use of medications (e.g. antidepressants in depressed patients). Psychiatrists have special expertise in the administration and management of treatment with psychotropic medications. However, not all psychiatrists have working familiarity with the administration of these medications to medically ill patients and one role of consultation-liaison psychiatrists must be the education of other psychiatrists, not just non-psychiatric physicians, in such issues. This topic could fill a chapter of its own, thus only general issues will be raised here, in relation to the process of choosing a psychotropic medication: (a) side-effects reasonably tolerated by general psychiatric patients may not be tolerated by already physically symptomatic medical patients; (b) medications may aggravate a medical problem (e.g. liver function); (c) it is not uncommon for patients to refuse one more tablet on top of the large numbers they may already be taking; (d) drug interactions are a crucial issue: in addition to the usual pharmacodynamic and pharmacokinetic considerations when prescribing any drug (giving additional weight to the effects of the concurrent medical illness on these considerations), the consultation-liaison psychiatrist needs to be aware of such other issues as protein-binding competition and cytochrome P450 interactions, about which there is a burgeoning literature and which is not without controversy (e.g. Nemeroff et al 1996; Preskorn 1998).

Psychologists also use interventions that target biological processes. For example, work from experimental psychology has provided the basis for the practice of applied psychophysiology. Biological targets can include muscle tension for headache patients, peripheral temperature for those with Raynaud's disease, anal sphincter control for patients with fecal incontinence and resting blood pressure for those with hypertension. Other symptoms commonly treated by psychological interventions include pain and anticipatory nausea. Interactive effects of treatments in this domain must always be understood (e.g. the effect of minor tranquilizers on muscle tension).

Affective Targets

Emotions such as depression and anxiety are often targets of treatment. Psychotropic medications can be very effective, as can cognitive-behavioral programs for depression, anxiety and anger management. Often these are combined. The provision of emotional support is an intervention that accompanies most others used by clinicians in practice.

Too often in the past, psychiatrists have failed to treat patients whose depression is "understandable", such as cancer patients, pharmacologically. The trend has fortunately been reversed and psychiatrists are now using psychopharmacological intervention, when appropriate. In fact, the evidence is that cancer patients who are depressed and have the appropriate "biological" indicators for response to antidepressants, respond very well to pharmacotherapy (Craig & Abeloff 1974; Costa et al 1985; Evans et al 1988; Leibenluft & Goldberg 1988). Also, Ribeiro et al (1993) and McDaniel et al (1995) highlight the use of biological markers as predictors of such a response.

Cognitive Targets

Knowledge, attitudes and health beliefs are common targets of intervention. Examples of interventions include the provision of sensory and procedural information to promote coping with stressful medical procedures, examination of meaning in life when dealing with terminal illness, and various cognitive-behavioral therapies emphasizing cognitive restructuring and challenging irrational beliefs.

The patient's construct of the illness, which will have variables relating to development, personal experience, cultural issues and current events (including understood and misunderstood explanations), will be of fundamental importance in shaping the response to treatment. Therapy, especially psychological but also pharmacological, is likely to fail (a) if illness constructs provide an impediment to cognition shifts or (b) if patient and therapist do not have some common ground, including conceptual framework for the illness, on which to build therapy (Paoletti 1997).

Behavioral Targets

Using principles of behavior change, clinicians often target relevant patient behavior, e.g. compliance with medication, assertion skills, self-management skills, behavioral health habits (smoking, exercise, diet).

Again, "transcultural" issues, which may include the experience common to medical patients, will influence behavior in relation to adherence to medical regimens (Paoletti 1986, 1991).

Environmental Targets

In addition to interventions designed for the patient, targets for change can include the family, the health-care system, and the sociocultural context. Within these units, physical, affective, cognitive, or behavioral domains may be the focus of intervention.

Family. Referrals to social services are often necessary to deal with resource issues of the family. Family therapies can also be used to alleviate anxiety, promote realistic expectations, and prevent unwitting reinforcement of sick-role behavior.

Health-care system. Environmental interventions can be used to increase orientation, privacy, and supportive atmospheres for patients, although clinicians must often serve as patient advocates in attempts to bring about changes in health-care systems design. In the affective domain, the clinician may need to work with health-care providers to reframe their feelings about a patient and to facilitate the development of therapeutic relationships. In the cognitive realm, the clinician often assumes an educational role to increase the knowledge of other providers about the psychological aspects of health and illness. Clinicians also focus on health-care providers' behavior in developing communication skills and contingency management programs (e.g. fixed-interval medications for chronic pain patients versus an as-needed basis).

Sociocultural context. Many aspects of the sociocultural context are outside the scope of interventions available for specific patients. However, the social support network is not, and often can be improved by psychological intervention. In addition, consultations with employers can facilitate the patient's return to work, especially with disfiguring or culturally unpopular illnesses.

More long-term "interventions" for which psychologists have specific training involve contributions to knowledge through research on treatment outcome, health–behavior relationships, and health-care systems design. This research contributes to guidelines for practice as well as to health policy, which can significantly impact patient care.

INTERVENTION METHODS

Flexibility in the use of interventions is important. Some methods are very general, broadband in approach (e.g. maximizing the placebo effect, supportive counseling); others are designed to address narrower targets (e.g. biofeedback for fecal incontinence, relaxation training for pain control). Many methods are used in combination, and in fact the empirical support for some has been established only within multimethod treatment programs. Many methods are as useful with environmental targets (family members, health-care providers) as they are with the patient. Each intervention must be tailored to the individual situation.

No one clinician is expert in all possible interventions. There are systematic differences between psychiatrists and psychologists in that the former have significant training in the use of medications, whilst psychologists have substantial training with behavioral and applied psychophysiological strategies. The specific interventions relevant to particular problems will be more fully articulated in subsequent chapters of this book.

Huyse et al (1990), in a study of 820 operationalized interventions, found the following frequencies of recommendations: diagnostic action, 41%; medication, 69%; focus on the medical treatment (other than diagnostic and medication), 35%; obtaining additional psychosocial information, 30%; psychosocial management on the ward, 61%, specifically its organization; discharge planning, 41%; aftercare management, 24%. These authors highlight the importance of systematic recording of operationalized recommendations and evaluation of treatments recommended, given that consultee concordance with the consultant's recommendations is important to treatment outcome.

Placebo

The placebo effect refers to the changes in behavior that result from the patient's expectations and beliefs that a particular treatment will provide benefit. It influences all target domains, and comprises a significant proportion of all health-care interventions.

Supportive Counseling

Health-care providers generally attempt to support their patients through reassurance. Supportive counseling may be on an individual, family, or group basis. Psychiatrists and psychologists often train other health-care providers and members of the patient's social support network to provide this method of intervention, and provide it themselves when other resources are not available. Support groups allow individuals with a similar illness or problem to interact with one another to obtain information, as well as to discuss concerns and coping strategies.

Education and Information

An essential aspect of treatment is education about the biopsychosocial model and its application to the individual and his/her illness. It seems obvious that information is fundamental to all interventions, and of course the informed consent process itself. In addition, how and when information is presented can be crucial. As a specific intervention, both procedural and sensory information are used in preparation for stressful medical procedures, an area of significant psychological research (Johnston & Vogele 1993). However, clinicians must understand individual differences regarding response to information, as some individuals can initially do worse with more information. It is also important to remember that information is often a necessary but insufficient ingredient for behavior change.

Medications

Psychiatrists have special expertise with psychotropic medications, but there are considerations specific to C-L psychiatry. It is outside the scope of this chapter to comprehensively cover medication that may be used in this setting and space only allows an exploration of general principles. Some of the general issues relating to medication have already been covered under the headings of biological and affective targets of intervention. An important role of the C-L psychiatrist is to use judiciously or guide physicians in the use of psychotropic medication, running a fine line between inappropriate sparing and unnecessary use, as well as between cautioning on problems (side-effects and interactions) and avoiding the frightening of physicians away from appropriate use. Depression, anxiety and delirium are three common conditions that may require pharmacotherapeutic intervention.

Depression

The newer antidepressants, including serotonin-selective reuptake inhibitors or SSRIs (e.g. sertraline, citalopram, paroxetine, fluvoxamine, fluoxetine), serotonin and noradrenaline reuptake inhibitors or SNRIs (e.g. venlafaxine), reversible inhibitors of MAO or RIMAs (e.g. moclobemide) and post-synaptic 5-HT2 inhibitors (e.g. nefazodone), have added new dimensions to the treatment of depression, particularly certain issues of safety. Data are still accumulating on safety in some specific areas of use (e.g. the immediate post-infarct period, post-stroke, post-transplant), but, in general, these drugs are supplanting the tricyclics in consultation-liaison psychiatry.

The diagnosis of major depression in the medically ill is made difficult by the overlap of biological symptoms of depression and symptoms of the medical illness itself, but such symptoms as inappropriate feelings of guilt and anhedonia, as well as pervasiveness of depressed mood and psychomotor retardation or agitation are clues to the presence of biological depression.

Consideration must then be given to interaction of the illness and medical treatments with the candidate antidepressants. In general, in the C-L psychiatry situation, desirable attributes include short half-life (in case of interaction), low protein binding (e.g. if the patient is already or likely to be on protein-bound drugs, such as warfarin or digoxin), low P450 cytochrome interaction (especially in a situation where polypharmacy already exists), simplicity of dosage, low physical side-effect profile and safety in the co-morbid condition.

One factor not to be overlooked is discussion with the physicians of replacement, where possible, of medical treatments that may be contributing to the depression, such as centrally acting antihypertensives, immunosuppressants and progestogens.

Anxiety

This is perhaps the most overlooked psychiatric diagnosis in medical patients, possibly because it is so obviously expectable, even more than depression. While education about the illness, support and cognitive-behavioral techniques may go a long way to reduce anxiety, some patients will require tranquilizing. Short-acting benzodiazepines are probably the most commonly used drugs. This is one situation where the term "short-term use" need not be a cliché. Unless there are indications for longer-term use, it is desirable to try to stop the benzodiazepines before the patient leaves hospital or at the first outpatient review. When using these drugs, consideration needs, again, to be given to the co-morbid condition and other medication (e.g. to avoid compounding of sedation in patients already on other sedative medication; e.g. to avoid respiratory depression in pulmonary conditions, in patients on other respiratory suppressants such as opioids, and in neonates if the drug is being used in the final phase of pregnancy).

Delirium

The American Psychiatric Association has recently published guidelines on the treatment of delirium (APA 1999). In addition to the treatment of the medical condition causing the delirium and to general medical and psychological support measures, the use of psychotropic medication in delirium remains indicated. Low-dose haloperidol remains "most frequently used because it has few anticholinergic side effects, few active metabolites, and a relatively small likelihood of causing sedation and hypotension" (APA 1999, p. 2). However, newer antipsychotics like risperidone, olanzapine and quetiapine, are starting to be used (p. 2). Benzodiazepines are used in "delirium caused by withdrawal of alcohol or sedative hypnotics" (p. 2).

Verbal Psychotherapy

A variety of psychotherapies have been used with medical patients, including analytic, cognitive-behavioral, interpersonal, rational-emotive, directive, existential, and systems-oriented approaches. Psychotherapy can occur in individual, marital, family or group formats. Very brief interventions are utilized in inpatient settings, and both short-term and longer-term approaches are used with outpatients. All clinicians need expertise in crisis intervention, especially with problems related to illness, injury and death.

Relaxation Training

Relaxation training is perhaps the best researched health psychology intervention. Originally proposed as a physiological intervention, effects have been well documented in the affective and cognitive realms as well (e.g. decreased anxiety, perceived mastery). Specific strategies include diaphragmatic breathing, progressive muscle relaxation and autogenic training.

Hypnosis and Imagery

Through the use of focused awareness, imagination and created images, interventions can be designed to promote relaxation, reduce unpleasant affect (e.g. anxiety), target specific symptoms (e.g. pain), and promote behavior change. Specific strategies include guided imagery, covert sensitization, self-hypnosis and Ericksonian methods.

Biofeedback

The principal goal of biofeedback is to teach voluntary control over physiological processes. The most commonly used forms of biofeedback are skin electrical resistance, electromyographic (EMG) and skin temperature, although others, such as ear oximetry, heart rate, airway resistance and electroencephalography (EEG), have also been utilized. Biofeedback has been helpful in the treatment of bruxism, tension headache, anxiety, migraine headache, Raynaud's disease, chronic pain, torticollis, fecal incontinence, irritable bowel syndrome and essential hypertension.

It is important to note that biofeedback is not just a physiological treatment, as effects have also been documented in affective and cognitive domains. For example, in discussing the treatment of chronic back pain, Belar & Kibrick (1986) highlight several reasons why clinicians might choose EMG biofeedback: (a) to reduce spasm or equalize paraspinal muscle tension; (b) to train in general relaxation (and thus promote increased pain tolerance and decreased distress); and (c) to facilitate "physiological insight" about relationships between physiological and psychological processes.

Systematic Desensitization

Systematic desensitization is often used to reduce fears concerning medical procedures (e.g. needle phobias, ventilator weaning) and to help patients cope with initial public exposure after disfigurement. This procedure can be performed imaginally or in vivo, and usually involves a combination of both.

Modeling

Observational learning can facilitate the acquisition of adaptive behaviors and help decrease anxiety. Coping models viewed through doll play or videos are used with children in preparation for stressful medical and dental procedures. Post-organ transplant patients have served as coping models for adults prior to transplantation. And modeling is an especially important method in the teaching of self-care skills.

With respect to modeling, an interesting issue arises for the behavior of clinicians in relation to medical patients. Is it appropriate to provide consultations with a pack of cigarettes in one's pocket, or to be significantly overweight? In psychology, ethical principles hold that personal behavior is private, as long as it does not undermine professional practice. Yet personal health habits, or their consequences, are quite visible to consumers. Clinicians must be aware of their own stimulus value to patients.

Skills Training and Behavioral Rehearsal

Modeling, role-playing, and behavioral rehearsal can be incorporated into skills-training interventions. Skills in assertion and communication are perhaps most frequently addressed, as patients are often intimidated when dealing with health-care professionals. Patients are often encouraged to write down relevant questions prior to meeting with their physicians.

In targeting the skills of health-care providers, a common recommendation is for the provider to request that patients repeat their understanding of the problem and the recommended treatment plan. Since it has been shown that patients lose up to 50% of information provided during an office visit (Ley 1982), this simple procedure can eliminate many miscommunications, enhance compliance and improve satisfaction with the interaction.

Contingency Management

Contingency management is conducted through the use of various procedures such as positive and negative reinforcement, punishment, response cost, extinction and shaping. A major advantage to these methods is that other professionals and family members can implement them in their day-to-day contacts with patients. A major disadvantage is that they can be implemented poorly, thus an assessment of how well controlled the conditions for implementation are is essential. Contingency management is a hallmark of pain management rehabilitation programs, and has been used with difficult ward behavior, adherence in pediatric hemodialysis, ruminative vomiting in infants, and in health habit change programs.

Self-Monitoring and the Use of Cues

The use of diaries can be an effective intervention because of its reactive nature and its ability to promote self-awareness. Self-monitoring requires self-discipline and can be useful in assessing adherence to treatment. It also provides a record of progress during treatment. The use of cues can enhance self-monitoring programs, e.g. audible alarms to signal medication taking, colored dots to prompt internal scanning for tension, use of cue-controlled relaxation methods.

Other Cognitive Strategies

Other methods such as distraction, calming self-statements, and cognitive restructuring, can affect symptom perception and promote behavior change. A variety of cognitive strategies are combined in programs such as stress inoculation training.

Paradoxical Interventions

Paradoxical interventions, although not well researched, may be useful in cases of patient resistance, or when attempts to decrease symptoms actually result in increased levels. Paradoxical approaches have been used with problems such as insomnia and encopresis.

PROFESSIONAL ISSUES

All clinicians working with medical patients must be aware of a number of professional issues, some of which can differentially impact on psychiatrists and psychologists. For example, with their behavioral science background, psychologists are not physicians. To the extent that a physician is professionally chauvinistic, problems in professional collaboration might ensue. Yet being outside of the medical hierarchy has been at times beneficial for psychologists; the discipline has independent professional status with expertise medicine does not have, but is not viewed as sufficiently threatening, or competitive, to thwart communication. Moreover, psychologists must often seek medical information from consultees, and in the interchanges that result both disciplines can become students in the biopsychosocial understanding of the patient. Psychologists never have to prove themselves as "real physicians", which is a problem psychiatrists can sometimes face with their medical colleagues, despite their extensive medical training background.

Both psychologists and psychiatrists must deal with the mind–body dualism that is pervasive in social attitudes and much of health care. Patients are often resistant, if not hostile to referrals, thinking that it means their physician believes their problem is "all in the head" or that they are "crazy". And, if significant psychopathology is present, consultees often want to "dump" the patient onto psychiatric wards that are not well suited to deal with complex medical-surgical problems. To provide more integrated care, specialized treatment units and programs have been developed (e.g. medical psychiatric and behavioral wards within general hospitals for patients with significant comorbidity, multidisciplinary rehabilitation programs for patients with chronic pain, inpatient behavioral management programs for children with unstable diabetes). Many behavioral medicine programs are headed by psychologists, although in our experience medical-psychiatric units tend to be headed solely by psychiatrists.

Although the base rate of psychopathology is significant in medical patients, clinicians working in this area must be knowledgeable about normal development, stress and coping, and other behavioral health issues that are not "psychopathology". They must be skilled in working with disciplines other than mental health-care professionals, and understand the sociopolitical aspects of the health-care system.

Psychologists and psychiatrists must also be comfortable working with patients with significant medical problems. Issues related to loss, disfigurement and death and dying are common, yet the desire to avoid such problems may have been the reason some helping professionals were drawn to psychological or psychiatric practice.

Psychologists and psychiatrists must be able to tolerate the role of the consultant, which at times means that recommendations go unheeded or patients are discharged without notice. They must recognize that they serve as bridges between their core discipline and the rest of health care, and are thus not mainstream in either, as they attempt to serve an integrative function in a society that is mind–body dualistic in nature. They need to view themselves as health professionals and not just as mental health professionals.

Clinicians must also communicate appropriately. Decades ago, Lipowski, a major leader in consultation-liaison psychiatry, bemoaned physicians' perceptions of the psychiatrist as "a scientifically unsophisticated, medically ignorant, and impractical man, given to sweeping statements about other people's motives based on abstruse theories of questionable validity" (Lipowski 1967, p. 158). Given some of the psychological and psychiatric consultation reports we have seen, some evidence for this perception still remains. Psychologists and psychiatrists need to avoid "psychobabble" in communications, whether it be analytic or behavioral, and be sure to offer recommendations that are pertinent to the consultee's behavior and specify the plans for follow-up. Tips for written communications can be found in Table 3.2.

Special ethical issues can arise in settings where team approaches can lend themselves to a diffusion of responsibility for patient care. Clinicians need to be alert to issues of follow-up and follow-through. These must be documented as well. When patients are seen on an outpatient basis, psychiatric and psychological records are often kept separate from the medical chart in an effort to protect patient confidentiality. This practice can lead to a perception by consultees that their patients disappear "down a rabbit hole" when referred to mental health professionals. To provide integrated care, appropriate documentation and recommendations need to be made in the records regularly reviewed by other health-care professionals, without revealing unnecessary sensitive information in the more open medical chart.

TABLE 3.2 Tips for Written Communications

---

1. Be prompt.
2. Avoid jargon.
3. Be concise.
4. Provide information relevant to the consultee's behavior (i.e. practical suggestions).
5. Avoid including personal information regarding the patient that is unnecessary to respond to the referral question.
6. Specify plans for follow-up.
7. Follow the facility's rules and regulations regarding medical chart entries (for example, write in black ink; never obliterate an entry, but correct errors with an initialled single line strike-through; do not leave spaces between entries; date and time entries; use only approved abbreviations).

Other ethical issues arise when working with patients from different cultural or ethnic backgrounds whose customs and health belief models may differ substantially from those of the majority culture. Insensitivity to issues of diversity with respect to age, ethnicity, race, religion, sexual orientation, gender and other cultural issues could result in poor rapport, inadequate communication, misinterpretation of assessment results, and the design of inappropriate interventions.

Knapp & VandeCreek (1981) have highlighted the risk for malpractice should psychologists inadvertently practice medicine without a license (e.g. as patient symptom management skills increase, recommending a decrease in medication without consultation with the prescriber). Psychiatrists without a substantial background in psychometrics might have risks using psychological tests. Both psychologists and psychiatrists must practice within their limits of training and of competence, and provide full information to patients concerning alternative treatments available, even if not within their own professional expertise. Other malpractice risks relate to the nature of the consultant role. In this role, clinicians often do not have the ongoing relationships with patients that may provide a protective function against malpractice claims. Moreover, the input to medical decisions that are made (e.g. organ transplant) can have significant consequences to the physical health of the patient. Sensitivity regarding these issues is an important component of obtaining informed consent to consultation.

In the United States, the disciplines of psychology and psychiatry have each recognized that specialized training and expertise is fundamental to practice with medical patients. Board certification processes are overseen by the American Board of Professional Psychology or the American Board of Medical Specialties. How these services should be administratively organized is another matter and multiple models currently exist. However, a leading psychiatrist has argued that the long-term development of the field depends upon its independence from traditional departments of Psychiatry, with their primary focus on mental illness (Agras 1992). He recommends independent, multidisciplinary departments of behavioral medicine to best serve both research and patient-care activities in this fast growing field.

THE FUTURE

Consultation-liaison psychiatry has come a long way from its "psychosomatic medicine days" (Levy 1989; Smith 1993). It is encouraging that in an era of managed care (present in some countries and emergent in others), the role of C-L psychiatry and clinical health psychology is being recognized, not only in its own right, but also in its utility in reducing expenditure budgets (Goldberg & Stoudemire 1995; Gonzales & Randell 1996). Similarly, clinical health psychologists are increasingly making a contribution to the health-care system with a focus not only on individual assessment and treatment but systemic interventions such as improving information communication to patients. Psychologists' expertise in outcomes assessment and research is very useful in the design and evaluation of health-care services as well.

With shorter lengths of stay, it is becoming important to increase the focus of psychiatry and psychology on outpatient work (Dolinar 1993; Gonzales & Randell 1996). The increasing need to collaborate with primary health-care physicians is also highlighted (Huyse & Hengeveld 1989).

Furthermore, the need to substantiate the effectiveness of our interventions and our value in the system, through research, is imperative (Goldberg & Stoudemire 1995; Wright et al 1996; Belar 1997).

Research needs to focus on cogent issues: e.g. (1) evaluation of outcomes; (2) the required length of treatment with antidepressants, as people who become depressed in a medical setting may have different medium- and long-term requirements than other depressed patients (and the relative usefulness of medication versus cognitive-behavioral approaches); (3) understanding of psychophysiologic processes, e.g. in delirium; (4) the development of psychological treatment strategies relevant to particular medical disorders; (5) improvement of psychometric methods in predicting response to treatment; (6) understanding the impact of the health-care environment and improving provider–patient communication.

REFERENCES

Agras WS: Some structural changes that might facilitate the development of behavioral medicine. *J Consult Clin Psychol* **60**: 499–504, 1992.

APA (American Psychological Association): *Guidelines for Computer-Based Tests and Interpretations.* American Psychological Association: Washington, DC, 1986.

APA (American Psychiatric Association): Practice guidelines for the treatment of patients with delirium. *Am J Psychiatry* **156** (5): Supplement, 1999.

Antonowicz JL: Missed diagnoses in consultation-liaison psychiatry. *Psychiatr Clin N Am* **21**: 705–714, 1998.

Barsky AM: Hidden reasons some patients visit doctors. *Ann Intern Med* **94**: 492–498, 1981.

Beck AT: *Depression: Causes and Treatment.* University of Pennsylvania Press: Philadelphia, 1972.

Belar CD: Training the clinical psychology student in behavioral medicine. *Professional Psychol* **11**: 620–627, 1980.

Belar CD: Collaboration in capitated care: Challenges for psychology. *Professional Psychol: Research and Practice,* **26**: 139–146, 1995.

Belar CD: A proposal for an expanded view of health and psychology: The integration of behavior and health. In RJ Resnick and RH Rozensky (eds): *Health Psychology Through the Life Span: Practice and Research Opportunities.* American Psychological Association: Washington, DC, 77–81, 1996.

Belar CD: Clinical health psychology: A specialty for the 21st century. *Health Psychol* **16**: 411–416, 1997.

Belar CD and Deardorff WW: *Clinical Health Psychology in Medical Settings: A Practitioner's Guidebook.* American Psychological Association: Washington, DC, 1995.

Belar CD and Kibrick S: Biofeedback in the treatment of chronic back pain. In A Holzman and D Turk (eds): *Pain Management: A Handbook of Psychological Treatment Approaches.* Pergamon Press: New York, 131–150, 1986.

Belar CD, Deardorff WW and Kelly KE: *The Practice of Clinical Health Psychology.* Pergamon Press: New York, 1987.

Clayson D and Mensh IN: Psychologists in medical schools: The trials of emerging political activism. *Am Psychol* **42**: 859–862, 1987.

Collins D, Dimsdale JE and Wilkins D: Consultation/liaison psychiatry utilization patterns in different cultural groups. *Psychosom Med* **54**: 240–245, 1992.

Costa E, Mogos I and Toma T: Efficacy and safety of mianserin in the treatment of depression in women with cancer. *Acta Psychiatrica Scandinavica* **72**: 85–92, 1985.

Craig TJ and Abeloff MD: Psychiatric symptomatology among hospitalized cancer patients. *Am J Psychiatry* **131**: 1323–1327, 1974.

Derogatis LR: The Psychosocial Adjustment to Illness Scale (PAIS). *J Psychosom Res* **30**: 77–91, 1986.

Dolinar LJ: A historical review of out-patient consultation-liaison psychiatry. *Gen Hosp Psychiatry* **15**: 363–368, 1993.

Engel GL: The need for a new medical model: A challenge for biomedicine. *Science* **196**: 129–136, 1977.

Evans DL, McCartney CF and Haggerty JJ: Treatment of depression in cancer is associated with better life adaptation: a pilot study. *Psychosom Med* **50**: 72–76, 1988.

Folstein MF, Folstein SE and McHugh PR: "Mini-mental state": A practical method for grading the cognitive state of patients for the clinician. *J Psychiatr Res* **12**: 189–198, 1975.

Freyne A, Buckley P, Larkin C and Walsh N: Consultation liaison psychiatry within the general hospital: Referral pattern and management. *Irish Med J* **85**: 112–114, 1992.

Goldberg RJ and Stoudemire A: The future of consultation-liaison psychiatry and medical-psychiatric units in the era of managed care. *Gen Hosp Psychiatry* **17**: 268–277, 1995.

Gonzales JJ and Randell L: Consultation-liaison psychiatry in the managed care arena. *Psychiatr Clin N Am* **19**: 449–466, 1996.

Hamilton M: The assessment of anxiety status by rating. *Br J Med Psychol* **32**: 50–55, 1959.

Hathaway SR and McKinley JC: *The Minnesota Multiphasic Personality Inventory Manual.* Psychological Corporation: New York, 1967.

Huyse FJ and Hengeveld MW: Development of consultation-liaison psychiatry in the Netherlands: Its social psychiatric heritage. *Gen Hosp Psychiatry* **11**: 9–15, 1989.

Huyse FJ, Strain JJ and Hammer JS: Interventions in consultation/liaison psychiatry. Part I: Patterns of recommendations. *Gen Hosp Psychiatry* **12**: 213–220, 1990.

Johnston M and Vogele C: Benefits of psychological preparation for surgery: a meta-analysis. *Ann Behav Med* **15**: 245–256, 1993.

Kamerow DB, Pincus HA and MacDonald DI: Alcohol abuse, other drug abuse and mental disorders in medical practice. *JAMA* **255**: 2054–2057, 1986.

Knapp S and VandeCreek L: Behavioral medicine: Its malpractice risks for psychologists. *Prof Psychol* **12**: 677–683, 1981.

Leibenluft E and Goldberg RL: The suicidal, terminally ill patient with depression. *Psychosomatics* **29**: 379–386, 1988.

Leigh H and Reiser MF: *Biological, Psychological and Social Dimensions of Medical Practice.* Plenum: New York, 1980.

Levenson JL, Hamer RM and Rossiter LF: A randomized controlled study of psychiatric consultation guided by screening in general medical inpatients. *Am J Psychiatry* **149**: 631–637, 1992.

Levy NB: Psychosomatic medicine and consultation-liaison psychiatry: Past, present and future. *Hosp Commun Psychiatry* **40**: 1049–1056, 1989.

Ley P: Studies of recall in medical settings. *Human Learning* **1**: 223–233, 1982.

Lipowski, ZJ: Review of consultation psychiatry and psychosomatic medicine: I. General principles. *Psychosom Med* **29**: 153–171, 1967.

McDaniel JS, Musselman DL, Porter MR, Reed DA and Nemeroff CB: Depression in patients with cancer: diagnosis, biology, and treatment. *Arch Gen Psychiatry* **52**: 89–99, 1995.

Melzack R: The McGill Pain Questionnaire: Major properties and scoring methods. *Pain* **1**: 277–299, 1975.

Meenan RR, Gertman PM and Mason JH: The Arthritis Impact Measurement Scales: Further investigation of a health status measure. *Arthr Rheumatol* **25**: 1048–1053, 1982.

Millon T: On the nature of clinical health psychology. In T Millon, CJ Green and RB Meagher (eds): *Handbook of Clinical Health Psychology*. Plenum: New York, 1–27, 1982.

Millon T, Green CJ and Meagher RB: *Millon Behavioral Health Inventory Manual*. National Computer Systems, Minneapolis, MI, 1982.

Moos RH: *Work Environment Scale Manual*. Consulting Psychologists Press: Palo Alto, CA, 1981.

Moos RH and Moos B: *Family Environment Scale Manual*. Consulting Psychologists Press: Palo Alto, CA, 1981.

Neehall J and Beharry N: The pattern of inpatient psychiatric referrals in a general hospital. *West Indian Med J* **42**: 155–157, 1993.

Nemeroff C, DeVane C and Pollock B: Newer antidepressants and the cytochrome P450 system. *Am J Psychiatry* **153**: 311–320, 1996.

Ormont MA, Weisman HW, Heller SS, Najara JE and Shindledecker RD: The timing of psychiatric consultation requests. Utilization, liaison and diagnostic considerations. *Psychosomatics* **38**: 38–44, 1997.

Paoletti N: Transcultural aspects of antidepressant therapy. Proceedings of Symposium on Recent Trends in the Treatment of Depression: Melbourne, Australia, pp 36–41, 1986.

Paoletti N: Fasi di sviluppo collettivo in gruppi omogenei di emigrati. In G Bartocci (ed): *Psicopatologia, cultura e pensiero magico*. Liguori Editore: Naples, pp 65–72, 1990.

Paoletti N: Farmaci e tranculturalismo. In: GG Rovera, S Fassino and D Munno (eds): *Psicopatologia e farmaci*. Centro Scientifico Editore: Turin, pp 113–125, 1991.

Paoletti N: Cultural construction of Self and therapy: Models of illness. Paper presented at the 1997 International Symposium on Transcultural Psychiatry, World Psychiatric Association, Transcultural Psychiatry Section: Rome, 3–9 October 1997.

Preskorn SH: Debate resolved: there are differential effects of serotonin selective reuptake inhibitors on cytochrome P450 enzymes. *J Psychopharmacol* **12**: S89–S97, 1998.

Ribeiro SCM, Tandon R, Grunhaus L and Greden JF: The DST as a predictor of outcome in depression: a meta-analysis. *Am J Psychiatry* **150**: 1618–1629, 1993.

Rosensky RH, Sweet JJ and Tovian SM: *Psychological Assessment in Medical Settings*. Plenum Press: New York, 1997.

Sadock BJ and Sadock VA (eds): *Kaplan and Sadock's Comprehensive Textbook of Psychiatry*, 7th Edition. Lippincott, Williams and Wilkins: Philadelphia, 2000.

Smith GC: From psychosomatic medicine to consultation-liaison psychiatry. *Med J Aust* **159**: 745–749, 1993.

Wright M, Samuels A and Streimer J: Clinical practice issues in consultation-liaison psychiatry. *Aust NZ J Psychiatry* **30**: 238–245, 1996.

4

Management of Medical and Surgical Patients: Consultation-Liaison (C-L) Psychiatry and Clinical Health Psychology

James J. Strain
Department of Psychiatry, Mount Sinai – NYU Medical Center/Health Service, New York, USA

and

David J. de L. Horne
University of Melbourne, Australia

SECTION A: CONSULTATION-LIAISON (C-L) PSYCHIATRY
James J. Strain

INTRODUCTION

Consultation-liaison (C-L) psychiatry has evolved over the last 50 years from basically employing the psychosomatic model of mind–body problems, to a systematic approach to the patient who experiences psychiatric-social-psychological as well as medical morbidity (Axis I and/or II as well as Axis III morbidity concomitantly; DSM-IV, American Psychiatric Association 1995). In this evolution, several key domains have been foci for its development: (1) historical antecedents; (2) universal psychological stresses of medical illness and hospitalization; (3) instrumentation to measure psychiatric morbidity in the medically ill; (4) epidemiological studies of the occurrence of psychiatric-psychological dysfunction in diverse medical settings; (5) outcome studies of psychiatric interventions in the medical setting; (6) C-L models of mental health training for non-psychiatric physicians; (7) the electronic record of clinical database management; (8) literature search strategies for the C-L setting; (9) psychotropic–medical drug interactions; (10) new models of

Psychology and Psychiatry: Integrating Medical Practice.
Edited by J. Milgrom and G. D. Burrows © 2001 John Wiley & Sons, Ltd.

health-care delivery, e.g. psychiatry-medical inpatient hospital units; and (11) guidelines for training C-L psychiatrists. Each of these areas will be discussed in the following pages. The C-L psychiatrist and ethics will not be discussed in this chapter (Moros et al 1987; Kornfeld et al 1997).

HISTORICAL ANTECEDENTS

C-L psychiatry had its roots in "psychosomatic medicine", the mind having effects over bodily function. Engel (1962, 1967a), on the other hand, has conceptualized a "somatopsychic phenomenon" in which the body has influences over the mind, e.g. steroid psychosis, delirium secondary to pulmonary infections, anxiety states as a result of hypoxia, etc. Here the body processes are the mechanisms for the effects seen on mental behavior. Much of the early conceptual framework was based on the work of Franz Alexander (see Pollock 1964), and later that of Flanders Dunbar (Dunbar 1934), which hypothesized that psychological processes in predisposed individuals could make them vulnerable to certain diseases, e.g. peptic ulcer, ulcerative colitis, hypertension, asthma, etc. These were psychiatrists working with patients with medical illness who often used the psychoanalytic model, from which they deduced conclusions as to the psychological stresses which impacted on a vulnerable body.

As time passed it became clear that these formulations were burdened by inadequate scientific rigor; often the psychological state was a result of the physical illness, rather than the other way around, a psychological personality giving rise to a specific physiological state. Many of the illnesses studied, such as ulcerative colitis, were heterogeneous diseases, which in time would have to be dissected out and studied separately, reminiscent of "consumption", which eventually was partitioned into cancer, infectious disease, asbestosis, emphysema, etc. Today current work in "*psychosomatics*" is concerned with much more discrete physiologic entities and examines three distinct phases of physical illness: (1) pre-illness; (2) initiation of illness; and (3) maintenance of illness. Each phase has its own psychological and physiological risk factors which need to be separately addressed depending upon which phase a particular patient is in. Current research is much more specific, and outcome studies are underway to examine, using randomized controlled trials, the effectiveness of psychiatric/psychological interventions with the medically ill (see below).

At the same time, in the United States there has been an evolution underway to move psychiatric inpatients, and outpatients, to acute care general hospitals, in the communities where patients lived and worked. This evolution has had such enormous support that in 1998 most general hospitals have psychiatric inpatient units and offer ambulatory psychiatric care to psychiatric and medical patients. In fact, it was anticipated that by the year 2000 approximately 90% of psychiatric inpatients would be cared for in acute general hospitals. Only 10% (those with chronic disabilities, or aggressive disturbances, who cannot at this time return to the community) will continue to be hospitalized in long-term chronic mental hospitals often separate from a medical facility.

This revolution in the delivery of mental health care to psychiatric patients in the hospitals of the medically/surgically ill provided psychiatry a unique opportunity to relate to other medical disciplines and have access to their patients. As a result, psychiatrists were given access to medical, surgical, obstetric and other patients, not only to care for psychosomatic disorders, but to deal with issues around the management of illness, such as noncompliance, coping, and disease state management. Psychosomatic was the term used in the 1930s and 40s for those medical illnesses which could be initiated, exacerbated, or maintained by psychosocial mechanisms. It was the original focus of psychiatrists working in the general hospital and with the medically ill. C-L took a much broader view of the cohort of interest, including within its borders illnesses not regarded as psychosomatic, e.g. neoplasia, cardiac conditions and infections. At the same time C-L addressed behavioral disorders of the medically ill, as well as the more traditional mental disorders, e.g. depression, anxiety, delirium, obsessionality, psychoses, and personality disorders that were co-occurring with medical disorders, but did not necessarily precipitate the medical morbidity. Psychiatrists could now offer diagnosis, treatment, and follow-up for these primary psychiatric disorders, that hitherto had not been diagnosed and treated on medical and surgical wards. Finally, this placement of psychiatry squarely in the province of the acute care general hospital afforded the unique opportunity to teach and develop the mental health skills of primary care physicians, as well as teaching tomorrow's medical students and residents.

With the final step of moving from the consultation model—waiting for a referral from medicine and then dealing only with the referred population (the numerator)—psychiatry advanced to the liaison model whereby the psychiatrist became part of the medical/surgical ward team, made rounds, and was able to have contact with the entire population of a ward (the denominator). This overcame the obstacle of the primary care physician's inability to detect, assess, diagnose, treat, and offer follow-up mental health care to patients where they would not have suspected the presence of such morbidity. In a sense, psychiatry and the psychiatrist had moved back into medicine, so that the acute care general hospital became also a *de facto* mental health center. By broadening the scope of psychiatry to survey the scene and not wait for the occasional call for help, psychiatry re-entered the stream of medicine as a crucial and essential medical specialty.

Furthermore, such placement gave psychiatry the opportunity to examine the effects of psychiatric and medical comorbidity on our *taxonomy* (DSM-IV, American Psychiatric Association 1995); our *instruments* (e.g. the Hamilton Depression Scale, Beck Depression Inventory); the *outcome measures* (functional status measures, e.g. Medical Outcomes Scale assessing both psychiatric, quality of life as well as physical functional status); *costs* (health resource utilization with and without comorbidity, and before and after treatment of the psychiatric component); and the *ethical issues* when mental status affects the medical condition (whether a dying candidate receives a liver transplant if it is evaluated that he/she may not be able mentally to manage the treatment requirements to maintain and preserve a scarce resource).

UNIVERSAL STRESSES OF MEDICAL ILLNESS AND HOSPITALIZATION

The sick and hospitalized patient is vulnerable to eight categories of psychological stress (Strain & Grossman 1975; Strain 1978). An important function of the C-L psychiatrist is to address these stresses, attenuate their pernicious effects, and teach the caretakers how they may ameliorate these universal concerns of their patients.

The Basic Threat to Narcissistic Integrity

Sudden illness, hospitalization, and the threat of death challenge the individual's belief that he is indestructible, that he is the master of his destiny.

These events also challenge the infantile fantasy, which may persist in adult life, that our omnipotent parents (and, later, the physician) can ensure our pain-free, pleasurable, and protected existence—and our immortality.

Fear of Strangers

When the patient enters the hospital, they feel that they have put their life into the hands of a group of strangers to whom they have no close personal ties, and who may or may not be competent to assume responsibility for their survival.

This feeling is reminiscent of the fear of strangers which can first be observed in the human infant from the third to the sixth month of life—when the sight of an unfamiliar face produces a startle response, body tension, and tearfulness.

Separation Anxiety

The hospitalized patient experiences anxiety because they are separated from important persons and things—from the environment that provided the support and gratification necessary for their effective functioning and sense of intactness.

This anxiety mimics the anxiety that characterizes the separation-individuation phase of development, which occurs between the ages of six and 30 months. The toddler's ability to separate from his/her mother is a crucial first step toward the achievement of autonomy. But the individual is always "vulnerable" in this regard; the anxiety surrounding separation may be reactivated, to varying degrees, in later life whenever there is a need to separate from the familiar and confront the unknown.

Fear of Loss of Love and Approval

This stress may be prominent, for example, in the patient who has undergone a mutilating surgical procedure, or in the patient who, because of a debilitating illness, is unable to return to work, and fears that their passive dependence on others may incur the disapproval of their family and friends—and the loss of their esteem.

The fear of loss of love and approval can be observed or inferred from the behaviour of the two-year-old, and it persists to varying degrees throughout life. This fear has its onset when the child realizes that his/her needs may not be gratified automatically by his/her mother, and that their fulfillment is contingent upon his/her ability to please her.

Fear of the Loss of Control of Developmentally Achieved Functions

Severe illness may temporarily undo previously mastered physical and mental functions. Some patients agonize over the transient loss of these functions, and remain convinced, despite assurances to the contrary, that they will never be regained.

Concurrent with their fear of the loss of love and approval, a young child fears the loss of previously achieved physical and mental functions. Specifically, they are aware that their movement from passivity to activity, via the achievement of new skills—standing, walking, talking, etc.—evokes pleasure in the mother. Thus, they equate the loss of these functions with loss of her love and approval and, carried to its worst possible outcome, the loss of mother herself.

Fear of Injury or Loss of Body Parts

Once a patient enters the hospital, their body becomes the property of the physicians, to do with what they will. Bodily fluids are drained; the patient is exposed, probed, and weakened. These routine hospital procedures require the patient to assume a passive-submissive stance vis-à-vis the physician, which may stir up frightening sexual and aggressive fantasies.

Specifically, these fantasies may reactivate the fears of bodily damage that typically arise in the child at about the age of two-and-a-half, and reach their peak at five—during the period when the child is moving from an ambiguous to a definite sense of sexual identity. This fear of injury to body parts, which is one of the most persistently potent psychological forces in childhood, is readily reactivated in any potentially traumatic situation (either perceived or actual), and particularly by acute illness and hospitalization.

Guilt and Fear of Retaliation

Feelings of guilt and shame, which may be revived by physical illness, and the patient's fantasy that illness and hospitalization are punishment for previous "sins" of omission or commission are a major source of psychological stress.

Although they do not identify it as such, the three-year-old child feels ashamed when, for a variety of reasons, they regress to an earlier stage in their development—when, for example, they lose previously achieved sphincter control, or are unable to control their unacceptable behavior and impulses. Characteristically, when they get sick, they believe their illness to be a consequence of these "sins". Despite the acquisition of logic, intelligence and experience, the perception of illness and hospitalization as retaliation by a "higher being" for one's transgressions persists in the unconscious of the adult.

Fear of Pain

The fear of pain cuts across all of the stresses listed above. In the vulnerable patient, each of these stresses may compound the basic painful experience, and, conversely, severe pain may increase the magnitude of each of these stresses.

Pain—in the guise of physical discomfort, hunger, or the like—is part of the human condition from birth. The fear of pain is never fully overcome, for once eased, the concern that it may recur remains. The individual copes with pain differently at different stages in their development. The neonate's total organismic reaction to the pain of discomfort or hunger, demands for immediate relief, and total dependence on the mother as the source of such relief, give way in the course of normal development to the child's increasing capacity to tolerate discomfort, to a growing ability to separate from mother, to respond favorably to strangers, to be more confident about their ability to control their body, and, in time, to guard the body against injury. Moreover, they are better able to separate mind from body, so that mental pain is less likely to be translated into physical pain.

Although these stresses are present to varying degrees in every medical patient, inevitably they take on different forms at different phases of disease.

Doctor–Patient Relationship

In addition the C-L psychiatrist needs to address the stresses on the physician. Understanding of the doctor–patient relationship hinges on recognition of the role of stress as an inherent feature of human growth and maturation (Leigh & Reiser 1992). In the course of their own emotional development, internists have been exposed to the same conflicts as their patients, and they bring these unresolved (albeit quiescent) conflicts to the clinical setting (Lin et al 1995). The patient's attitudes and behavior, and the nature and outcome of the illness, may revive these conflicts in their medical caretakers. And, as is true of the patient, the internist's vulnerability to the patient's reaction to stress will depend on the quality of their object relationships, past and present, and the degree to which they have resolved their own childhood conflicts. For example, the patient who fails to get better may threaten the doctor's sense of narcissistic integrity. Contact with new patients and their families may revive the internist's strong feelings of stranger anxiety. Medical caretakers may react adversely when they are not loved or admired by their patients (even as they may resent being cast in the role of all-caring, all-accepting parent). They may identify with patients who must undergo mutilating procedures, and experience the same degree of stress. And, as might be expected, the dying patient frequently evokes feelings of guilt and shame in their medical caretakers, who berate themselves for not keeping an adequate vigil or for not knowing enough about the illness to help the patient.

Thus, the internist is charged with a dual responsibility. Clearly, if they are to provide adequate medical and psychosocial care for the patient, they must understand the nature of the psychological stresses provoked in the patient by illness and hospitalization, and be able to help the patient to cope with these stresses (Lin et al 1995). But they must also possess sufficient self-knowledge to recognize and cope with the stresses under which they are operating. Otherwise these stresses may adversely affect their relationship with and attitudes toward the patient, with the result that they may become either too involved with or too remote from the patient.

The internist's problem is further compounded by the fact that the posture they assume in their interactions with the patient (and the patient's attitudes toward the caretakers) does not remain static. The sequence of becoming ill, being treated, and then recovering implies a constantly changing doctor–patient relationship. Each stage has its own stresses. The patient who has just suffered a myocardial infarction must remain completely passive during the initial, critical stage of their illness (Frasure Smith et al 1993). As the patient recovers, their autonomous activities increase in extent and power. Similarly, the surgical patient is considered a "good" patient if they are able to remain quiet and follow orders for the first few hours immediately following their operation. At this stage it is most important that they are able to regress sufficiently to assume a completely dependent role. Later on, however, the patient's role changes. Once they have recovered from the initial trauma of surgery, the patient must try to sit up, walk, and cough against pain, if they are to be regarded as a "good" patient. Actually, this transition from passivity to activity, from total dependence to relative independence, may take place in just a few hours, but it signals the beginning of physiological and psychological recovery. The doctor plays a crucial role in the implementation of these adaptive changes in the patient's behaviour and attitudes. They must be flexible to achieve a delicate balance, catering to the patient's dependency needs even while encouraging independence. But, most important, medical caretakers must be sufficiently flexible to accept the fact that their patients may not always be able to fulfill the prerequisites of the "good" patient or to adhere to a prescribed timetable in making the transition from passivity to activity (Lin et al 1995).

Within this conceptual framework we have found it useful to evaluate the doctor–patient relationship in terms of three interrelated dynamic "systems":

1. The stage of patient's illness (or convalescence).
2. The patient's personal reaction to their illness and to their internist.
3. The internist's reaction to their patient and to their patient's illness.

The goal of the psychiatrist is to detect discordance in these systems. Any one, or all three, may be out of phase, producing an angry, disruptive patient, or an anxious, withdrawn doctor.

A 75-year-old man who had suffered a stroke, but had recovered sufficient motor capacity for limited self-care, was extremely angry with the resident because he hadn't been washed and fed. The patient's behavior evoked a counterdefensive reaction in the resident, who challenged him by saying, "Do more for yourself", after which he turned his back and abruptly walked away. To make matters worse, on his way out he murmured an aside to a colleague (which was overheard by the patient) to the effect that he couldn't stand patients like that. After this episode, the patient said, "I wish I were dead."

The doctor's response to this patient was out of phase with the stage of the patient's illness and its meaning to him. The patient's needs (which, admittedly, were somewhat unrealistic), as well as his resultant anger, should have been understood as an attempt to compensate for his feelings of being damaged and helpless, and they should have been dealt with directly. Instead, and inevitably, this confrontation produced feelings of guilt and shame in doctor and patient alike. The patient's stated wish that he would die seemed to stem from his feelings of mortification and guilt, and, of course, it was also an attempt to punish the doctor. But, perhaps because of the staff's own guilt, the patient's statement was interpreted by them as evidence of his suicidal tendencies, and a request for a psychiatric consultation was promptly initiated.

CONFOUNDS IN ASSESSING COMMON PSYCHIATRIC DISORDERS IN THE MEDICALLY ILL

For the physician, diagnosis proceeds along a continuum that begins with: (1) understanding the stated reason for the patient's visit or consultation (e.g. problems, complaints, signs, symptoms); (2) assessment of the reason for the contact (e.g. establishing disorders, diseases, syndromes); and (3) formulation of a diagnosis, hopefully the etiology of the disorder, and the prognosis. Management can flow from any level of this continuum. For example, a patient who presents with acute chest pains will be "managed", e.g. hospitalized, even before the underlying problem and diagnosis are established. And the definitive diagnosis may never be derived.

Diagnosis of the most common psychiatric disorder—depressive disorder—is confounded in the medically/surgical ill in that four of the vegetative symptoms that constitute the algorithm, i.e. eating, sleeping, energy, libido, may all be affected by medical illness (Cohen-Cole & Kaufman 1993). For example, the cancer patient may experience all of these vegetative symptoms secondary to their neoplasia. The ideation symptoms that constitute the algorithm, e.g. feelings of helplessness, hopelessness, guilt, suicidality also may accompany physical illness. The two major symptoms, persistent dysphoria, anhedonia (for two to four weeks), are also commonplace in the seriously medically ill. If the symptom is secondary to physical illness it is not to be "counted" in the algorithm for depression. Therefore, depression is often overdiagnosed in the medical setting if all the symptoms are "counted" or a standard depression measurement scale is employed, e.g. the Hamilton or Beck Depression Inventories; and if they are not "counted", then depression will be underdiagnosed. Similar confounders obtain for the anxiety disorders in which many of the key symptoms that constitute the diagnosis also derive from medical illness, e.g. diaphoresis, tachycardia, tachypnea, palpitations. Therefore, symptoms that can be accounted for by other medical conditions do not necessarily justify a diagnosis (or treatment) of a depressive or anxiety disorder. However, for the organic mental disorder—delirium—which emanates from physiological sources and is a product of physical process, the symptoms physiologically produced are "counted" toward its psychiatric diagnosis. The development of new instruments for the measurement of psychiatric disorders in the medically ill are essential to advance the C-L field in the 21st century. Until this is done appropriate screening strategies and epidemiological studies in primary care and inpatient hospital settings will be compromised (but see Field & Lohr 1992; Spitzer et al 1994; Broadhead et al 1995).

EPIDEMIOLOGICAL STUDIES OF OCCURRENCE OF PSYCHIATRIC–PSYCHOLOGICAL DYSFUNCTION IN THE MEDICALLY ILL

Psychosocial disability and psychiatric disorders are prevalent in the population and are more often encountered in medical and outpatient settings. Researchers have used one-month and point prevalence studies to demonstrate that 16% of community cohorts exhibit psychiatric morbidity. It is estimated that 21–26% of medical outpatients have psychiatric disorders. The age- and sex-adjusted prevalence of mental disorders in those patients with a chronic medical condition was 25% compared to 17.5% without. Lifetime presence of a mental disorder in the chronic physically ill reached 42.0% (most often substance abuse, affective or anxiety disorders) compared to 33.0% who did not have long-term disability. Finally,

30–60% of those in acute general medical/surgical inpatient settings have significant psychosocial/psychiatric morbidity (Regier et al 1993; Katon & Gonzales 1994; Katon et al 1990; Morris et al 1993).

Medical patients have a much higher morbidity for specific disorders than is encountered in the population at large: delirium (15–30% of those hospitalized); depression (two to three times greater); panic and somatization (10–20 times more frequent); and, substance abuse (three to five times more likely). This indicates that the medical setting—where patients have already put themselves within a medical facility—is an excellent venue to initiate screening, triage, and commence some effort to confront the psychiatric morbidity. In fact, as indicated previously, the medical setting is an important "*de facto*" mental health setting from which to launch an effort to ameliorate mental suffering (Smith et al 1986; Levenson 1992).

In addition, psychiatric morbidity is associated with high utilization of general medical services and increased health services utilization in several parameters (Smith 1994; Smith et al 1995). Researchers observed that 50% of high utilizers had psychiatric morbidity: major depression or dysthymia (40%), anxiety (21.8%), somatization (20%), panic (12%), alcohol or substance abuse (5%). Depressed patients in the medical setting use three times more health resources, encounter twice the costs, and make seven times more visits to the emergency facilities than those not depressed (Johnson et al 1992). Patients with panic disorder visit the emergency room 10 times more often than those without (70% of those with panic disorders encounter 10 or more doctors until a correct diagnosis is achieved). In addition, the need for acute care hospitalization can triple when asthma patients experience comorbid anxiety disorders.

Patients with alcohol abuse or dependent disorders have twice the total health-care costs of those without, and too often are not identified during an inpatient hospitalization (Regier et al 1993). Patients with depression have increased health-care costs: $4246 versus $2371 for nondepressed; patients with anxiety disorders versus without, $2390 against $1397. Mean rehospitalization costs in those patients with cardiac disease and psychological distress versus those without were $9504 and $2146 respectively. It has repeatedly been shown that an association exists between increased length of patient stay in the acute care medical hospital and the presence of psychiatric morbidity (Johnson et al 1992; Hall & Wise 1995; Katon et al 1990, 1995). This increase in the utilization of health-care resources persisted for at least four years after the first hospital discharge (Saravay & Lavin 1994).

Finally, the Medical Outcomes Study has demonstrated that the presence of depressive morbidity is related to profound physical impairment equivalent to that observed in several other chronic medical conditions: diabetes, hypertension, arthritis, coronary artery disease, and that the social impairment is even greater (Wells 1995; Hays et al 1995). Clearly, it is essential to have enhanced methods of detection for psychiatric comorbidity in the medical setting (Cohen-Cole & Kaufman 1993).

OUTCOME STUDIES OF PSYCHIATRIC INTERVENTIONS IN THE MEDICAL SETTING

Inpatients

C-L intervention studies for acutely hospitalized medical patients demonstrated improved patient status and decreased costs (Fuller 1995; Hall & Wise 1995). For a cost of $20 000.00, a C-L intervention with elderly hip-fracture patients that screened for and treated psychiatric morbidity saved $167 000.00 in decreasing length of hospital stay (Strain et al 1991). In addition, over half of the studied population: (1) had significant diagnosable DSM-IV disorders (most commonly organic mental and affective disorders—56%); (2) were discharged with decreased psychiatric morbidity; (3) had fewer rehospitalizations; and (4) needed fewer re-habilitation treatment days.

Outpatients

The prevalence of somatization disorder in the outpatient medical setting has been reported to be 9%, three times more frequent than in the general population (Smith et al 1986). Somatization disorder is also described as Briquet's Disease (Yutzy et al 1994). It encompasses eight symptoms in four systems, e.g. pain, genito-urinary, neurological and gastro-intestinal systems. It is more common in women, begins before the age of 30, and leads to a life of medical disorders and physician visits, out of all keeping with the degree of physical disability. This somatization population consumes three times more hospitalization, increased outpatient visits, and two to nine times the US per capita for health-care resources of those patients who are not somatizers. Smith et al (1995) demonstrated improved psychiatric status and decreased utilization of medical resources after a C-L intervention with primary care physicians and with the patients themselves (Smith et al 1986; Rost et al 1994).

Spiegel et al (1989) demonstrated that women with metastatic breast cancer (stage IV) who were treated in an ongoing group therapy protocol lived 18 months longer than controls, and had a better quality of life. This important study is now under replication at several national and international sites (Spiegel et al 1989). Fawzy et al observed that patients with metastatic melanoma who were treated with group and educational protocols survived longer, and with better quality of life than matched controls (Fawzy et al 1993).

Studies indicate that undetected psychiatric morbidity in the medical setting utilizes more health resources and produces more impairment of functional status than medical illness alone. Minimal intervention, e.g. notifying the primary care physician of psychiatric morbidity, is inadequate to effect change. Structural change in the pattern of health care provided by primary care must be undertaken to ensure that adequate C-L involvement occurs at every phase of treatment: assessment, treatment, and follow-up.

C-L MODELS OF MENTAL HEALTH TRAINING

In order to identify how primary care physicians, internists—general practice internists, family practitioners—are trained in mental health knowledge and skills, the National Institutes of Mental Health undertook three studies in a random selection of training programs in the United States (Strain et al 1985; Strain et al 1994). It was identified that there were six models of mental health training, each of which had a different impact upon the competencies of the trainee to identify and treat mental health morbidity in the primary care setting. These models were:

1. *Consultation*—having the C-L psychiatrist see referred patients on the medical wards, the teaching being mainly accomplished through the medical chart note. Unless house officers asked for psychiatric consultations they received no training.
2. *Liaison*—ongoing structured teaching time usually on the medical wards was provided by the C-L psychiatrist in addition to offering consultations.
3. *Bridge*—a C-L psychiatrist would join the medical team, usually in the outpatient setting.
4. *Hybrid*—any of several mental health professionals could serve as teacher to the primary care physician, e.g. social worker, psychologist, anthropologist, offering a variation in the focus of the teaching.
5. *Post-graduate training*—a primary care physician would spend two years learning psychiatric care of their particular patient cohort (Engel 1967b).
6. *Dual trained*—primary care physicians had full training in medicine and psychiatry and could refer patients to themselves for psychiatric care.

These models constitute the majority of mental health training for primary care physicians after their graduation from medical school in the United States. In some specialties, e.g. surgery, there may be no mental health training during the residency. Each model employed a different amount of training time, different disciplines of teachers, and different expectations of what the physician should be able to do after training.

THE ELECTRONIC RECORD—THE USE OF THE COMPUTERIZED CLINICAL DATABASE

Software applications have been designed for the C-L setting which allow studies to proceed within an institution, among institutions, within a city, and throughout a country—MICROCARES (Strain et al 1996). The software has been translated into Portuguese and Spanish and a German version is planned. In addition, international studies may be undertaken using a structured universal database that is systematically employed using commonly defined variables. This system would give the C-L psychiatrist access to data to make clinical, administrative, research, and educational decisions not available from the current handwritten consultation notes that are commonly employed in most teaching hospitals today. The software program allows the C-L psychiatrist to have in his/her portable laptop computer at the side of the patient the entire archive of consultations seen by that institution, menu-driven computerized printed chart notes, consultant logs on all patients seen, letter to the referring doctor, use of screening devices, study of specific cohorts of patients, and transfer of electronic data to spreadsheets or statistical packages. That is, every patient seen by the C-L psychiatrist may become part of a central C-L database for developing further knowledge and approaches to the psychiatric disorders of the medically ill. Prototypic international-multiple institutional studies have been reported (Smith et al 1995; Strain et al 1996a). It is anticipated that all medical records will be electronic in the early part of the 2lst century and that the handwritten consultation form will be obsolete (Shortliffe et al 1990; Piemme 1998).

Literature Database in C-L Psychiatry

Treatment needs to be influenced by pertinent research reports at the patient's side for the enhancement of instantaneous clinical decision-making. To achieve this end, a C-L psychiatry literature database with ongoing updates has been developed along with its software: MICROCARES—Literature Search System. First, the most common psychosocial/psychiatric problems encountered by the C-L psychiatrist were determined by examining three years of data from over 2000 consultations at a major teaching hospital (Strain et al 1994). This set of common issues was confirmed by 12 additional teaching hospitals. Second, world experts ($n = 100$) were asked to examine the literature in an area of their expertise with a selection focused on reports germane to the C-L psychiatrist, e.g. cancer (Jimmie Holland, Memorial Sloane-Kettering Cancer Center) and to identify from the studies extant those regarded as most important for residents, fellows, and attendings, offering psychosocial/psychiatric care to patients having this specific medical disorder. From thousands of studies 50–100 were selected for each designated problem area as essential to the knowledge base of the C-L practitioner. Third, the experts were asked to denote within their selections those most important papers—the "five star" "creme de la creme"—choices which were essential reading for clinical decision-making. Over 500 000 papers were identified, from which 2700 were selected as the expert list of essential references in C-L psychiatry. Then another selection was made from these 2700 of the very most important papers which were regarded as required and seminal reading for trainees. Fourth, the experts were requested to develop a *commentary/annotation* as to why the study selected was so important, and how its results compared with other findings in the literature, to serve as a teaching synopsis for the consultant and consultee. Fifth, the citations, their abstracts and the commentaries were imported into a software program—MICROCARES LITERATURE DATABASE—which was initially based on a Windows 95 platform that can operate on a Window Pen Entry laptop notebook that mimics the physician's writing pad and pen or on any computer with Windows 3.1, 95, or 98 configurations, employable at the bedside or in the ambulatory clinic (The MICROCARES clinical data management and literature database software systems may be obtained by contacting: James J. Strain, MD, The Mount Sinai–NYU Medical Center/Health System, 1 GL Levy Place, New York, New York 10029, USA.) This is available for Windows 95–98 systems and is fully described (including hardware requirements) in Hammer et al (1995). Studies demonstrate that patients are not offended by the computer technology of the pen-entry laptop, and in many cases appreciated that their information was being handled in such a careful manner.

Psychotropic Drug–Medical Drug Interactions

It is essential that the C-L psychiatrist know and understand psychotropic–medical drug interactions and the pharmacokinetics as they relate to end-organ dysfunction—kidney, liver, lung, heart—and the aging process (Strain et al 1996b). Over 25 000 psychotropic–medical drug interaction publications were perused to select the 83 that were eventually selected for the C-L Literature Database. A further refinement identified 15 of the 83 as "five star" or essential reading for the C-L psychiatrist, and as seminal teaching tools for residents and fellows. These articles can be available at the patient's side to enhance clinical decision-making in the use of psychotropic drugs in the medically ill (Strain et al 1996b).

It is certain that this drug database will be substantially altered in the next five years; this underscores the need for the C-L psychiatrist to have methods to keep sufficiently informed and updated on a timely basis (see Strain et al 1996b).

Computerized methods of accessing this pharmacological literature exist. MICRO-MEDEX is a computerized database that has been compiled from multiple drug information systems. DRUG-REAX is a subsection of MICROMEDEX which searches multiple drugs simultaneously for drug–drug, drug–food, and drug–disease interaction data. DRUGDEX is a software system that contains drug monographs with drug interactions obtained from case reports and drug interaction references. In addition, there are many journals, services, and current advances that include information on drug–psychotropic drug interactions: *Pharmacotherapy*; *Annals of Pharmacotherapy*; *Clinical Pharmacology and Therapeutics*; *Drug Safety*; *Drugs*. Monitoring services include:

Clin-Alert; *Reactions, Clinical Abstracts/Current Therapeutic Findings*; *Current Contents/ Adverse Reactions* and *Excerpta Medical/Adverse Reactions*; and *American Journal of Health-System Pharmacy, Current Literature* (a section of the *Journal of the American Society of Health-System Pharmacists*). The majority of these resources are not known or employed by psychiatrists, but are the information systems of pharmacists and consultants. Most large institutional settings, e.g. university teaching hospitals, have established Drug Information Centers within their pharmacy departments. Trained pharmacists with access to the information sources above are more adept at determining potential drug–psychotropic drug interactions, or can provide the best advice given the state of current knowledge. Pharmaceutical companies also have information services and can often assist on potential or reported interactions on their manufactured products. These in-house information services cull data from the published literature, clinical trials, foreign databases, and unpublished spontaneous case reports from medical professionals.

NEW MODELS OF HEALTH-CARE DELIVERY

Several new models of health-care delivery have developed in which the C-L psychiatrist has an unusual opportunity to participate. The Psychiatry–Medical Units in some hospitals accommodate those patients too medically ill to be treated by psychiatry and too psychiatrically ill to be treated in medical wards. They have nurses equipped to manage both psychiatric and medical conditions. Pain Management Units often employ psychiatrists for evaluation and treatment. Organ Transplantation Services routinely have psychiatrists attached for the assessment and management of their patients. Invitro Fertilization and High Risk Pregnancy services have found it useful to have the input of psychiatry.

The concept of the "Center" has permitted the employment of psychiatrists as members of the team, e.g. Cancer, Diabetes, Cardiac, Trauma, Gastro-Intestinal, Neurological, etc. At the Mount Sinai Hospital in New York City there are now 12 distinct care services managing illnesses that are grouped by systems. In these are "Centers" that aim to provide both inpatient and outpatient care with continuity throughout the illness. The ubiquity of primary and secondary psychiatric disorders, problems of coping, noncompliance, psychotropic drug–drug interactions, etc. often require the services of a psychiatrist to ensure that appropriate medical care can be supplied. Outcome data on the management of these diverse disorders where the presence of a psychiatrist as member of the team occurs versus those without, will help determine the fiscal support that can be gained for the C-L psychiatrist.

GUIDELINES FOR C-L PSYCHIATRY

In recent years guidelines have been developed based on the best evidence available, many specifically for mental states, and in the medical setting.

The United States Department of Health and Human Services, Public Health Service, Agency for Health Care Policy and Research (AHCPR) has sponsored over 19 guidelines for treatment, many of which are of particular importance to the C-L psychiatrist. For example, *Management of Cancer Pain, Acute Pain Management in Adults: Operative Procedures, Managing Early HIV Infection, Acute Low Back Pain, Post Stroke Rehabilitation, Cardiac Rehabilitation, Smoking Cessation, Alzheimer's Disease, Anxiety and Panic Disorder,* and *Chronic Headache Pain* were constructed incorporating these same attributes. One of the most important attributes is scheduled review including constant updating and reconsideration of the strength of the evidence.

This means that guidelines can become the textbook of tomorrow, incorporating new findings and published in a few weeks to months for rapid updating, almost in the way medical journals are now distributed, but in an even more efficient manner. Amendments can be distributed "overnight" to update diagnostic and treatment approaches with new findings in the form of electronic alerts to facilitate the best therapeutic strategy and tactics for the clinician on the strength of the most recent evidence. The C-L psychiatrist needs not only to be aware of these guidelines, but to provide feedback to developers and promoters with observations to enhance their utility. Many guidelines have a paucity of psychiatric and/or behavioral statements/ recommendations. Therefore, guidelines that are not specifically geared to psychiatry, e.g. *Diagnosing and Managing Unstable Angina, Urinary Incontinence in Adults, Benign Prostatic Hyperplasia: Diagnosis and Treatment* may benefit from the input of C-L psychiatrists to augment the psychosocial/psychiatric morbidity component that may be lacking. Specialty organizations, e.g. the American Psychiatric Association (2000) have also developed important guidelines to be employed for comorbidity in the medical setting, e.g. *Practice Guideline for Major Depressive Disorder in Adults*. These guidelines developed with the "pure" psychiatric patient must be amended by incorporating conditions/modifications for those individuals who have psychiatric and medical comorbidity. Like the assessment instruments described above, they are too often lacking in the dimensionality considerations that concurrent medical illness superimposes on psychiatric morbidity. Tomorrow's guidelines for psychiatric morbidity must include algorithms and parameters to account for the contingencies of medical illness which may confound and add risks and injunctions to recommendations and treatment in the medical setting.

The strength of the evidence for treatment has been codified and enhanced by the efforts of the Cochrane Collaboration—Oxford University, Oxford, England—funded by the United Kingdom's National Health Service which has established criteria for the assessment of validity of random control trials–treatment trials. This is the highest level of assessment and has been promulgated in the Cochrane Database of Systematic Reviews (1995) and includes for example, *Stroke Unit Trialists' Collaboration. A Systematic Review of Specialist Multidisciplinary Team (Stroke Unit) Care for Stroke Inpatients*; *Elective versus Caesarean Delivery of the Small Baby*; *The Effects of Family Intervention for Those with Schizophrenia*; *Support from Caregivers for Socially Disadvantaged Mothers* (see Cochrane Database of Systematic Reviews for any of these reviews). These meta-analytic studies by clinical experts in a given discipline offer the C-L psychiatrists a cross-comparison among studies which heightens the strength of the evidence, and thereby should have the most important impact on their treatment and clinical decision-making (Chalmers et al 1992). New reviews are continually being developed, and in time, such efforts will help move the world's repository of the random control trials to a more refined and "truer" definition of reality than is extant in most medical treatment areas to date. This effort goes well beyond one research team or one finding. These reviews are labor-intensive as they require hand examination of journals, since MEDLINE and other on-line search methods do not include many critical studies.

Finally, guidelines have been developed for the teaching of C-L psychiatry (Stoudemire et al 1998). A Task Force of the Academy of Psychosomatic Medicine has formulated the training requirements for the teaching of C-L psychiatry at three levels: medical student, house officer, and fellow. These guidelines will enhance the standardization of instruction across teaching hospitals throughout the country and permit the improvement of the pedagogic effort as new knowledge is developed.

According to the Institute of Medicine *Guidelines for Clinical Practice*, developers of guidelines should incorporate eight attributes: (1) Validity—including strength of the evidence and estimated outcomes; (2) reliability/reproducibility; (3) clinical applicability; (4) clinical flexibility; (5) clarity; (6) multidisciplinary process; (7) scheduled review; and (8) documentation. These attributes were incorporated into the guidelines for the treatment of *Depression in Primary Care* (Rush et al 1993).

Attribute (6) in this list brings to notice that the C-L team consists of several members, each of whom has an essential role. Although most of the information provided to date in this chapter describes the characteristics of the patient cohort served, and the process of the C-L psychiatrist's role at the medical/surgical behavioral interface, it has not presented the functions of many other members of the team who provide C-L services in the acute care general hospital setting. The psychologist is not only an important member of the team, but in many settings coordinates the C-L activities of the institution. The advantages of psychology and psychiatry on some liaison teams are discussed at the end of the chapter, preceded by a section highlighting the perspective of the psychologist working in the medical setting. The psychologist's role in patient evaluation, treatment, and working in a liaison role with medical/surgical physician and nursing staff in many settings is similar to the psychiatrist's. An additional and important role is the psychologist's provision of psychological testing, and this is essential in several medical arenas: rehabilitation medicine, neurosurgery, neurology, and poorly diagnosed mental disorders in any medical/surgical setting. Often the psychologist's testing will not only help clarify diagnostic formulations, it also assists in treatment planning, by assessing cognitive strengths and weaknesses that suggest optimal therapeutic interventions. The role of the psychologist on the C-L team is also to serve as teacher and consultant to all other members of the team. Finally, the role of the psychologist to foster research in so many sectors, diagnoses, treatment/outcome effectiveness, and alternative approaches, all of which brings an important and essential element to the C-L setting.

CONCLUSION

C-L psychiatry has an unusual opportunity to enter the arena of medicine and be the ambassador for the specialty of psychiatry in an attempt to improve the plight of the medically ill who have concurrent psychiatric comorbidity. Since behavioral issues are ubiquitous in medicine, e.g. noncompliance, anxiety, depression, assisting the physician and his/her patient with this comorbidity will not only enhance the psychiatric status of the patient, but their functional status, and perhaps medical status as well. With the concern about utilization of health-care resources, any measure to decrease costs will be welcome: Treatment of psychiatric and medical comorbidity is one method to decrease unnecessary consumption of limited resources. In a similar vein it is important to ascertain which mental health professional should be doing which functions. If a psychiatrist is not required, as evidenced from random control studies, then a less expensive mental health professional can be employed. If a medically trained mental health professional is required, e.g. in the intensive care units, severe end-organ dysfunction, utilization of medical and psychotropic medication, the assessment and adjudication of drug side-effects, then a psychiatrist should be employed by the health system for this function.

As the majority of patients with mental health disorders seek their health care in the ambulatory medical arena, and primarily by primary care physicians, psychiatric knowledge and skills must be imparted to this essential cadre of physicians, so that they may more effectively play the role of triage officer of the mentally ill that are in their purview. Screening, diagnosis, treatment, understanding psychotropic–medical drug interactions, assessing outcome, and the provision of follow-up must either be taken on by them, or assigned to other capable mental health care workers. The standard with which these functions are undertaken must incorporate the fact that medical illness places the patient with mental morbidity in a vulnerable position, and that integrated assessment of mind and body and their interaction cannot be compromised by employing health-care workers who are not up to this task. Even the combination of primary care physician and a nonpsychiatric mental health-care worker may not collectively have the skills and knowledge for the intensive confounds that present with psychiatric and medical comorbidity. Guidelines for training and standards of care must dictate who can care for whom in the medical setting. Clearly the opportunity prevails to optimize care for this vulnerable population.

SECTION B   CONSULTATION-LIAISON (C-L) PSYCHOLOGY OR CLINICAL HEALTH PSYCHOLOGY?

A commentary by David J. de L. Horne

INTRODUCTION

The previous section of this chapter has presented a broad picture of how consultation-liaison (C-L) psychiatry has developed and what constitute some of the major contemporary concerns of this field. Of course, the way C-L services work and the issues to be tackled do vary from country to country, even if we confine ourselves to purely English-speaking countries. If C-L psychiatry, as a well developed service, is a relatively new phenomenon, then C-L clinical psychology as a regular component of medical and surgical care is even more embryonic (Bieliauskas 1991). Certainly, since the 1980s there has been a rapidly increasing body of psychological knowledge that is relevant to the treatment and management of patients with primary physical illness, rather than psychiatric disturbance. This is reflected in a variety of journal titles such *Behavioral Medicine*, *Journal of Behavioral Medicine*, *Health Psychology*, *The British Journal of Health Psychology*, etc. and also in a number of textbooks (e.g. Weinman 1981; Sweet et al 1991; Baum et al 1997 and, of course, the present volume).

Thus, it could be said that C-L psychology parallels C-L psychiatry, in bringing relevant aspects of scientific psychological knowledge and clinical skills to bear on any medical or surgical problem within the general hospital or medical setting. A more recent term, "clinical health psychology", has also been proposed to best describe the specialized field combining knowledge from clinical psychology and health psychology (Belar 1997). The clinical psychologist is an expert in the application of clinical assessment and treatment skills to change an individual's maladaptive behavior, thoughts and emotions. Health psychology provides an expanding knowledge base regarding psychological factors in health and illness within a biological and sociological context. The clinical health psychologist draws on expertise from both clinical and health psychology to work as a practitioner in a medical/healthcare setting.

Given this background, the conclusion at the end of the last section about the importance of collaboration between psychologists and psychiatrists, and the content of the rest of this book, I propose to focus on a few common but key issues particularly well-managed by psychologists. These are of interest not only to psychologists practicing in a C-L setting, but to their health colleagues (especially psychiatrists) and most importantly, to the patients at the receiving end of their care. These are:

- Clinician–patient communication
- Factors in compliance and adherence to treatment
- Dealing with medical anxieties and phobias in patients and clinicians
- Preparing patients for invasive medical and surgical procedures.

Clinician–Patient Communication

Good interpersonal skills are part of being a good clinician. This could sound like a motherhood statement, but unfortunately good communication between healthcare professionals themselves and between such professionals and their patients or clients, is not universal and may sometimes be actually bad, even though everyone may have good intentions. James Strain, on page 100, has given a beautiful example of how clinician miscommunication led to a 75-year-old man suffering from a stroke being assessed as suicidal when, in fact, he was actually misunderstood by one of the doctors and was consequently angry. So, avoiding creating unnecessary feelings of guilt and anger in clinical settings is crucial for optimal care. Psychology has much to teach about interpersonal skills in communication and this has now been recognized in all medical schools in the UK and Australia, where the teaching of communication skills to all undergraduate medical students has become an important, compulsory and examinable part of the curriculum. In my own teaching I often remind students that if information is not received and processed by those for whom it is intended, then it is not information but noise. Where there are patients and health-care staff from different cultural and language backgrounds this complex process of communication becomes even more difficult to negotiate. Some excellent research and clinical practice are now developing around serious consideration of these transcultural issues. For example, there is a Centre for Cultural Studies in Health, associated with the University of Melbourne, which produces both research and practical information for clinicians wishing to be better equipped in working with people from a range of cultural backgrounds. This is most important in many places today where immigration has led to huge cultural diversity (Minas 1999).

The psychologist in a hospital and clinic setting may well be able to use his or her skills to identify barriers to communication between staff and patients and help people to more successfully negotiate these. For example, some research I am currently involved in, on an oncology ward, reveals that patients and staff may have different perceptions of the atmosphere of a ward and that an individual's self-concept of locus of control can be a key factor in influencing these perceptions (Black et al 1999; Moos 1996). Such findings are important. They can help all concerned with patient care to understand better what patients' experiences are like and facilitate changes in communication and procedures that enhance feelings of well-being and ability to cope with difficult treatments, such as chemotherapy.

A number of common barriers to effective communication in clinical settings have been identified. These include: language; culture; religious beliefs; age; gender; education; personal and practical resources; health beliefs and expectations; current state of health; values; impact of possible outcomes; subjectivity/objectivity; differing agenda for patient and clinician.

Recognizing such barriers and successfully negotiating them involves skills that can be learned and improved upon by appropriate training. This communication between doctor/clinician and patient has often been referred to as the art of therapy or medicine, but it is, in fact, a set of socially skillful behaviors that are amenable to psychological investigation and understanding. There are now many texts on how to improve communication skills in clinical practice (e.g. Burman 1992).

The above discussion of communication issues in medical settings sets the scene for a discussion of how to optimize the chances of recovery from illness, or disease, through patients actually carrying out the treatments that are prescribed for them.

Factors in Compliance/Adherence to Treatment

It is well known that patient noncompliance is a major concern in medicine and costs communities millions of dollars. Before discussing how to improve compliance, a few words about terminology and underlying concepts are needed.

Compliance is the most predominantly used term today but there are problems with it, and adherence may be a better term. Compliance has been defined as, "complying with a request, demand...a tendency to give in to others", whereas adherence is defined as, "to stick fast... *stay firm in supporting*" (my italics—Krebs 1985).

Thus, compliance has connotations of authoritarian power so that if a person fails to comply they may be seen as somehow wilful, negative, rebellious and, in fact, "a difficult patient". The term "a difficult patient" is interesting. The question has to be asked "difficult" for whom? (Di Matteo & Di Nicola 1982, pp 242–243). Any clinical consultation, be it ever so routine or a prolonged diagnostic or therapeutic session, is a complex social psychological phenomenon. In fact, whether a patient actually takes the treatment prescribed depends upon a range of factors. Patients may make perfectly rational decisions, in their own eyes, not to comply, or they may simply forget to take the medicine due to memory problems, being distracted and a host of other reasons. It is now well established that if compliance occurs through a process of negotiation between practitioner and patient then adherence to the regimen is much more likely. Higginbotham et al (1988) point out that "all clinical practice is fundamentally interpretive" and "from individual's standpoint, 'illness' represents a configuration of personal trauma; life stresses; fears and expectations about the illness; social reactions of friends and authorities; and therapeutic experiences" (p 106). Therefore, failure on the part of the clinician to understand the patient's conceptual framework and beliefs about illness and health is likely to result in less than optimal adherence to treatment (Benjamini et al 1997). It is far better to understand patients' explanatory concepts of disease and illness and help them to make informed choices about treatment, although this is not always an easy process (Perkins & Repper 1999).

Because effective treatment needs to be based on a negotiated contract that takes into account both clinician and patient belief systems (either implicitly or explicitly), I believe the term "adherence to treatment" is more appropriate. It has less authoritarian connotations, and if failure occurs then renewed problem-solving is required rather than blaming the patient. For example, mapping out memory difficulties (Ley 1982), instituting self- or other monitoring programs (France & Robson 1997), and providing meaningful rewards to reinforce success (acknowledgment and praise often suffice) can all be highly successful.

Monitoring of behaviors, and even thoughts and feelings, can be especially important and in the hospital setting can be facilitated by appropriately trained staff. Here nursing staff often play a key role. Where a ward atmosphere is good there will be strong cohesiveness, a sense of belonging and working together, amongst staff of all disciplines. Where it is bad, and it can be measured (Moos 1996), there will be confusion, anger and friction with attendant negative effects on patient care (Moos & Schwartz 1972). It is the nursing staff that have ongoing, frequent close contact with patients whilst other staff, especially the more senior of them, tend to drop in to monitor, control and advise on how things are going.

Thus, in monitoring adherence to treatment it is crucial to know whether certain behaviors have or have not occurred, from taking medicines, to getting out of bed, walking, etc. Accurate behavioral charts are quite easy to devise. When things are not working the charts can be reviewed, preferably with the patient, who is a partner in the whole process, and reasons for non-adherence determined.

This will involve ascertaining what the patient believes and feels about what is going on (their health belief system) and what they are capable of doing about it, influenced by their locus of control. Psychology has made an important contribution to methods of behavior change by introducing cognitive-behavioral therapies and the methods which are very effective in helping understand how all of thoughts, feelings and behaviors interact. Not only can actual behaviors be recorded, e.g. time patient got up and took himself to the bathroom unaided, but, if necessary to overcome barriers to adherence, the strength of a patient's feelings and beliefs can also be recorded, as well as their content. Thus, for example, if a patient fails to go to the bathroom unaided, when they might normally be expected to do so, their fear or anxiety can be quantified, perhaps using simple analogue measures (McCormack et al 1988), and their beliefs and thoughts mapped out as a basis for further systematic therapeutic intervention.

Thus, successful adherence to treatment acknowledges that the patient is an idiosyncratic person who is focused on their own needs. These needs can only be met through good communication, which as Di Matteo and Di Nicola remind us (1982, p 271) has to occur in, "...a manner that (as much as possible) both emphasizes the patient's personal responsibility and reduces his or her anxieties, confusions and dissatisfactions."

This model of adherence to treatment (Meichenbaum & Turk 1987) that I am advocating very much complements James Strain's conceptualization of three dynamic systems influencing the patient's transition through stages, from passivity to activity in their illness, that was described earlier in this chapter.

There is another issue in the adherence/compliance debate: the failures of doctors, nurses and other health practitioners to comply with health procedures (O'Brien 1997). This form of noncompliance is widespread, complex in its manifestations but important in its implications. Health-care professional inertia is a major factor in such noncompliance (Meichenbaum & Turk 1987). It would seem education alone is not enough to improve this situation (e.g. Gerberding 1991) but that, as for patients, more proactive interventions such as cognitive-behavioral programs incorporating specific feedback can improve adherence to professional procedures (e.g. De Vries et al 1991).

Dealing with Medical Anxieties and Phobias in Patients and Clinicians

This important topic is a natural progression from discussion of communication and adherence. Anxieties suffered by patients have received an enormous amount of attention from psychologists over the years, but those of clinicians rather less so.

Medical phobias are extremely common, and this is not the place to review the vast relevant literature. However, it is useful to be reminded why people turn to clinicians for help. Most often they come because of pain, changes in bodily function and appearance, depression and anxiety. All of these may be associated with fear. For the clinician, illness, disease, clinics and hospital environments are a normal, everyday part of working life. For the patient this is not usually the case. Anxiety may manifest itself in many ways and there is a huge armamentarium of treatments psychologists can draw upon. Knowledge about the effectiveness and specificity of psychological treatments is improving all the time (Roth & Fonagy 1996). Some common patient fears likely to be encountered in those who are physically ill include fear of pain; fear of being touched (for some, a normal medical examination may resemble an assault, e.g. a vaginal examination in a woman who has been sexually assaulted); fear of being dependent; fear of wasting the clinician's time; fear of asking questions; fear of being trapped (claustrophobia); fear of injections and fear of the sight of blood.

Cognitive behavioral therapies can offer quick and effective interventions for many of these medical fears; for example, this 61-year-old man was referred to me by his surgeon following cardiac surgery.

When the patient regained consciousness from his anesthetic he pulled out all his leads and tubes and leapt through a glass window on the ward, fortunately onto a balcony (since he was several storeys above street level). It emerged he had a longstanding history of claustrophobia which had not been identified during his pre-surgery preparation. As he required further surgery, urgent help was sought from me as the consultation-liaison clinical psychologist. A program of systematic desensitization, using both imaginal and invivo scenes, combined with relaxation incorporating patient self-produced imagery ("driving an open top sportscar, wind in face and speeding along" [*sic*]) was implemented with complete success. Seven treatments over ten weeks saw him able to cope well with subsequent treatments, as well as having improved quality of life in other areas, e.g. he was able to ride underground trains and other forms of public transport with no anxiety symptoms at all.

When it comes to clinician anxieties and fears the picture is less clear because these are less well researched. Feelings of fear concerning failure, loss of emotional control and being helpless to do anything very effective are probably quite common. An enhanced awareness of professional ethics and increasing use of codes of conduct for many kinds of professionals underline the fact that powerful psychological forces are at work in carers as well as the cared for. Perhaps all clinicians, and not just those involved in directly dealing with emotional problems and mental health, need better education and psychological preparation for being a clinician. Issues of transference and counter-transference and how they affect professional boundaries are always there in any interaction with patients. Knowing one's limitations and competencies is important. There will be clashes in values between professionals from different disciplines, such as surgeon, physician, psychiatrist, physiotherapist and nurse. The psychologist and psychiatrist may well be able to help other professionals identify these clashes and the emotions associated with them; for example, applying knowledge about anger and its resolution (Novaco 1994; Chemtob et al 1997) can be very useful. Professional burnout is a concern but the sensible use of psychological principles means its effects can be minimized, for example by acknowledging clinician needs and concerns with patient care, helping them cope with issues of control and ambiguity and providing social support (Maslach 1982, 1997).

Preparing Patients for Invasive Medical and Surgical Procedures

This is also an area where the application of psychological research has produced significant benefits in recent years. A comprehensive overview has been provided by Horne et al (1994 a, b) and Wilson-Barnett (1994). The theme of preparation follows logically from the previous discussion about medical phobias and anxieties and can be regarded as a secondary, prophylactic level of intervention aimed at (1) better equipping patients to cope with invasive procedures they are about to have and, (2) preventing iatrogenically produced anxieties, phobias and depression.

Today, in developed countries with literate populations, medical and surgical procedures are generally explained to patients prior to being carried out. This is partly to improve patient response but it is also due to increased accountability of the professions in today's society. Failure to explain and obtain informed consent can lead to unpleasant professional and legal consequences. Of course, if the procedural information supplied is not understood, there is a clinician-to-patient communication problem of the kind already described.

There is another form of preparation—"sensory". It is useful for the patient to know what the *experience* of the procedure will be like and, even better, to know how to cope with unpleasant side-effects, such as transient pain. A wide range of studies involving such techniques as modelling (for example, using puppets with children, videotapes, etc.), listening to accounts by patients who have successfully coped with the procedures, relaxation training, stress inoculation and so on, have demonstrated clear benefits. These include a reduction in post-operative pain (e.g. Postlethwaite et al 1986), quicker and less complicated recovery from surgery carried out under general anesthetic, including less dependence on post-operative analgesics (e.g. Wells et al 1986; Holden-Lund 1988).

There are problems, including the fact that not all patients respond in the same way to all forms of both procedural and sensory pre-procedure information. As Janis (1958) noted long ago, both high and very low levels of pre-operative anxiety prognosticated more complex recovery from surgery, with best outcome resulting in those with moderate levels of anxiety.

Pre-procedural psychological assessment is required to determine what forms of preparation are likely to be optimal for an individual. Factors such as whether the patient is a high monitor or a blunter (Miller 1987; Miller et al 1988), whether he or she has high internal or external health locus of control in relation to health concerns (Wallston et al 1994), may all be useful parameters to assess so that coping strategies are based upon the individual's own needs and perceptions.

A simple checklist of steps in preparation can help the busy clinician optimize effective preparation. One such list has been developed by France and Robson (1997, pp 205–206). These steps can be summarized as follows:

1. Provide information about the procedure to be undertaken. However, this on its own has only a weak effect on post-procedure outcome.
2. Provide information about the physical sensations to be experienced.
3. Provide information about outcome. This needs to address a number of areas, such as life expectancy, functional restrictions, levels of pain, issues of disfigurement and levels of dependency or care required from others.
4. Provide specific behavioral instructions on how to cope.
5. Train in relaxation techniques. These can certainly make the patient feel better but, bearing in mind Janis's (1958) findings, can have equivocal effects on actual recovery processes.
6. Train in cognitive techniques. These can be highly effective in preventing post-operative anxiety and depression because the patient is able to detect irrational and exaggerated negative thoughts and feelings and come up with a more realistic assessment of their status.

CONCLUSIONS

This contribution has covered some key issues in consultation-liaison psychology. For these points to be effective it is necessary for the psychologist to be respected and for the advice offered to be appreciated before it will be implemented. It is important for the psychologist to be part of the clinical team; it is often not enough just to consult, there must be true liaison. With limited, and perhaps shrinking, health-care resources for psychological and psychiatric services in medical and surgical settings, this is a difficult task. A minimum requirement is that medical, nursing and other health staff need to know whom to call upon automatically. Services such as oncology and burns units have very clear-cut needs for a C-L service and ideally should have specific psychologists and psychiatrists allocated to them. Failing this, regular contact between the psychologist and medical and nursing staff is a quick and effective way of keeping in touch and showing they are serious in wanting to be part of the service. This strategy can also gain allies from a variety of professions who may help lobby for better psychological resources for their service, with resultant better outcomes for patients and clinicians alike.

SECTION C   ADDENDUM FOR INTEGRATION OF PSYCHOLOGY AND PSYCHIATRY ON THE SAME TEAM

James J. Strain and David J. de L. Horne

An issue that has not been sufficiently addressed is the benefit from having a psychiatrist and psychologist on the same consultation-liaison team. Whilst the two disciplines describe their unique contributions in the acute care center medical/surgical setting, they frequently do not work side by side. There are distinct advantages to having the expertise of psychologist and psychiatrist on the same team, even evaluating the same patient, and certainly for measurement of behavioral components and research pursuits. The detailed discussion of the precepts of the alliance model of psychiatry presented below is intended to highlight potential areas of collaboration between the psychologist and the psychiatrist working in concert, as part of an alliance team.

1. The practice of primary, secondary, and tertiary prevention.
2. The fostering of diagnostic accuracy (with particular emphasis on case detection).
3. Clarification of the status of the caretaker.
4. Provision of ongoing education to the nonpsychiatric staff to promote autonomy.
5. The development of core biopsychosocial knowledge.
6. Promotion of structural changes in the medical setting to promote the psychological care of the medically ill.

PRIMARY, SECONDARY AND TERTIARY PREVENTION

Liaison psychiatry enhances the quality of psychological care for the medically ill by using Caplan's (1961) longstanding model of prevention—anticipating and preventing the development of psychological symptoms that may adversely effect the initiation of medical illness, e.g. stress and coronary heart disease (primary prevention); treating such symptoms after they have developed so that they will not maintain illness, e.g. smoking cessation following a myocardial infarction (secondary prevention); and rehabilitating patients who have manifested such symptoms in order to prevent their recurrence (tertiary prevention). Psychologists and psychiatrists can work in each phase to decrease the opportunity for the initiation, maintenance, or recurrence of disease secondary to psychological precipitants.

FOSTERING OF DIAGNOSTIC ACCURACY

In the acutely medically/surgically ill patient, there is a need to assess pharmacological effects of both the medical drugs and the co-administered psychotropic medications. This is a twofold task: First there is a need to know if the behavioral components are related to the effects of the medical drugs on the patient. It is known that the 17 drugs commonly administered to the patient with HIV—the antivirals, antineoplastics, anti-infection agents—can have important central nervous system (CNS) effects, resulting in anxiety, depression, psychosis, and impulse control problems. Steroids have an important effect upon the CNS and may result in mania, depression, or disordered behavioral control. Interferon may have profound CNS effects. Therefore it is essential to know and assess the impact of the medical drugs upon the patient's psychological state. Second, if one is to add psychotropic medication, it is essential to know the interactions that may occur if a psychotropic medication is added to a particular medical drug, or a medical drug is added to the regimen of a patient currently on psychotropics. For example, there are countless interactions between the prescriptions for cardiac drugs and commonly employed psychotropic medications (84 interactions at the last count) (Strain et al 1999). Third, in the medically/surgically ill, it is essential to evaluate the function of vital organs that can affect the CNS directly, or affect the metabolism of drugs that in turn can affect the CNS, e.g. liver, kidney, lungs. Such biological–somatic evaluation of vital organ/body system drug interactions on behaviors can be seen in patients experiencing symptoms such as delirium. In these three areas the psychiatrist with expert knowledge of biological bases of psychopathology can add to the assessment, the database, and the hypotheses underlying a particular patient's psychopathology.

On the other hand, the psychologist can bring to bear expertise in assessing behavioral changes in objective and reproducible ways, and such assessments can form important baselines of behavior for monitoring changes over time. The use of structured instruments to illuminate responses in cases of diagnostic uncertainty are of critical importance and not well understood, or sufficiently employed by the psychiatrist. An abundance of appropriate rating scales exist. Greater understanding of instrumentality in the assessment of behavior is a much needed tool for psychiatry that psychology can impart, teach, and practice as a member of the dual discipline team. The monitoring and assessing of behaviors require at least two important elements. One is to define and accurately measure the frequency of a behavioral event, such as fainting, vomiting, etc. The other is to measure the intensity of patient experiences, such as degree of nausea, anxiety, etc. Visual Analogue Scales (VAS) are extremely robust and reliable measures of intensity and are easy to design to meet an individual patient's need (McCormack et al 1988). Even when relevant rating scales are available, it may still be important to design and implement individually tailored behavioral assessments and measures of intensity.

The organic brain syndromes are an excellent example of this type of collaboration in the alliance model of liaison psychiatry. A structured assessment of the patient's cognitive capacity will not only supply elements to enhance diagnostic accuracy, but also indicate mental strengths and capacities for specific intellectual functions. For example, clinical neuropsychological approaches to diagnosis of the organic mental disorders may be categorized as (1) "fixed battery", involving the administration of a comprehensive, invariant series of tests, and (2) "branching or adjustive", calling for selection of tests according to the reason for referral, background data, and findings obtained during an interview which may suggest the presence of specific deficits and gauge the patient's ability to cooperate (Levin 1981). The development of screening devices for organic mental disorders, cognitive dysfunction, anxiety, depression and suicidality are important collaborative developments for the medical/surgical setting.

CLARIFICATION OF THE STATUS OF THE CARETAKER AND THE PROVISION OF ONGOING EDUCATION TO THE NONPSYCHIATRIC STAFF TO PROMOTE AUTONOMY

The alliance model of liaison psychiatry incorporates the proposition that responsibility for the psychological care of the medically ill hospitalized patient cannot be relegated solely to the psychiatrist or the psychologist. Rather, optimal care of the patient is a consequence of joint efforts of those with whom he or she comes into daily contact—the doctor, nurse, important family members—and the psychological climate of the ward. It follows a collaboration by psychologist and psychiatrist to "measure" and "assess" the degree of stress the patient evokes in medical caretakers and family; their capacity to adapt to the patient and to his or her illness (and to the interventions of psychological caretakers); and the capacity of the caretakers to understand and offer psychological work. Here the collaboration between psychiatry and psychology can have a major impact on the training of all ward staff and family members to more adequately assess and manage behavioral needs.

DEVELOPMENT OF CORE BIOPSYCHOSOCIAL KNOWLEDGE

Research Pursuits

This assessment rigor is especially important for samples or cohorts which will be used for clinical research. Not nearly enough research is conducted in the typical Consultation-Liaison psychiatry service, and much of the clinical care is lost to hypothesis generation and testing. Furthermore, the level of the assessment would not qualify for meaningful research, not being at a standard much higher than that from a medical chart review. The psychologist as team member can impart this added dimension to the common skills both disciplines employ, e.g. psychotherapy, conflict resolution, counseling, family therapy, etc. Observing a patient from two points of view can be enlightening to both professions, and especially for the students who observe. This mutual education and strengthening of skills and knowledge by interdisciplinary exchanges enriches both professions, and allows a more synergistic assessment and treatment plan formation for the patient. In most liaison settings there is a strong need for the psychiatrist to be assisted in research design, appropriate and rigorous documentation of findings assisted by systematic reliable and valid instruments, data analysis, and hypothesis generation and testing. The assemblage of knowledge in the ill medical and surgical patient with co-morbid mental morbidity, is essential if the psychological care of the medically ill is to be improved. This involves the development of reliable and valid screening, and diagnostic assessment measures suitable for the medically ill who are perplexed by the occurrence of vegetative signs that can confound the diagnosis—the attribution of symptoms as emanating from the body or the mind, e.g. sleep disorder, dysphoria, lack of energy, diminished libido, all of which may be symptoms of medical or psychiatric illness, or both. It indicates the need for systematic treatment algorithms and an assessment of outcome. Psychiatry could be assisted in so many of these pursuits by an active collaboration with psychology and a merging of skills and competence from both disciplines to garner new knowledge from all the clinical work which is performed in every general hospital every day—thousands of psychiatric/psychological consultations.

PROMOTION OF STRUCTURAL CHANGES IN THE MEDICAL SETTING

The need for new models to promote mental health care in the acute general hospital setting, e.g. medical-psychiatry units, substance abuse units, if dealing with physical symptoms of unknown etiology, means all can benefit from a collaboration of the two disciplines of behavioral science on the medical wards: psychology and psychiatry. The management of pain, transplantation (with its welter of psychological concerns), and rehabilitation would all be enhanced by psychologists and psychiatrists striving to create a milieu that addresses the psychological care of the medically ill. Combined teaching rounds with medical staff, nurses, and ward caretakers would promote attitudes, knowledge, and skills toward enhanced psychological care around the clock. This would be a giant step forward from the psychiatric or psychological consultant who appears from time to time to care for the patient. It would foster a milieu that automatically includes psychological evaluation, treatment, and assessment of outcome in every patient. Such an alliance between the two disciplines would significantly enhance the ambience of the acute care general hospital medical/surgical setting.

REFERENCES

American Psychiatric Association: *Diagnostic and Statistical Manual (Fourth Edition)*. American Psychiatric Press: Washington, DC, 1995.

American Psychiatric Association: Practice guideline for the treatment of patients with major affective disorders (revision). *Am J Psychiatry* **157**(4) (Suppl): 1–45, 2000.

Baum A, Newman S, Weinman J, West R and McManus C (Eds): *Cambridge Handbook of Psychology, Health and Medicine*. Cambridge University Press: Cambridge, England, 1997.

Belar CD: Clinical health psychology: A speciality for the 21st century. *Health Psychol* **16**: 411–416, 1997.

Benjamini Y, Leventhal E and Leventhal H: Attributions in Health. In Baum A, Newman S, Weinman J, West R and McManus C (Eds): *Cambridge Handbook of Psychology, Health and Medicine*. Cambridge University Press: Cambridge, England, p 72, 1997.

Bieliauskas LA: Critical issues in consultation and liaison-adults. In Sweet JJ, Rozensky RH and Tovian SM (Eds) *Handbook of Clinical Psychology in Medical Settings*. Plenum: New York, pp 187–199, 1991.

Black C, Horne DJ de L and Green M: Health Locus of Control and perception of Ward Atmosphere of patients and staff in an in-patient oncology ward: A preliminary investigation. (Submitted for publication.) Department of Psychology, University of Melbourne: Melbourne, Australia, 1999.

Broadhead WE, Leon AC, Weissman MM, Barrett JE, Blacklow RS, Gilbert TT, Keller MB, Olfson M and Higgines ES: Development and validation of the SDDS-PC screen for multiple mental disorders in primary care. *Arch Family Med* **4**: 211–219, 1995.

Burman P: *Effective Communication Skills for Health Professionals*. Chapman & Hall: London, 1992.

Caplan G: *Principles of Preventive Psychiatry*. Basic Books: New York, 1961.

Chalmers I, Dickersin K and Chalmers TC: Getting to grips with Archie Cochrane's agenda. *BMJ* **305**: 786–788, 1992.

Chemtob CM, Novaco RW, Hamada RS and Gross DM: Cognitive-behavioural treatment for severe anger in posttraumatic stress disorder. *J Consult Clin Psychol* **65**: 184–189, 1997.

Cochrane Database of Systematic Reviews: *The Cochrane Collaboration, Issue 2, Oxford, Update Software, 1995*. British Medical Journal Publishing Group: London, 1995.

Cohen-Cole SA and Kaufman K: Major depression in physical illness: Diagnosis, prevalence and antidepressant treatment. (A ten year review: 1982–1992.) *Depression* **1**: 181, 1993.

DeVries JE, Burnette MM and Redmon WK: Improving nurse compliance with glove wearing through performance feedback. *J Appl Behav Analysis* **24**: 705–711, 1991.

Di Matteo MR and Di Nicola DD: *Achieving Patient Compliance: The Psychology of the Medical Practitioner's Role*. Pergamon: New York, 1982.

Dunbar HF: Physical–mental relationships in illness: trends in modern medicine and research as related to psychiatry. *Am J Psychiatry* **91**: 541–562, 1934.

Engel GL: *Psychological Development in Health and Disease*. Saunders: Philadelphia, 1962.

Engel GL: The concept of psychosomatic disorder. *J Psychosom Res* **11**: 3–9, 1967a.

Engel GL: Medical education and the psychosomatic approach. A report on the Rochester experience 1946–1966. *J Psychosom Res* **11**: 77–85, 1967b.

Engel GL: The need for a new medical model: a challenge for biomedicine. *Science* **196**: 129–136, 1977.

Fawzy I, Fawzy N, Hyun CS, Elashoff R, Guthrie D, Fahey L and Morton D: Malignant melanoma: effects of an early structured intervention, coping and effective state on recurrence and survival 6 years later. *Arch Gen Psychiatry* **50**: 681–689, 1993.

Field MJ and Lohr KN: *Guidelines for Clinical Practice: From Development to Use*. National Academy Press: Washington, DC, 1992.

France R and Robson M: *Cognitive-Behavioural Therapy in Primary Care: A Practical Guide*. Jessica Kingsley: London, 1997.

Frasure-Smith N: Depression and 18 month progress after myocardial infarction. *Circulation* **91**: 999–1005, 1995.

Frasure-Smith N, Lesperance F and Talajic M: Depression following myocardial infarction: Impact on 6 months survival. *JAMA* **270**: 1819–1825, 1993.

Fuller MG: More is less: Increasing access as a strategy for managing health care costs. *Psychiatric Services* **46**: 1015–1017, 1995.

Gerberding JL: Does knowledge of Human Immunodeficiency Virus infection decrease the frequency of occupational exposure to blood? *Am J Med* **91**: 308–311, 1991.

Hall CW and Wise MG: The clinical and financial burden of mood disorder: cost and outcome. *Psychosomatics* **36** (Suppl): 11–18, 1995.

Hammer JS, Strain JJ, Friedberg A and Fulop G: Operationalizing a bedside Pen Entry notebook clinical database system in Consultation-Liaison psychiatry. *Gen Hosp Psychiatry* **17**: 165–172, 1995.

Hays RD, Wells KB, Sherbourne CD et al: Functioning and well-being outcomes of patients with depression compared with chronic general medical illness. *Arch Gen Psychiatry* **52**: 11–19, 1995.

Higginbotham HN, West SG and Forsyth DR: *Psychotherapy and Behavior Change: Social, Cultural and Methodological Perspectives.* Pergamon: New York, 1988.

Holden-Lund C: Effects of relaxation with guided imagery on surgical stress and wound healing. *Res Nursing Health* **11**: 235–244, 1988.

Horne DJ de L, McCormack HM, Collins JP, Forbes JF and Russell IS: Psychological treatment of phobic anxiety associated with adjuvant chemotherapy. *Med J Aust* **145**: 346–348, 1986.

Horne DJ de L, Vatmanidis P and Careri A: Preparing patients for invasive medical procedures: Adding behavioral and cognitive interventions. *Behav Med* **20**: 5–13, 1994a.

Horne DJ de L, Vatmanidis P and Careri A: Preparing patients for invasive medical procedures: Using psychological interventions with adults and children. *Behav Med* **20**: 15–21, 1994b.

Janis IL: *Psychological Stress—Psychoanalytic and Behavioral Studies of Surgical Patients.* Wiley: New York, 1958.

Johnson J, Weissman M and Klerman GL: Service utilization and social morbidity associated with depressive symptoms in the community. *JAMA* **267**: 1478–1483, 1992.

Katon W and Gonzales J: A review of randomized trials of psychiatric consultation-liaison studies in primary care. *Psychosomatics* **35**: 268–278, 1994.

Katon W, VonKorff M, Lin E et al: Distressed high utilizers of medical care: DSM-III-R diagnosis and treatment needs. *Gen Hosp Psychiatry* **12**: 355–362, 1990.

Katon W, VonKorff M, Lin E et al: Collaborative management to achieve treatment guidelines: Impact on depression in primary care. *JAMA* **273**: 1026–1031, 1995.

Kornfeld DS, Youngner SJ, Steinberg MD, Powell T and Lederberg MS: Clinical ethics. An important role for the Consultation-Liaison psychiatrist. *Psychosomatics* **38**: 307–308, 1997.

Krebs WA (Ed): *Collins Australian Pocket English Dictionary.* Collins: Sydney, 1985.

Leigh H and Reiser M: *The Patient: Biological, Psychological and Social Dimensions of Medical Practice.* Plenum Book Co.: New York, 1992.

Levenson JL: Psychosocial intervention in chronic medical illness: an overview of outcome research. *Gen Hosp Psychiatry* **14**: 43S–49S, 1992.

Levin HS: Clinical neuropsychological testing. I: Description of test background. Personal communication, 1981.

Ley P: Studies of recall medical settings. *Human Learning* **1**: 223–233, 1982.

Lin E, VonKorff M, Katon W et al: Primary care physician behavior and patient's adherence to antidepressant therapy. *Medical Care* **33**: 67, 1995.

Maslach C: *Burnout: The Cost of Caring.* Prentice-Hall: Englewood Cliffs, NJ, 1982.

Maslach C: Burnout in health professionals. In Baum A, Newman S, Weinman J, West R and McManus C (Eds): *Cambridge Handbook of Psychology, Health and Medicine.* Cambridge University Press: Cambridge, England, pp 275–278, 1997.

McCormack HM, Horne DJ de L and Sheather S: Clinical applications of visual analogue scales: a critical review. *Psychol Med* **18**: 1007–1019, 1988.

Meichenbaum D and Turk DC: *Facilitating Treatment Adherence: A Practitioner's Guidebook*. Plenum Press: New York, 1987.

Milgrom J and Hardardottir D: Clinical health psychology—a specialty in its own right. *Bull Aust Psychol Soc*: 13–18, 1995.

Miller SM: Monitoring and blunting: Validation of a questionnaire to assess styles of information seeking under threat. *J Personal Soc Psychol* **52**: 345–353, 1987.

Miller SM, Summerton J and Brody S: Styles of coping with threat: Implications for health. *J Personal Soc Psychol* **54**: 142–148, 1988.

Minas HI: Cross-cultural training for health professionals. In Dimopoulos M and Antonios Z (Eds): *The Distinctiveness of Australian Cross-cultural Education*. Human Rights and Equal Opportunity Commission: Sydney, 1999.

Moos RH: *Ward Atmosphere Scale Manual: Development, Applications, Research* (3rd edn). Mind Garden: Redwood City, CA, 1996.

Moos RH and Schwartz J: Treatment environment and treatment outcome. *J Nerv Ment Dis* **154**: 265–275, 1972.

Moros D, Rhodes R, Baumrin S and Strain JJ: Thinking critically in medicine and its ethics: relating applied science and applied ethics. *J Appl Philosophy* **4**: 229, 1987.

Morris PLF, Robinson RG, Andrzejewski P et al: Association of depression with 10-year poststroke mortality. *Am J Psychiatry* **150**: 124–129, 1993.

Novaco RW: Clinical problems of anger and its assessment and regulation through a stress coping skills approach. In O'Donohue W and Krasner L (Eds): *Handbook of Psychological Skills Training: Clinical Techniques and Applications*. Allyn & Bacon: Boston, USA, 1994.

O'Brien MK: Compliance among health professionals. In Baum A, Newman S, Weinman J, West R and McManus C (Eds): *Cambridge Handbook of Psychology, Health and Medicine*. Cambridge University Press: Cambridge, England, pp 278–281, 1997.

Perkins RH and Repper JM: Compliance or informed choices. *J Ment Health* **8**: 117–129, 1999.

Piemme TE: Computer-assisted learning and evaluation in medicine. *JAMA* **260**: 367–372, 1988.

Pollock G: Franz Alexander: a tribute. *Arch Gen Psychiatry* **11**: 229–234, 1964.

Postlethwaite R, Stirling G and Peck CL: Stress inoculation for acute pain: a clinical trial. *J Behav Med* **9**: 219–227, 1986.

Regier DA, Narrow WE, Rae DS et al: The de facto US mental and addictive disorders service systems: Epidemiologic Catchment Area prospective 1-year prevalence rates of disorders and services. *Arch Gen Psychiatry* **50**: 85, 1993.

Rost K, Kashner TM and Smith GR: Effectiveness of psychiatric intervention with somatization disorder patients: improved outcomes at reduced costs. *Gen Hosp Psychiatry* **16**: 381–387, 1994.

Roth A and Fonagy P: *What Works for Whom? A Critical Review of Psychotherapy Research*. Guilford: New York, 1996.

Rush AJ, Golden WE, Hall GE et al: *Depression in Primary Care: Volume 1. Detection and Diagnosis. Clinical Practice Guidelines: Agency for Health Care Policy and Research*. AHCPR publication No. 93–0550. US Department of Health and Human Services: Rockville, MD, April 1993.

Saravay SM and Lavin M: Psychiatric comorbidity and length of stay in the general hospital: a critical review of outcome studies. *Psychosomatics* **35**: 233–252, 1994.

Shortliffe EH, Perreault LE, Fagan LM and Wiederholds G (Eds): *Medical Informatics Computer-Applications in Health Care*. Addison-Wesley Publishing Company: Reading, MA, 1990.

Smith GR Jr: The course of somatization and its effects on utilization of health care resources. *Psychosomatics* **35**: 263–267, 1994.

Smith GR Jr, Monson RA and Ray DC: Psychiatric consultation in somatization disorder: a randomized controlled study. *N Engl J Med* **314**: 1407–1413, 1986.

Smith GR Jr, Rost K and Kashner TM: A trial of the effect of a standardized consultation on health outcome and costs in somatizing patients. *Arch Gen Psychiatry* **52**: 238–243, 1995.

Spiegel D, Bloom JR, Kraemer HC et al: Effects of psychosocial treatment on survival of patients with metastatic breast cancer. *Lancet* **ii**: 888–891, 1989.

Spitzer RL, Williams JBW, Kroenke K et al: Utility of a new procedure for diagnosing mental disorders in primary care: the PRIME-MD 1000 study. *JAMA* **272**: 1749–1756, 1994.

Stoudemire A, Bronheim H and Wise TN: Guidelines for the training of C-L psychiatrists. *Psychosomatics* **39**: S3–S7, 1998.

Strain JJ: *Psychological Interventions in Medical Practice*. Appleton-Century-Crofts: New York, 1978.

Strain JJ and Grossman S: *Psychological Care of the Medically Ill: A Primer in Liaison Psychiatry*. Appleton-Century-Crofts: New York, pp 24–27, 1975.

Strain JJ, Pincus HA, Gise LH and Houpt J: Models of mental health training in primary care. *Psychosom Med* **47**: 95–110, 1985.

Strain JJ, Lyons JS, Hammer JS et al: Cost offset from a psychiatric consultation-liaison intervention with elderly hip fracture patients. *Am J Psychiatry* **148**: 1044–1049, 1991.

Strain JJ, Hammer JS and Fulop G: APM task force on psychosocial interventions in the general hospital inpatient setting. *Psychosomatics* **35**: 253–262, 1994.

Strain JJ, Hammer JS, Himelein C, Caliendo G, Mayou R, Smith GC, Malt U, Lyons J and Kurosawa H: Further evolution of a literature database: content and software. *Gen Hosp Psychiatry* **18**: 294–299, 1996a.

Strain JJ, Caliendo G and Himelein C: Drug–psychotropic drug interactions and end organ dysfunction: clinical management recommendations, selected bibliography, and updating strategies. *Gen Hosp Psychiatry* **18**: 300–375, 1996b.

Strain JJ, Caliendo G, Alexis JD, Lowe RS III, Karim A and Loigman M: Part II: Cardiac drug and psychotropic drug interactions: significance and recommendations. *Gen Hosp Psychiatry* **21**: 408–429, 1999.

Sweet JJ, Rozensky RH and Tovian SM: Clinical psychology in medical settings: past and present. In Sweet JJ, Rozensky RH and Tovian SM (Eds): *Handbook of Clinical Psychology in Medical Settings*. Plenum Press: New York, 1991.

Wallston KA, Stein MJ and Smith CA: Form C of the MHLC scales: A condition-specific measure of locus of control. *J Personal Assessment* **63**: 534–553, 1994.

Weinman J: *An Outline of Psychology as Applied to Medicine*. John Wright: Bristol, England, 1981.

Wells JK, Howard GD, Nowlin WF and Vargas MJ: Presurgical anxiety and postsurgical pain and adjustment: Effects of stress inoculation procedure. *J Consult Clin Psychol* **54**: 831–835, 1986.

Wells KB: Cost containment and mental health outcomes: experiences from US studies. *Br J Psychiatry Suppl* **27**: 43–45, 1995.

Wilson-Barnett J: Preparing patients for invasive medical and surgical procedures: Policy implications for implementing specific psychological interventions. *Behav Med* **20**: 23–26, 1994.

Yutzy SH, Cloninger CR, Guze SB, Pribor EF, Martiun RL, Kathol RG, Smith CR, Kane F, Remmerl RR and Strain JJ: DSM-IV field trial: testing a new proposal for somatization disorder. *Am J Psychiatry* **152**: 97–101, 1994.

5

Management of Acute and Chronic Pain

Michael K. Nicholas and Murray Wright
University of Sydney Pain Management and Research Centre, Sydney, Australia

INTRODUCTION

The evolution of the role of psychiatry in the management of pain essentially reflects the development of consultation-liaison psychiatry (Lipowski 1986) which had its beginnings in models of psychosomatic medicine in the late 1950s. Clinical psychologists have also become increasingly involved in the field of pain, from basic research through to clinical management. Their role was given particular impetus by the development of the gate control theory (Melzack & Wall 1965) in the mid-1960s and by the developments in Behavioural Medicine and Medical Psychology in the 1970s (Boudewyns & Keefe 1982; Pearce & Wardle 1989; Prokop & Bradley 1981). It is now common to find psychiatrists and clinical psychologists working alongside each other in the same pain clinic, although the two disciplines have reached the pain field from different directions. Not surprisingly, our colleagues in the other health-care professions wonder how we differ and which patient should be seen by which discipline.

This chapter will review evidence of the ways in which psychological factors can contribute to clinical pain problems and it will also explore the ways in which clinical psychologists and psychiatrists can help in the assessment and management of both acute and chronic pain problems. Differences in the roles of the two disciplines will be outlined and the implications for clinical practice will be discussed.

BACKGROUND

Clinical Pain

The classification of pain remains a disputed arena (Chaplan & Sorking 1997). However, there is general agreement that clinical pain may be divided into two

Psychology and Psychiatry: Integrating Medical Practice.
Edited by J. Milgrom and G. D. Burrows © 2001 John Wiley & Sons, Ltd.

main categories: acute (short-lived) pain and chronic (persistent or intractable) pain (Loeser & Cousins 1990). Their causes vary, as do their patterns. Typically, acute pain is associated with surgery or recent injury. It is expected to abate with the process of healing. Acute pain is normally attributed to nociception (i.e. the activation of nociceptive nerve endings by noxious stimuli such as tissue damage and inflammation). Chronic pain, in contrast, persists beyond the expected healing period and may persist for years with fluctuating intensity and resistance to treatment. Chronic pain may be attributed to nociception, but it can also be caused by neuropathic mechanisms (Siddall & Cousins 1997). In many cases, chronic pain may have no clear physiological or pathological basis and is referred to as "pain of unknown origin" (Merskey & Bogduk 1994). Some writers and clinicians differentiate between chronic pain due to malignant disease and chronic pain of either unknown origin or noncancer disease. Others, however, see no difference between chronic pain of different origins, apart from the obvious differences in possible consequences (Staats 1996).

In clinical settings, it has typically been argued that clinical psychologists and psychiatrists have little to offer in the management of acute pain, especially post-surgical pain, which is normally left to medical and nursing personnel to ensure adequate analgesia is provided (Barratt 1997). The fact that this is not always achieved, however, has given rise to calls for a greater involvement of clinical psychologists and psychiatrists in this area, although resources are often limited (Cousins 1989). In contrast, in the management of chronic pain, clinical psychologists and psychiatrists have often been regarded as essential personnel, either as members of multidisciplinary teams or as a means of moving troublesome patients out of the medical domain (Long 1996).

Conceptual Underpinnings

The publication of the gate control model of pain in 1965 (Melzack & Wall 1965) provided the major impetus to the conceptualization of pain as an experience which was the end-product of a number of interacting physiological and psychological mechanisms. In the gate control model, psychological factors such as attention, past experience and emotion were considered to influence pain perception and response by influencing descending inhibitory processes in the central nervous system. A direct result of this model was the demise of the notion that pain could be neatly divided into summary categories, such as "organic" or "psychological". The task this set clinicians and researchers was to determine the contribution made by both domains to the experience of pain. The subsequent adoption by the International Association for the Study of Pain of a definition of pain as "an unpleasant sensory and emotional experience associated with actual or potential tissue damage, or described in terms of such damage" (1979) added further weight to the conceptualization of pain as a psychological phenomenon which had a variable relationship to tissue damage.

While the details of the gate control model have evolved with subsequent research, many of the actual mechanisms by which psychological factors influence pain perception remain to be fully described. Nevertheless, evidence has accumulated to support the original concept that psychological factors play an integral role in pain perception (see Flor et al 1990, and Birbaumer et al 1995, for comprehensive reviews of experimental and clinical studies). Particular examples include acute pain induced in the laboratory where forewarning about painful stimulation has been shown to reduce the aversive aspects of pain, especially if the subject perceives a degree of control over the aversive stimulation (Averill 1973; Thompson 1981).

Experimental studies have also shown that psychological factors are involved in chronic pain phenomena in two main ways: as a modulating or mediating factor and as a maintenance factor (Birbaumer et al 1995; Gamsa 1994a, b; Turk 1996). For example, a number of studies have shown that the level of disability in chronic pain patients is associated more with psychological variables, such as distress and maladaptive cognitions, than with pathophysiology (Burton et al 1995; Keefe et al 1989; Main et al 1992). Fordyce (1976) and others (e.g. Brena & Chapman 1985; Ross et al 1988) have also argued that many of the problems experienced by chronic pain patients are due to the effects of learning. That is, behaviours such as pain complaints, limping, resting and taking medication may persist because they have been reinforced by their consequences or by the contingencies existing in the patient's current environment. The assertion that psychological factors can be a cause of chronic pain is less well supported by empirical studies (Gamsa 1994a), although there is evidence that psychological and social factors may increase a person's vulnerability to developing maladaptive responses to persisting pain (Gatchel 1996).

The practical consequence of these developments is that psychological factors can no longer be seen as primarily consequences of pain, but rather an integral element in understanding clinical pain phenomena.

MODELS OF PAIN AND IMPLICATIONS FOR TREATMENT

Biopsychosocial Model of Pain and DSM-IV

The original biopsychosocial model of illness enunciated by Engel (1977) posited that symptoms should be conceptualized as the result of a dynamic interaction between psychological, social and pathophysiological variables. Engel's model has since been elaborated in the pain context and a review of the empirical support for this model in relation to pain can be found in Turk (1996) and Turk & Flor (1999). In essence, the model incorporates the notion that biological factors can initiate and influence physiological changes; psychological factors are reflected in the appraisal and perception of internal physiological phenomena; and these appraisals and behavioural responses are in turn influenced by social factors. At the same time, the model also posits that psychological and social factors can influence biological factors, such as hormone production, activity in the autonomic nervous system and physical deconditioning (Flor et al 1990). For example, behavioural responses, such as avoidance of activity due, say, to fear of pain or expectation of further injury, can result in physical deconditioning which over time is likely to be reflected in greater disability (e.g. Bortz 1984; Troup & Videman 1989). The clinical implication of the biopsychosocial model indicates that to assess a patient's pain complaint adequately the clinician(s) must address not only the possible biological basis of the patient's symptoms, but also the range of psychological and social/environmental factors that have been found to influence pain, distress, and disability. These factors, in turn, can then be the subject of targeted interventions.

The biopsychosocial model of pain may be contrasted with the approach taken to pain by DSM-IV (American Psychiatric Association 1994). When pain is the predominant focus of the clinical presentation, DSM-IV names it "pain disorder", which is included within the group of Somatoform Disorders. The criteria for the diagnosis are that (A) the pain must involve one or more anatomical sites and be the predominant focus of the clinical presentation; (B) the pain must cause clinically significant distress and impairment in important areas of functioning, such as occupation and social activities; and (C) psychological factors must play an important role in the onset, severity, exacerbation or maintenance of the pain. Furthermore, three subtypes of the disorder were identified according to the assessed nature and degree of their association with psychological factors. While mental health professionals have generally regarded the more operational approach of DSM-IV as an improvement over the earlier DSM versions, a number have been critical of its handling of pain. Fishbain (1995), for example, concluded that the pain disorder category "has little utility for the pain clinician" (p 18). Fishbain (1995) also pointed out that the diagnosis is overinclusive (almost all patients attending a pain clinic would meet the criteria), and that criterion C not only requires a value judgement by the clinician but the assessment of the relationships between pain report, psychological variables and medical status is of doubtful validity. In many ways the criticisms by Turk and Rudy (1986) of the criteria for Psychogenic Pain Disorder in DSM-III also apply to criterion C of Pain Disorder in DSM-IV—that it contains an implicit assumption that the cause of all pain syndromes is known, as well as an implicit acceptance of a unidimensional model of pain: that pain is either physical or psychogenic. In the light of experimental studies and clinical research, the diagnosis "pain disorder" makes little useful contribution to either treatment planning or prognosis.

This analysis of the pain disorder category does not mean that other conditions commonly associated with pain should be overlooked. The presence of depression is particularly important. But here, too, simple application of DSM-IV criteria for major depressive episode, dysthymic disorder, sleep disorder, adjustment disorder and conversion disorder could result in the diagnosis being applied to most chronic pain patients (Fishbain 1995). For example, a number of the criteria for major depressive episode, such as sleep disturbance and loss of energy, can equally be associated with persisting pain as with underlying depression. In this context it should be mentioned that a strong school of thought has maintained that chronic pain is actually a variant of a depressive disorder (e.g. Blumer & Heilbronn 1982). However, the weight of empirical evidence is that depression is more likely to be a consequence of chronic pain than a cause and the two conditions may co-exist (Gamsa 1994a; Romano & Turner 1985; Turk & Salovey 1984). Discriminating between DSM-IV diagnoses and the phenomena of pain syndromes is inevitably controversial, but the authors would argue that clinical decision-making in pain cases would be aided by more precise identification of the different factors contributing to the features of a particular case, rather than a reliance on a global category, such as pain disorder or major depressive episode, to account for the presenting problems.

No one clinician is likely to possess all the skills required for a comprehensive biopsychosocial assessment and formulation. It has been found more fruitful to employ a multidisciplinary team of clinicians, each making their contribution to the assessment and formulation of the case (Loeser et al 1990). Ideally, the outcomes of their assessments should be discussed in a case conference format as soon as possible after the individual assessments. At this meeting a formulation of the problems presented by a given patient can be arrived at and further investigations or treatment plans can be established. This coordinated approach has a number of advantages, including the increased likelihood of consistency of application of agreed intervention and the reduced chance of splitting of staff by patients. In addition, interventions can be applied in a manner designed to maximize their effectiveness (and avoid the situation where one section of the treatment team is telling the patient she/he has to learn to live with their pain while another section is conducting tests to determine which medication or operation could relieve it—the patient, not surprisingly, is likely to be confused and adherence to any self-management therapy is jeopardized).

At the Centre where the authors work, for example, all new patients are seen only after receipt from the referring physician of adequate background material (previous reports, results of scans, tests, etc.). On the day of assessment each patient is assessed separately by a physician (usually an anesthesiologist), a clinical psychologist or psychiatrist (used interchangeably), and by a physiotherapist (all of whom have specialized in pain management). The patients also complete a battery of questionnaires during the morning. These questionnaires are designed to complement the areas covered by the staff interviews, and include measures of mood, disability, pain-related cognitions, health status/quality of life, and perceived spousal responses (see case histories reported on page 146). Each member of the assessment team presents their findings at a lunch-time meeting and these are then discussed by the multi-disciplinary group, along with a consideration of the patient's questionnaire results. The team develops a working formulation of the case, a plan for treatments (or further investigations), and a set of goals considered by the team to be realistic for each patient. Following the staff meeting, the physician who assessed the patient then sees the patient again to provide feedback from the meeting, to deal with any questions the patient may have and to arrange the next steps in the plan. A date for a file review of progress towards these goals is also set (usually two to three months from assessment). This is intended to ensure that a check is made on the degree of progress of all patients being treated and a decision is made at these reviews about the effectiveness of the treatment plan, any modifications that may be indicated are made or, if appropriate, the patient may be discharged from the centre.

While this model is typically applied to the assessment of chronic pain conditions, it can equally be appropriate, in modified form, for acute pain cases. Clearly, the time-frame for the assessment of acute pain cases will be much shorter, as will the length of contact with the pain clinicians who may work in an advisory manner with the ward staff. A number of studies have demonstrated that such a multidisciplinary approach can be useful in cases of post-surgical pain, preparation for surgery and acute episodes of cancer pain (Johnston & Vogele 1993; Jay et al 1986).

ASSESSMENT OF PAIN

The focus of an assessment of pain will depend on whether it is an initial or diagnostic assessment or an outcome assessment. In the first instance, the psychological assessment will be concerned with assessing the ways in which psychological factors are contributing to the presenting case and whether or not the features could be better explained by a psychiatric diagnosis. The initial assessment should also identify suitable targets for any proposed treatment. For example, at the authors' clinic, specific treatment goals are identified for all new patients assessed and the clinic team later reviews progress towards these goals. The specific goals are subsumed under such headings as pain, activities, work, sleep, mood, medication, and family/significant others. The initial assessment should also identify any issues, such as clarifying a surgical opinion or testing the patient's responsiveness to a particular agent, which need to be resolved before treatments commence.

In contrast to initial assessments, outcome assessments are concerned with determining the extent to which particular goals or outcomes have been achieved after an appropriate interval or trial of treatment. These will vary according to expectations. For example, a trial of responsiveness to a new agent (e.g. a medial branch nerve block) should show a result on a pain rating almost immediately. On the other hand, a goal such as return to work may well take months to achieve and may involve the cooperative efforts of a number of health-care and rehabilitation professionals. Ideally, just as initial assessments inform the development of a treatment plan, outcome assessments should inform a review, and possible revision, of the treatment plan, which would then be further reviewed at a later date.

Issues of particular relevance to clinical psychologists and psychiatrists working in this field include the relationship between diagnosis and case formulation, comorbidity, the use of questionnaires and psychological tests, and integrating the medical and psychological findings to develop a coordinated treatment plan. Useful references on the assessment of pain may be found in Karoly & Jensen (1987), Turk & Melzack (1992) and Williams (1999).

Comorbidity

The psychiatric assessment of a person with chronic pain is no different to the psychiatric assessment of any person with a medical problem and must be based on a complete description of the presenting symptoms, the history of present illness, past history (medical and psychiatric, including treatments and their efficacy) and family and personal history. Depression is the most common comorbid condition, but there are a number of other important disorders also to be considered. Post Traumatic Stress Disorder is likely to occur in a number of chronic pain patients, particularly those who have acquired their conditions as a result of industrial or motor vehicle accidents (Eisendrath 1995; Tyrer 1992). The focus on physical injuries and their treatment can result in this condition being overlooked, even though it can significantly contribute to the overall disability.

Substance abuse is another difficult area to be addressed in assessment and treatment of the chronic pain sufferer (Krishnan et al 1988b). Understanding the significance of the patient's use of narcotics and other psychoactive substances, and their contribution to the overall clinical picture, becomes very important in treatment planning which might set goals towards more rational use of psychoactive drugs or even their withdrawal. Substance abuse might involve recreational drugs, or prescribed drugs including narcotics, antidepressants, or anxiolytics. Understanding the effects of these substances on the overall presenting symptoms (physical and psychological), the potential interactions with other forms of treatment and the likely consequences of an attempt to rationalize or withdraw such drugs becomes very important in the assessment and treatment of pain sufferers.

The assessment of comorbid personality disorders or prominent personality traits strongly influencing a person's response to chronic pain is also an important part of the formulation (Gatchel 1996; Keefe et al 1992). Naturally, such issues should be approached with caution as a cross-sectional assessment of any person in distress is likely to lead to a somewhat biased assessment of personality. A longitudinal history dating back before the onset of the medical condition and also the use of reliable informants is significantly likely to enhance confidence in the assessment. It is of course important to incorporate any such prominent personality traits or personality disorders into a diagnostic formulation, because this will influence the treatment approach. On occasion it may be productive to deal with such personality problems with individual psychotherapy, and this may assist compliance with other components of treatment, but it has also been observed that the group approach to cognitive behavioural treatment, which is widely used in pain clinics, can assist the personality-disordered patient to make significant gains (Roth & Fonagy 1996).

Diagnosis Versus Case Formulation

One of the difficulties confronting clinicians managing the patient presenting with pain is that of incorporating the symptoms and signs into a diagnostic formulation which can be used to develop a rational management plan. Ideally, the formulation should include a description of the individual's behavioural response to pain (e.g. active or passive), as well as the response of relevant environmental agents (spouse, family, work, treating physicians) and the apparent interactions between the different domains (e.g. the cognitions of the patient, their behaviours, affective responses, the current environmental and historical contexts). The "diagnosis" may or may not be the target of specific treatment. It has been our experience that holistic management using an integrated cognitive-behavioural treatment program targeted at identified cognitions and behaviours, such as catastrophic cognitions and activity patterns which aggravate pain, will often lead to improvement in the symptoms and signs contributing to that "diagnosis" (e.g. Maruta et al 1989). This assessment and management of comorbidity is perhaps one of the more complex issues pertaining to pain management, but is of critical importance because of the potential to be inappropriately focused on an aspect of the patient's presentation at the expense of the whole.

Nowhere is this more apparent than in the assessment of depression. It is well recognized that some form of affective disturbance very commonly accompanies chronic illness of any kind, and this is certainly true of the chronic pain population (Fishbain et al 1986; Krishnan et al 1988a; Merskey & Spear 1967; Ward 1990). The difficulty arises when one attempts to interpret the significance of symptoms and signs of depression in this group. Considering some of the key symptoms on which the diagnosis of depression is based helps to illustrate this difficulty. Sleep disturbance is a common symptom of depression, but is also almost invariable in the sufferer of chronic pain. The precise nature of the sleep disturbance should be clarified—is it simply disturbed because of pain, because the person is anxiously ruminating about their predicament, or does the person complain of an "early morning awakening" pattern? It is also often the case that the person complaining of a sleep disturbance has frequent naps during the day (or other problems of sleep hygiene) which contribute more to their complaints than does the pain or depression per se.

The individual with chronic pain has often experienced numerous losses (function, role, relationships, finances) which contribute to a sense of dysphoria, and the targeting of certain of these areas through a cognitive-behavioural program will reduce the feelings of dysphoria. An appetite disturbance is also a prominent symptom of depression, but can be found in patients with chronic pain who are not depressed. Of course, there are some patients who have developed a major depression which does require treatment in its own right, and a failure to recognize and treat this illness is likely to impair a person's response to other components of treatment. The importance of attempting to understand the causal or functional relationship between components of comorbidity cannot be overemphasized, and we believe that such causal hypotheses should be addressed in the formulation. This will set the scene for planning an appropriate intervention in which the targets are likely to include different classes of behaviours or problems (e.g. excessive daytime resting, low daily activity levels, excessive use of analgesics) as well as specific diagnostic categories like depression.

Use of Tests and Questionnaires

While there is no substitute for a careful clinical interview with the patient in the comprehensive assessment of his/her pain problem, there are a number of self-report tests or questionnaires that can greatly enhance the completeness of a clinical interview. It is critical to bear in mind when using questionnaires in this context that their results are as subject to bias as any verbal responses made by a patient during an interview. Equally, there would be no point in administering questionnaires simply to replicate a clinical interview. Rather, as Matarazzo (1990) pointed out, the best use of questionnaires is to test or raise hypotheses. Their strength lies in their known psychometric properties, and those tests with established norms (relevant to the clinical population) can provide a useful gauge when considered alongside other clinical information.

Given the overwhelming number of instruments now available, it is also important to define carefully the domains of interest to assess when determining which questionnaires to use. This applies not just to whether it is an initial assessment or a treatment outcome measure, but also to the variables measured. One of the principal errors of much early pain outcome research, and some not so early, was that only simple visual analogue scales for assessment of pain severity were used (Waddell & Turk 1992). This approach overlooks much potentially important clinical data and makes little sense when pain is conceptualized as a multidimensional phenomenon.

Utilizing a multidimensional conceptualization of pain, a number of instruments with established psychometric properties are available to assess the following domains:

1. Pain severity levels (e.g. a simple 0–10 numerical scale, where 0 = no pain and 10 = unbearable pain).
2. Degree of interference in daily life due to pain (e.g. Sickness Impact Profile (Bergner et al 1981); Roland & Morris—Short SIP (Roland & Morris 1983); Oswestry Low Back Pain Disability Questionnaire: Fairbank et al 1980).
3. Mood (Beck Depression Inventory: Beck et al 1961; Modified Zung Self-Rating Scale for Depression: Main & Waddell 1984; Hospital Anxiety and Depression Scale: Zigmond & Snaith 1983).
4. Cognitions, such as self-efficacy beliefs, locus of control, and beliefs about pain (e.g. Pain Locus of Control: Main & Waddell 1991; Pain Self-Efficacy Questionnaire: Nicholas et al 1992; Pain Beliefs and Perceptions Inventory: Williams & Thorn 1989; Survey of Pain Attitudes: Jensen & Karoly 1992; Pain-Related Self Statements: Flor et al 1993).
5. Use of pain coping strategies (e.g. Coping Strategies Questionnaire: Rosenstiel & Keefe 1983; Vanderbilt Pain Management Inventory: Brown & Nicassio 1987).

For a more complete review of these instruments see Williams (1999). These dimensions can be addressed equally in initial assessment and outcome evaluation contexts. Some measures, such as those assessing pain coping strategies and cognitions, as well as specific rating scales assessing targeted behaviours (e.g. length of sitting time or distance walked) can also be useful in process assessment during treatment (to gauge whether targeted behaviours or cognitions are changing). In some countries comprehensive personality measures are also commonly used. The best example is the Minnesota Multiphasic Personality Inventory (MMPI). However, there is considerable debate about the value of this approach (see Main & Spanswick 1995, for an extensive discussion), and it can be argued that the time required to complete such an instrument could be better used in employing shorter and more focused instruments to measure the dimensions of interest.

A more summary approach can be achieved using the West Haven Yale Multidimensional Pain Inventory (WHYMPI) (Kerns et al 1985), which samples some of the domains referred to earlier (pain severity, interference in daily life, mood, and sense of control), with additional scales assessing the perceived nature of the patient's interactions with their significant others or spouse. These additional scales can add useful information for formulating the case and identifying potential treatment targets or issues to investigate further. In this context, if time and availability permit, it can also be useful to use the spouse version of the WHYMPI which can provide additional information on the same domains as the patient version, but from the spouse's perspective (see Sharp & Nicholas 2000).

PSYCHOLOGICAL TREATMENT OF PAIN

Options and Evidence

Acute Pain

At least four psychological interventions have been shown to be useful in achieving improvements on pain measures, reduced use of analgesics in the postoperative period, mood, and recovery in postoperative pain. These are: relaxation training, procedural information, cognitive coping methods, and behavioural instructions (for systematic reviews see Johnston & Vogele 1993; Suls & Wan 1989).

While hypnosis shares many features of relaxation and imagery, it has a long history of use in acute pain conditions (Syrjala & Abrams 1996). Although much of the literature on the use of hypnosis in acute pain has often been at the levels of evidence of uncontrolled studies and expert opinion, recent papers have displayed more experimental rigour. Syrjala et al (1992), for example, described a study involving cancer patients undergoing bone marrow transplantation and found that those subjects who received hypnosis training reported reduced oral pain compared to those who received cognitive-behavioural coping skills training, treatment as usual and therapist contact. A fuller description of hypnosis in the management of pain can be found in Barber (1996) and Syrjala & Abrams (1996).

Psychological interventions for children in acute pain is an area that has long been neglected, but the field has received increasing attention in the past 15 years (for more detailed information see McGrath 1990). Recent work by Jay and colleagues (Jay et al 1991; Jay et al 1995) has supported the use of cognitive-behavioural therapy in children undergoing painful procedures and Zeltner et al (1990) in their report of the Subcommittee on the Management of Pain Associated with Procedures in Children with Cancer, recommended that both psychological interventions and general anesthesia should be offered as viable alternatives, or in combination, to patients and their parents.

Chronic Pain

Antidepressant medication. While this section is more concerned with psychological interventions, a brief comment on the use of antidepressant medication is warranted, given its widespread use. The most commonly used antidepressants are the tricyclics, whose role in the management of chronic pain has been reported in the literature for some years (Max et al 1995; Watson et al 1982). In the context of chronic pain the antidepressants are often used for their adjunctive analgesic properties rather than their antidepressant activity, and are often used in lower than normal antidepressant doses (Polatin 1996). The sedating qualities of many tricyclic antidepressants are advantageous to many pain patients who suffer from a sleep disturbance and this may also limit the role of some of the newer antidepressants, particularly SSRIs. The literature on the role of newer antidepressants is at this stage sparse; however, there is good evidence for the effectiveness of tricyclics in chronic pain populations. A recent systematic review of the randomized treatment outcome studies with tricyclic antidepressants used with subjects experiencing chronic neuropathic types of pain reported the number of patients needed to be treated (NNT) in order for one to benefit, relative to a control or placebo condition, in terms of pain reduction was of the order of 2.5 (NNTs between 2 and 4 are generally considered to be effective) (McQuay et al 1997). Of course, with the use of such agents there will also be the questions of tolerance of side-effects as well as whether the advantages of these drugs outweigh those of the more psychological and self-management strategies described below. To date, there has been only one randomized controlled trial comparing amitriptyline with cognitive-behaviour therapy for chronic noncancer pain (Pilowsky et al 1995) but methodological shortcomings limit the conclusions that can be drawn from this study (Williams et al 1996a). Nevertheless, numerous studies have revealed that patients participating in cognitive-behavioural pain management programs have withdrawn from antidepressants during these treatments and their reports of depressive symptoms have substantially declined (e.g. Maruta et al 1989; Williams et al 1999). This issue is considered further in the following sections.

Psychological treatments. In the main, psychological treatments are intended to improve mood, function (restoration of normal activities of daily life), reduce the use of unhelpful medication and to increase self-reliance despite persisting pain. Reduction in pain severity is usually seen as an indirect outcome, but it is often reported. Psychological interventions typically occur in the context of multidisciplinary treatments or programs, however, they can be performed in isolation. A consideration of the issues raised by these different modes of operating will be discussed in a later section. While the use of a range of psychological treatments has been reported in the management of chronic pain, few have been subjected to randomized controlled trials. Accordingly, sound empirical evidence for many commonly used psychological treatments, especially in clinical populations, is limited.

The most extensively studied treatments include operant- and cognitive-behavioural methods and relaxation strategies, usually in combination (Fordyce 1976; Gil et al 1988). Hypnotic techniques have also been extensively reported, but more in the context of acute and experimental pain rather than chronic pain (Barber 1996). The use of psychodynamic treatments has also been reported (e.g. Bassett & Pilowsky 1985; Grezesiak et al 1996; Lakoff 1983), but there are insufficient randomized controlled studies to draw meaningful conclusions about their effectiveness, which therefore remains to be established. Biofeedback methods received considerable attention when first introduced; however, their effectiveness relative to other treatments, such as relaxation training and cognitive-behavioural methods, has not been established although there is evidence of differential utility of biofeedback in different pain sites (e.g. Arena & Blanchard 1996). As is the case for most, if not all, treatments, it is always possible to find that some patients respond, but that is not sufficient to make claims about the utility for a particular intervention. It remains the case that, apart from the cognitive-behavioural methods, the effectiveness of most psychological treatments for chronic pain has not been reliably demonstrated.

A systematic review of 35 randomized controlled studies on cognitive-behavioural treatments (CBT) for chronic pain patients, excluding those treating headache patients, concluded that the high-quality studies demonstrated large and sustainable changes for the targeted outcomes (e.g. increased activity levels, improved mood, reduced use of analgesic medication), but less impressive results in lower-quality studies (McQuay et al 1997). More recently, a meta-analysis of 25 of these randomized controlled studies by Morley et al (1999) concluded that there was good evidence that cognitive-behavioural treatments were effective relative to waiting-list controls on all domains of measurement. Relative to alternative treatments (of which there were fewer available) the cognitive-behavioural treatments were significantly superior on measures of pain experience, cognitive coping and appraisal (positive coping measures) and reduced behavioural expression of pain. On measures of mood, negative coping strategies and social role functioning the differences were not significant. An earlier and broader meta-analysis of 65 randomized and nonrandomized multidisciplinary treatments, all of which incorporated behavioural or cognitive-behavioural components, found that even at long-term follow-up patients treated in this way were "functioning better than 75% of a sample that is either untreated or that has been treated by conventional, unimodal treatment approaches" (Flor et al 1992).

It is beyond the scope of this chapter to describe in detail cognitive-behavioural treatments for chronic pain, but broadly they utilize the principles of learning developed originally in operant laboratories and emphasize learning by doing and the use of response-contingent reward or reinforcement to encourage changes in specified behaviours such as exercises, or work-related tasks. Cognitive-behavioural treatments also explicitly attempt to help the patients identify and change the unhelpful beliefs or cognitions and coping strategies which have been shown to contribute to many of the problems commonly experienced by chronic pain patients. The critical features of CBT programs include reconceptualizing the problems faced by the patient (e.g. from pain causing all the problems and an expectation that others should resolve it to the view that the treatments options are limited and the patient must play an active role if desired outcomes are to be achieved). Skills training (for dealing with pain, stress, setbacks, sleep, depression/ anxiety, and significant others) and practice of the skills are also emphasized, and all staff must adhere to the principles of the program in their interactions with the patients (Bradley 1996; Harding & Williams 1998; Nicholas 1995).

Rather than continuing to target the pain for treatment in those cases for which there is no realistic cure available, CBT interventions are targeted at each specific problem area (e.g. behavioural deficits and excesses, such as resting too much, taking too many drugs, not engaging in daily household chores, as well as depressed mood and unhelpful beliefs) identified in the assessment process. Reduction in pain severity is usually seen as an indirect outcome, but it is often reported (Morley et al 1999).

A comprehensive review of psychological treatments for pain may be found in Gatchel & Turk (1996) and useful references for descriptions of cognitive-behavioural treatments may be found in Hanson & Gerber (1990) and Philips (1988).

Psychological Considerations in Treatment Planning and Implementation

In most multidisciplinary pain clinics, psychological treatments are often given at the same time as the physical methods, such as medication, nerve blocks, physiotherapy, and acupuncture. The assumption underlying this approach is that if pain can be ameliorated by treating it at the somatic level then distress and disability will be resolved or at least easier to manage (e.g. Wallis et al 1997). The psychological input in this context is usually aimed at addressing psychological or interpersonal issues identified at the initial assessment, such as excessive distress, unhelpful behaviour patterns, and over-protective spouses.

While this approach can appear attractive and potentially efficient, it does entail a risk. In particular, the nature of the medical and somatic therapy input risks maintaining the patient in a passive role whereby s/he expects the doctor to "fix" the problem for him/her (e.g. Fordyce 1988; Loeser 1996). In turn, this may limit the chances of success of the psychological treatment, especially where it is attempting to encourage greater self-reliance on the part of the patient. Thus, the two approaches (i.e. the medical and psychological) could appear to the patient to be in conflict, which could well compromise the effectiveness of the overall intervention.

Nevertheless, when this simultaneous approach to treatment is taken, it is critical that all components are coordinated and their purpose fully understood by the patient. As with most, if not all, medical and psychological treatments, better results are likely to be achieved if the patient is fully informed about his/her condition, the treatments proposed, their likely outcome and the patient's role. The patient should also play an active role in treatment decisions.

An alternative to the simultaneous approach to interventions is to give them in a planned sequence, also with an informed patient. In this approach, the medical or somatic interventions may be given initially with the expectation (held by both patient and doctor) that some reduction in pain severity could result, and this in turn would lead to improved mood and disability. When these interventions have been completed and if the desired outcomes have not been fully achieved, the patient could then be introduced to the more psychologically based treatments, such as a cognitive-behavioural pain management program, where the goal would shift from pain reduction to improved adjustment and self-management of pain. The advantage of this approach is that it is made clear to the patient that they have reached the end of medical technology and if they are to improve it will have to be through their own efforts, with the assistance of the pain management program.

As with the simultaneous approach, the sequenced approach also requires that the patient be kept fully informed about the treatments being given, and an opportunity is made to discuss his/her concerns about the process. It is crucial that the patient not be allowed to gain the impression that because the initial (physical) treatments have failed s/he is being relegated to psychological treatments. The obvious corollary, in the patient's mind at least, would be that s/he is being told their pain is "all in their head" (e.g. Merskey 1986). It is not difficult to predict poor adherence by the patient to any psychological treatment if this impression is not addressed adequately. It is helpful if, in preparing a patient for psychological treatment, it is made clear that, while the physical treatments have not been successful, there is no implication that the cause of the pain is mental. It should be emphasized that there are no other effective physical treatments currently available and that the patient is faced with the choice of either continuing to seek out further medical treatments, despite having completed adequate assessments and trials of appropriate treatments, or accepting that their pain is chronic and finding the most effective ways to live with it. Cognitive-behavioural treatment is aimed at teaching such patients how to live with pain. Thus, selecting such a treatment option should be construed as a positive step forward rather than an admission of failure.

An alternative scenario concerns the patient who is severely depressed and thought to be at risk of attempting suicide. The question arises as to whether the patient should be commenced on a pain management program in the belief that it will help the depression anyway (e.g. Maruta et al 1989), or should undergo treatment, including possible admission to a psychiatric ward, aimed at reducing the depression and stabilizing his/her mental state before entering the program. A recent study relevant here (Mynors-Wallis et al 1995) found that in a sample of patients with major depression in a primary care setting, brief problem-solving treatment (six sessions of basically cognitive therapy) was as effective as amitriptyline and more effective than placebo, even when given by a general practitioner (as opposed to a psychiatrist or clinical psychologist). Thus, for many chronic pain patients who are depressed, admission to a CBT pain management program may well be enough to deal with both the depression and pain-related problems. But, in general, caution should prevail and it is a matter for judgement on a case-by-case basis. Where the patient is severely depressed and unresponsive to environmental input or the suicide risk is high, normally it would be safer to treat the depression and stabilize the patient before admitting them to a pain management program.

Treatment Setting

To date, the treatment outcome literature in the pain field has been almost totally based on multidisciplinary group programs. To the best of the authors' knowledge, there have been no published controlled outcome trials comparing the effectiveness of a psychiatrist or clinical psychologist seeing patients individually with that of a comprehensive group program. Anecdotal accounts of successful outcomes achieved in individual practice settings do not, of course, provide reliable evidence, although they do show it is possible for good outcomes to be achieved in this setting, but they do not establish that it was due to the treating clinician.

However, in the experience of the authors, who have worked in both individual practice and group programs, the group programs, with multidisciplinary staff all applying cognitive-behavioural principles in the various aspects of the program, usually achieve greater changes more rapidly than is typical of patients seen individually (e.g. Williams et al 1996a, b; 1999). Group programs are also generally more economic to operate as 10 patients can be treated simultaneously versus only one when they are seen individually. Nevertheless, it is also the case that even in a group program some issues are best dealt with on an individual basis, especially where the patient is reluctant to discuss his/her concerns in front of the group or where there are long-standing issues such as marital problems which are not appropriate to explore in a group context.

When a group approach is not possible, for instance in an individual private practice or on a medical ward, an individual approach can still be a worthwhile option. This does mean less of the peer support and encouragement that group programs can provide, but it should also be possible to provide a more individually tailored treatment than feasible in group settings and this approach is also likely to be less intrusive on a patient's daily life (if s/he is an outpatient) than a group program, especially if the patient has young children or a job. If the patient is in a medical or surgical ward, the treatment can usually be arranged around his/her other appointments and the normal ward routine. In this context, a useful reference on cognitive therapy for inpatients can be found in Wright et al (1993), as well as in DeGood & Dane (1996).

Role-Specific Issues

The individual roles for clinical psychologists and psychiatrists in a pain treatment setting have significant areas of difference and overlap. Differences can be as much a product of an individual's background and experience as they are of the respective professional disciplines. However, it is the view of the authors that, apart from some specific issues, the question of which profession provides the service is less of an issue than who is able to provide the services required. In particular, these would include the ability to assess a patient within a biopsychosocial framework and to conduct evidence-based treatments.

There are, however, certain specific issues about which one can generalize. The psychiatrist by virtue of his/her biomedical background is especially qualified to comment on issues relating to psychotropic medication. These may include the effect and efficacy of previously attempted psychotropic treatments, the possible effect of current psychotropic treatment on the clinical presentation, and relevant options for future psychotropic treatment (see Polatin 1996 for a recent review). Other important issues in the pain setting include drug interactions, the effects of substance abuse, and strategies to rationalize medication, which also anticipate the effects of drug withdrawal on the clinical picture. Treatment of specific comorbidity may be more a reflection of individual training but the management of major depression or psychotic illness is likely to involve biological treatments more familiar to the psychiatrist.

Just as it will be generally accepted that the psychiatrist will usually be better qualified than the clinical psychologist in the use of psychotropic medication and the assessment of complications such as the contribution of other medical conditions to a patient's pain presentation, it can also be argued that the clinical psychologist will usually be better trained in the use of cognitive and behavioural treatment techniques as well as in developing both group and individually tailored interventions utilizing these psychological treatment modalities. It is also generally (but not universally) true that clinical psychologists are likely to be more familiar with (and expert in) the development and appropriate use of psychometric questionnaires and assessment measures.

It is of course an important aspect of both the psychiatrists' and psychologists' roles in pain management to identify and support the psychologically vulnerable patient. This may be an individual with psychiatric comorbidity or a past history of psychiatric illness, who may require a more integrated treatment plan and closer individual follow-up. Liaison with referring doctors and general practitioners to ensure that treatment modalities begun in the pain treatment setting can be carried through to the patient's normal environment can often be an important aspect, ensuring continuity of management and maintenance of treatment effects (Nicholas 1992). Whether it is the psychiatrist or clinical psychologist who provides this follow-up assistance will often depend more on third-party payers than on their professional discipline. However, if there are likely to be ongoing issues over the use of psychotropic medication then it would normally be more appropriate for the psychiatrist to remain involved with the patient.

TEAMWORK: PROFESSIONAL ISSUES

Multidisciplinary Versus Interdisciplinary

Working with a multidisciplinary team of health-care providers can sound attractive, with images of peer support for the providers and an array of skills being brought to bear for the betterment of the patient. However, the reality of health-care providers from different disciplines working together as a team can easily be at variance with the image. Consideration of team leadership will quickly reveal important issues for any team attempting to work in a cooperative manner. Traditionally, in the health-care systems of western industrialized countries, the head of most multidisciplinary teams in hospital settings has been a medically qualified physician. Predominantly, the physician takes responsibility for deciding on the treatment plan and designating who on "his/her team" should carry it out. This might be described as a "top down" approach. It is multidisciplinary in that members of several disciplines may be present, but due to the focus of power at the top, it risks overlooking potentially useful contributions by members of the team who may effectively be acting as technicians rather than as independent clinicians with a say in decision-making processes.

The traditional model has been challenged in recent years by the concept of interdisciplinary teams or multidisciplinary teams which operate in an interdisciplinary way (Loeser et al 1990). In this model, while there will usually be a team leader, s/he is not automatically a physician and s/he will operate more as a coordinator or overseer of a treatment plan worked out by discussion with the team members who will take responsibility for their component of the plan. For example, a physiotherapist will take responsibility for determining which exercises a patient should perform to assist him/her to reach functional goals identified at the initial multidisciplinary assessment. In this model, the individual team member is more responsible to the team for his/her performance, rather than just the team leader as in the "top down" model.

In the pain field, not surprisingly, most medical and surgical interventions typically involve the more traditional, multidisciplinary, "top down" team models. In contrast, multidisciplinary pain management programs, such as cognitive-behavioural programs, frequently operate along more interdisciplinary lines, often with a clinical psychologist rather than a physician in the role of team leader or a shared leadership between a physician and a clinical psychologist (e.g. Morgan et al 1979; Williams et al 1993). The team model which any clinic operates probably depends upon the treatment modalities offered by that clinic, but local regulations, traditions or power structures are also likely to influence the model utilized. Of course, many clinics can operate different models within their structure according to the treatments provided.

The discipline of the physician acting as team leader or medical director also varies between hospitals. Most commonly in the pain field it is an anesthesiologist (e.g. Williams et al 1993), but in others it is a psychiatrist (e.g. Houpt et al 1984) or, less commonly, a neurosurgeon (e.g. Bonica 1990). But regardless of the discipline of the director, almost all pain facilities are characterized by the use of a range of disciplines in the assessment and management of patients. In most instances, the director or team leader is really a role that is more dependent upon the skills required for the job than on membership of a particular discipline.

Team Dynamics

Inevitably, disagreements and tensions arise between all those working closely together in teams, especially when dealing with distressed patients who have complex problems. The temptation for members of any discipline under these conditions will often be to retreat to the familiar world of their own discipline. However, it is critical that mechanisms are available for all team members to deal effectively with disagreements within the team, as well as to provide sufficient support for team members to function with confidence. Responsibility for this would naturally lie with the team leader, who clearly should possess the appropriate skills to negotiate the possibly delicate concerns of individual team members (e.g. perceived loss of role or status within the team) while maintaining the team as an effective and functioning unit.

An essential ingredient in the context of effective teamwork is that the team is working according to an agreed model (Loeser et al 1990). For example, if some team members are dealing with the patient according to a biomedical model while others are taking a biopsychosocial approach, there is a high chance of conflict arising, not only among the staff but also between the patient and the staff. The same would apply if some team members took a cognitive-behavioural approach while others took a psychodynamic view. Although in an ideal situation, clinicians from all the involved disciplines might like to provide patients with an eclectic intervention combining features of different models, the risk of conflicting messages being given to the patient is very high and, consequently, there is an increased likelihood of confusing the patient to the detriment of their outcomes. The corollary of this is that all team members, regardless of discipline, should be adequately educated in the model on which the team is operating as well as sufficiently trained in the skills to implement it. This does not mean that all staff should become psychologists or see themselves as such, but rather they should be conversant enough with the model to apply it reliably in their interactions with the patients. Thus, if a cognitive-behavioural model underlies a pain management program, the multi-disciplinary staff should all receive training in cognitive-behavioural theory and its application in their work (Nicholas 1996). For example, while the clinical psychologist would induct the patient into the cognitive-behavioural approach, a physician or physiotherapist would use cognitive-behavioural principles in their interactions with the patient to ensure s/he makes and maintains the desired behavioural and cognitive changes relevant to their aspects of the program (e.g. medication reduction and regular practice of specified exercises) (see Harding & Williams 1998, for an example).

CONCLUSIONS: TO WHOM SHOULD WE REFER THIS PATIENT?

This chapter has attempted to outline the ways in which a psychological approach is relevant to the understanding, assessment and management of both acute and chronic pain. In the view of the authors the question of whether the work described should be done by a psychiatrist or clinical psychologist is of secondary importance to identifying the person from either discipline who can best perform the roles outlined. It is possible that there is as much variation within professions as between them. The critical variable for determining who should provide the service is an adequate background and training in the field of pain and its management in a multidisciplinary context, rather than whether s/he is a psychiatrist or clinical psychologist.

It has also been argued that some roles are best performed by a particular discipline. In the main these refer to the use of psychotropic medication, and where severe comorbidity issues, such as Major Depression and/or Personality Disorder with risk of suicide attempts, arise which are likely to require consideration of admission to a psychiatric ward at some stage. In these contexts, a psychiatrist is the more appropriate person to be involved. Typically, clinical psychologists are more conversant with the use of tests and questionnaires and cognitive-behavioural therapies. However, this is not universal.

In the authors' view, given the differences between the disciplines outlined above, it is likely that a service would benefit most from having representatives of both disciplines available. It is our experience that this can achieve more expert coverage of the essential areas than is likely to occur with only one of either discipline. This is exemplified by the case history of the pain management of Ms Z, with which we conclude this chapter.

Name: Ms Z
Age: 25 years
Sex: Female
Marital status: Married
Site of pain: Lower back, right leg
Date of injury: 1990
Admitted to ADAPT pain management program: March, 1998
Treatment prior to ADAPT: acupuncture, medication, hospital admissions

TABLE 5.1 Measures of Ms Z's Progress

	Pre-ADAPT	Post-ADAPT	6 months follow-up	12 months follow-up
Medication (per day)	450 mg morphine	Nil	Nil	Nil
BDI (Depression)	52	23	42	"much improved"
PSEQ (self-efficacy)	3	30	20	"much better"
DQ (Disability)	21	14	21	"much reduced"
Work status	Off	4 h (× 2 days)	4 h (× 5 days)	5 h (× 5 days)

Ms Z presented at RNSH Pain Management & Research Centre with an eight-year history of chronic lower back pain and right leg pain following a motor vehicle accident in 1990. She presented as extremely depressed, very passive in the management of her pain, and extremely fearful of causing further damage due to movement. She reported sleep problems and significant marital problems. Ms Z was taking 450 mg of morphine (MS Contin) per day to relatively little effect. A multidisciplinary assessment concluded that no further medical/surgical interventions were appropriate and that Ms Z would be suitable for the centre's cognitive-behavioural pain management program, known as ADAPT. ADAPT is a group program (10 patients per group) conducted from 9.00 a.m. to 5.00 p.m. each day, five days a week over three weeks. Patients do not stay at the hospital but may stay at nearby motels. The ADAPT program is based closely on the program described in Williams et al (1996) which was established at St Thomas's Hospital, London, with the first author (MKN) of this chapter as its initial program director.

Ms Z was admitted as an inpatient at RNSH for 1 week prior to the ADAPT program to "detox" under cover of a Ketamine infusion. She commenced ADAPT (as a day-patient) the following week on 120 mg per day of MS Contin, plus temazepam for sleep and Panadeine.

During Week 1 of ADAPT she continued to experience withdrawal symptoms as the medication was further reduced, and she exhibited marked pain behaviours, seeking attention frequently about her symptoms. These behaviours were generally ignored by the staff (after explanation of the reason for this and reassurance by the staff that the symptoms she was experiencing were related to withdrawal effects and to disuse effects, rather than to more damage). The pain behaviours subsequently subsided in frequency.

Although she completed the full three weeks, Ms Z felt she had made relatively few gains during that phase. She attributed this to her medication withdrawal. However, the staff considered that her appearance was greatly improved, and she was walking and moving more freely. Videotape of her walking before and after the program was consistent with the staff impressions. Her husband attended during the program, and after some joint sessions with the clinical psychologist, some improvement was reported in their relationship. During her attendance at ADAPT a rehabilitation meeting was conducted between clinic staff and the workplace rehabilitation coordinator and plans were developed for a graduated return-to-work (RTW) program.

Unfortunately, the rehabilitation coordinator had little understanding of chronic pain and was not confident that Ms Z could RTW until she was reporting less pain. A recommendation was made by the ADAPT rehabilitation counsellor for an rehabilitation provider external to the workplace (one who was conversant with the ADAPT approach and would agree to implement it) to be allocated to her case and assist her RTW. Another rehabilitation meeting was conducted with the new rehabilitation provider and clinic staff, to develop the RTW plan. At the meeting Ms Z demonstrated no pain behaviours, reported she was taking no medication and was extremely motivated to trial a RTW (despite her pain).

Meetings and education sessions were conducted at the workplace by the new rehabilitation provider, regular monitoring occurred, with frequent liaison with the pain centre. The employer made considerable efforts to facilitate the RTW plan and was very accommodating and patient.

Ms Z has had many difficulties since the completion of the program, especially early on. She asked her husband to leave when she returned home (something that could be seen as indicative of her regaining her self-respect as she had previously been blaming herself for his infidelities). She resumed taking MS Contin (she had a few tablets left at home from before the pain program) on an irregular basis (though in greatly reduced doses). Fortunately, her local doctor assisted the management plan by not prescribing more medication. She commenced abusing alcohol as a means of coping, and had many "flare-ups" in pain. Unfortunately, due to her high medication level early in the program, the staff felt that she had had difficulty in absorbing the cognitive coping strategies taught during ADAPT. As a result she was not able to implement these strategies as well as required and thus she suffered more than necessary from her increased pain (hence her tendency to fall back on her old stand-bys of MS Contin and alcohol). Despite all of this, however, Ms Z remained at work, gradually increasing her hours, and commenced local psychological therapy for a limited period aimed at improving her skills in applying the strategies taught at ADAPT, free of the medication haze.

Within six months of completing ADAPT, Z's husband had returned home, she had ceased all medication and alcohol consumption, and her overall function and activity levels had increased dramatically, as well as her mood. She began attending the local gym on a regular basis. One year after the program she is working five hours per day, five days per week in her old position as a supervisor in her workplace. Outside work, she reports she has increased her activity level and is much happier with her new lifestyle. She continues to keep in touch with her rehabilitation provider from time to time. She is also continuing to apply the pain management strategies taught at ADAPT—to the extent that recently she had her wisdom teeth removed and she declined the offer of Panadeine Forte for the pain, preferring instead to use her own strategies.

REFERENCES

American Psychiatric Association: *Diagnostic and Statistical Manual of Mental Disorders* (4th edn), APA: Washington, DC, 1994.

Arena JG and Blanchard EB: Biofeedback and relaxation therapy for chronic pain disorders. In *Psychological Approaches to Pain Management: A Practitioner's Handbook* (Eds RJ Gatchel and DC Turk), pp 148–178, Guilford Press: New York, 1996.

Averill JR: Personal control over aversive stimuli and its relationship to stress. *Psychol Bull* **80**: 191–215, 1973.

Barber J: *Hypnosis and Suggestion in the Treatment of Pain.* Norton: New York, 1996.

Barratt SMcG: Advances in acute pain management. In *Acute and Chronic Pain. International Anesthesiology Clinics Vol 35* (Eds AR Molloy and I Power), pp 27–48, Lippincott-Raven: Philadelphia, USA, 1997.

Bassett D and Pilowsky I: A study of brief psychotherapy for chronic pain. *J Psychosom Res* **29**: 259–264, 1985.

Beck AT, Ward CH, Mendelson M, Mock N and Erbaugh J: An inventory for measuring depression. *Arch Gen Psychiatry* **4**: 561–571, 1961.

Bergner M, Bobbitt RA, Carter WB and Gibson BS: The Sickness Impact Profile: development and final version of a health status measure. *Medical Care* **19**: 787–805, 1981.

Birbaumer N, Flor H, Lutzenberger W and Elbert T: The corticalization of chronic pain. In *Pain and the Brain: from Nociception to Cognition. Advances in Pain Research and Therapy*, Vol 22 (Eds B Bromm and JE Desmedt), pp 331–344, Raven Press: New York, 1995.

Blumer D and Heilbronn M: Chronic pain as a variant of depressive disease. *J Nerv Ment Dis* **170**: 381–406, 1982.

Bonica JJ: Multidisciplinary/interdisciplinary pain programs. In *The Management of Pain.* 2nd edn (Ed JJ Bonica), pp 197–208, Lea & Febiger: Philadelphia, USA, 1990.

Bortz W: The disuse syndrome. *Western J Med* **141**: 691–694, 1984.

Boudewyns PA and Keefe FJ: *Behavioral Medicine in General Medical Practice.* Addison-Wesley: Menlo Park, USA, 1982.

Bradley LA: Cognitive-behavioral therapy for chronic pain. In *Psychological Approaches to Pain Management: A Practitioner's Handbook* (Eds RJ Gatchel and DC Turk), pp 131–147, Guilford Press: New York, 1996.

Brena SF and Chapman SL: Acute versus chronic pain states: the "learned pain syndrome". In *Chronic Pain: Management Principles* (Eds SF Brena and SL Chapman), pp 41–55, WB Saunders: London, 1985.

Brown GK and Nicassio PM: Development of a questionnaire for the assessment of active and passive coping strategies in chronic pain patients. *Pain* **31**: 53–64, 1987.

Burton AK, Tillotson KM, Main CJ and Hollis S: Psychosocial predictors of outcome in acute and subacute low back trouble. *Spine* **20**: 722–728, 1995.

Chaplan SR and Sorking LS: Agonizing over pain terminology. *Pain Forum* **6**: 81–87, 1997.

Cousins MJ: Acute pain and the injury response: immediate and prolonged effects. *Regional Anesthesia* **14**: 162–179, 1989.

DeGood DE and Dane JR: The psychologist as a pain consultant in outpatient, inpatient, and workplace settings. In *Psychological Approaches to Pain Management: A Practitioner's Handbook* (Eds RJ Gatchel and DC Turk), pp 403–437, Guilford Press: New York, 1996.

Eisendrath SJ: Psychiatric aspects of chronic pain. *Neurology* **45**: S26–36, 1995.

Engel CL: The need for a new medical model: a challenge for biomedical science. *Science* **196**: 129–136, 1977.

Fairbank JCL, Couper J, Davies JB and O'Brien JP: The Oswestry low back pain Disability Questionnaire. *Physiotherapy* **66**: 271–273, 1980.

Fishbain DA: DSM-IV: implications and issues for the pain clinician. *Am Pain Soc Bul* **4**: 6–18, 1995.

Fishbain DA, Goldberg M, Meagher BR, Rosomoff RS and Rosomoff H: Male and female chronic pain patients categorised by DSM-III diagnostic criteria. *Pain* **26**: 181–197, 1986.

Flor H, Birbaumer N and Turk DC: The psychobiology of chronic pain. *Adv Behav Res Ther* **12**: 47–84, 1990.

Flor H, Fydrich T and Turk DC: Efficacy of multidisciplinary pain treatment centers: a meta-analytic review. *Pain* **49**: 221–230, 1992.

Flor H, Behle DJ and Birbaumer N: Assessment of pain-related cognitions in chronic pain patients. *Behav Res Ther* **31**: 63–73: 1993.

Fordyce WE: *Behavioral Methods for Chronic Pain and Illness.* Mosby: St Louis, 1976.

Fordyce WE: Pain and suffering: a reappraisal. *Am Psychologist* **43**: 276–283, 1988.

Gamsa A: The role of psychological factors in chronic pain. Part I. A half century of study. *Pain* **57**: 5–15, 1994a.

Gamsa A: The role of psychological factors in chronic pain. Part II. A critical appraisal. *Pain* **57**: 17–30, 1994b.

Gatchel RJ: Psychological disorders and chronic pain: cause-and-effect relationships. In *Psychological Approaches to Pain Management: A Practitioner's Handbook* (Eds RJ Gatchel and DC Turk), pp 33–52, Guilford Press: New York, 1996.

Gatchel RJ and Turk DC (Eds): *Psychological Approaches to Pain Management: A Practitioner's Handbook.* Guilford Press: New York, 1996.

Gil K, Ross SI and Keefe FJ: Behavioral treatment for chronic pain. Four pain management protocols. In *Chronic Pain* (Eds RD France and KRR Krishnan), pp 376–413, American Psychiatric Press: Washington, DC, 1988.

Grezesiak RC, Ury GM and Dworkin RH: Psychodynamic psychotherapy with chronic pain patients. In *Psychological Approaches to Pain Management: A Practitioner's Handbook* (Eds RJ Gatchel and DC Turk), pp 148–178, Guilford Press: New York, 1996.

Hanson RW and Gerber KE: *Coping With Chronic Pain: A Guide to Patient Self-Management.* Guilford Press: New York, 1990.

Harding VR and Williams ACdeC: Activities training: Integrating behavioral and cognitive methods with physiotherapy in pain management. *J Occup Rehab* **8**: 47–60, 1998.

Houpt JL, Keefe FJ and Snipes MT: The clinical specialty unit: the use of the psychiatry inpatient unit to treat chronic pain syndromes. *Gen Hosp Psychiatry* **6**: 65–70, 1984.

International Association for the Study of Pain: Pain terms: a list with definitions and notes on usage. *Pain* **6**: 249, 1979.

Jay SM, Elliott CH and Varni JW: Acute and chronic pain in adults and children with cancer. *J Consult Clin Psychol* **54**: 601–607, 1986.

Jay SM, Elliott CH, Woody P and Siegel S: An investigation of cognitive-behavior therapy combined with oral valium for children undergoing painful medical procedures. *Health Psychology* **10**: 317–322, 1991.

Jay SM, Elliott CH, Fitzgibbons I, Woody P and Siegel S: A comparative study of cognitive behavior therapy versus general anesthesia for painful medical procedures in children. *Pain* **62**: 3–9, 1995.

Jensen MP and Karoly P: Pain-specific beliefs, perceived symptom severity, and adjustment to chronic pain. *Clin J Pain* **8**: 123–130, 1992.

Johnston M and Vogele C: Benefits of psychological preparation for surgery: a meta-analysis. *Ann Behav Med* **15**: 245–256, 1993.

Karoly P and Jensen MP: *Multimethod Assessment of Chronic Pain*. Pergamon: Oxford, 1987.

Keefe FJ, Brown GK, Wallston KA and Caldwell DS: Coping with rheumatoid arthritis pain: catastrophizing as a maladaptive strategy. *Pain* **37**: 51–56, 1989.

Keefe FJ, Salley AN and Lefebre JC: Coping with pain: conceptual concerns and future directions. *Pain* **51**: 131–134, 1992.

Kerns RD, Turk DC and Rudy TE: West Haven-Yale Multidimensional Pain Inventory (WHYMPI). *Pain* **23**: 345–356, 1985.

Krishnan KRR, France RD and Davidson J: Depression as a psychopathological disorder in chronic pain. In *Chronic Pain* (Eds RD France and KRR Krishnan), pp 195–218, American Psychiatric Press: Washington, DC, 1988a.

Krishnan KRR, McCann UD and France RD: Substance abuse in chronic pain patients. In *Chronic Pain* (Eds RD France and KRR Krishnan), pp 220–227, American Psychiatric Press: Washington, DC, 1988b.

Lakoff R: Interpretive psychotherapy with chronic pain patients. *Can J Psychiatry* **28**: 650–653, 1983.

Lipowski ZJ: Consultation liaison psychiatry: The first half century. *Gen Hosp Psychiatry* **8**: 305–315, 1986.

Loeser JD: Mitigating the dangers of pursuing cure. In *Pain Treatment Centers at a Crossroads: a Practical and Conceptual Reappraisal* (Eds MJM Cohen and JN Campbell), Progress in Pain Research and Management, Vol 7, pp 79–100, IASP Press: Seattle, USA, 1996.

Loeser JD and Cousins MJ: Contemporary pain management. *Med J Australia* **153**: 208–216, 1990.

Loeser JD, Seres JL and Newman RI: Interdisciplinary, multimodal management of chronic pain. In *The Management of Pain* (2nd edn) (Ed JJ Bonica), pp 2107–2120, Lea & Febiger: Philadelphia, USA 1990.

Long DM: The development of the comprehensive pain treatment program at Johns Hopkins. In *Pain Treatment Centers at a Crossroads: a Practical and Conceptual Reappraisal* (Eds MJM Cohen and JN Campbell), Progress in Pain Research and Management, Vol 7, pp 3–26, IASP Press: Seattle, 1996.

Main CJ and Spanswick CC: Personality assessment and the Minnesota Multiphasic Personality Inventory. *Pain Forum* **4**: 90–96, 1995.

Main CJ and Waddell G: The detection of psychological abnormality using four simple scales. *Current Concepts in Pain* **2**: 10–15, 1984.

Main CJ and Waddell G: A comparison of cognitive measures in low back pain: statistical structure and clinical validity at initial assessment. *Pain* **46**: 287–298, 1991.

Main CJ, Wood PLR, Hollis S and Spanswick CC: The distress and risk assessment method (DRAM): a simple patient classification to identify distress and evaluate the risk of a poor outcome. *Spine* **17**: 42–52, 1992.

Maruta T, Vatterott MK and McHardy MJ: Pain management as an antidepressant: long term resolution of pain associated depression. *Pain* **36**: 335–337, 1989.

Matarazzo JD: Psychological assessment versus psychological testing. *Am Psychologist* **45**: 999–1017, 1990.

Max MB, Gracely RH, Walther DJ, Smoller B and Dubnet R: Antidepressant drugs as treatments for chronic pain: efficacy and mechanisms. In *Pain and the Brain: from Nociception to Cognition* (Eds B Bromm and JE Desmedt) *Advances in Pain Research and Therapy*, Vol. 22, pp 501–515, Raven Press: New York, 1995.

McGrath P: *Pain in Children: Nature, Assessment and Treatment.* Guilford Press: New York, 1990.

McQuay HJ, Moore RA, Eccleston C, Morley S and Williams ACdeC: Systematic review of outpatient services for chronic pain patient control. *Health Technology Assessment* **1**(6): 1997.

Melzack R and Wall PD: Pain mechanisms: a new theory. *Science* **150**: 971–979, 1965.

Merskey H: Traditional individual psychotherapy and psychopharmacology. In *Pain Management: A Handbook of Psychological Treatment Approaches* (Eds AD Holzman and DC Turk), Pergamon Press: New York, 1986.

Merskey H and Bogduk N: *Classification of Chronic Pain: Descriptions of Chronic Pain Syndromes and Definitions of Pain Terms*, 2nd edn, IASP Press: Seattle, USA, 1994.

Merskey H and Spear FG: *Pain: Psychological and Psychiatric Aspects.* Bailliere, Tindall & Cassell: London, 1967.

Morley S, Eccleston C and Williams A: Systematic review and meta-analysis of randomised controlled trials of cognitive behaviour therapy and behaviour therapy for chronic pain in adults, excluding headache. *Pain* **80**: 1–14, 1999.

Morgan CD, Kremer E and Gaylor M: The behavioral medicine unit: a new facility. *Comprehens Psychiatry* **20**: 79–89, 1979.

Mynors-Wallis LM, Gath DH, Lloyd-Thomas AR and Tomlinson D: Randomised controlled trial comparing problem solving treatment with amitriptyline and placebo for major depression in primary care. *BMJ* **310**: 441–445, 1995.

Nicholas MK: Chronic pain. In *Relapse Prevention in Cognitive-Behavioural Therapy* (Ed PH Wilson), Guilford Press: New York, 1992.

Nicholas MK: Compliance: a barrier to occupational rehabilitation? *J Occup Rehab* **5**: 271–282, 1995.

Nicholas MK: Theory and practice of cognitive-behavioral programs. In *Pain 1996—An Updated Review* (Ed JN Campbell), pp 297–304, IASP Press: Seattle, USA, 1996.

Nicholas MK, Wilson PH and Goyen J: Comparison of cognitive-behavioral group treatment and an alternative non-psychological treatment for chronic low back pain. *Pain* **48**: 339–347, 1992.

Pearce S and Wardle J: *The Practice of Behavioural Medicine.* Oxford University Press and BPS Books: Oxford, 1989.

Philips HC: *The Psychological Management of Chronic Pain: A Treatment Manual.* Springer: New York, 1988.

Pilowsky I, Spence N, Rounsefell B, Forsten C and Soda J: Out-patient cognitive-behavioural therapy with amitriptyline for chronic non-malignant pain: a comparative study with 6-month follow-up. *Pain* **60**: 49–54, 1995.

Polatin PB: Integration of pharmacotherapy with psychological treatment of chronic pain. In *Psychological Approaches to Pain Management: A Practitioner's Handbook* (Eds RJ Gatchel and DC Turk), pp 305–328, Guilford Press: New York, 1996.

Prokop CK and Bradley LA: *Medical Psychology.* Academic Press: New York, 1981.

Roland M and Morris R: A study of the natural history of back pain. Part I. Development of a reliable and sensitive measure of disability in low-back pain. *Spine* **8**: 141–144, 1983.

Romano JM and Turner JA: Chronic pain and depression: does the evidence support a relationship? *Psychol Bull* **97**: 18–34, 1985.

Rosenstiel AK and Keefe FJ: The use of coping strategies in chronic low-back pain patients: relationship to patient characteristics and current adjustment. *Pain* **17**: 33–44, 1983.

Ross SL, Keefe FJ and Gil KM: Behavioral concepts in the analysis of chronic pain. In *Chronic Pain* (Eds RD France and KRR Krishnan), pp 104–114, American Psychiatric Press: Washington, DC, 1988.

Roth A and Fonagy P: *What Works for Whom? A Critical Review of Psychotherapy Research.* Guilford Press: New York, 1996.

Sharp JJ and Nicholas MK: Assessing the significant others of chronic pain patients: the psychometric properties of significant other questionnaires. *Pain* **88**: 135-144, 2000.

Siddall PJ and Cousins MJ: Neurobiology of pain. In *Acute and Chronic Pain. International Anesthesiology Clinics* (Eds AR Molloy and I Power), Vol 35, pp 1–26, Lippincott-Raven: Philadelphia, USA, 1997.

Staats PS: Pain is pain: why the dichotomy of approach to cancer and noncancer pain? In *Pain Treatment Centers at a Crossroads: A Practical and Conceptual Reappraisal* (Eds MJM Cohen and JN Campbell), *Progress in Pain Research and Management*, Vol 7, pp 117–123, IASP Press: Seattle, USA, 1996.

Suls J and Wan CK: Effects of sensory and procedural information on coping with stressful medical procedures and pain: a meta-analysis. *J Consult Clin Psychol* **57**: 372–379, 1989.

Syrjala KL and Abrams JR: Hypnosis and imagery in the treatment of pain. In *Psychological Approaches to Pain Management: A Practitioner's Handbook* (Eds RJ Gatchel and DC Turk), pp 231–258, Guilford Press: New York, 1996.

Syrjala KL, Cummings C and Donaldson GW: Hypnosis or cognitive-behavioral training for the reduction of pain and nausea during cancer treatment: a controlled study. *Pain* **48**: 137–146, 1992.

Thompson SC: Will it hurt less if I can control it? A complex answer to a simple question. *Psychol Bull* **90**: 89–101, 1981.

Troup JDG and Videman T: Inactivity and the aetiopathogenesis of musculoskeletal disorders. *Clin Biomechanics* **4**: 173–178, 1989.

Turk DC: Biopsychosocial perspective on chronic pain. In *Psychological Approaches to Pain Management: A Practitioner's Handbook* (Eds RJ Gatchel and DC Turk), pp 3–32, Guilford Press: New York, 1996.

Turk DC and Flor H: Chronic pain: a biobehavioral perspective. In *Psychosocial Factors in Pain: Critical Perspectives* (Eds RJ Gatchel and DC Turk), pp 18–34, Guilford Press: New York, 1999.

Turk DC and Melzack R (Eds): *Handbook of Pain Assessment.* Guilford Press: New York, 1992.

Turk DC and Rudy TE: Assessment of cognitive factors in chronic pain: a worthwhile enterprise? *J Consult Clin Psychol* **54**: 760–768, 1986.

Turk DC and Salovey P: "Chronic pain as a variant of depressive disease": a critical reappraisal. *J Nerv Ment Dis* **172**: 398–404, 1984.

Tyrer S: Psychiatric assessment of chronic pain. *Br J Psychiatry* **160**: 733–741, 1992.

Waddell G and Turk DC: Clinical assessment of low back pain. In *Handbook of Pain Assessment* (Eds DC Turk and R Melzack), pp 15–36, Guilford Press: New York, 1992.

Wallis B, Lord S and Bogduk N: Resolution of psychological distress of whiplash patients following treatment by radiofrequency neurotomy: a randomised, double-blind, placebo-controlled trial. *Pain* **73**: 15–22, 1997.

Ward NG: Pain and depression. In *The Management of Pain*, 2nd edn (Ed JJ Bonica), Lea & Febiger: Philadelphia, USA, 1990.

Watson CPN, Evans RJ and Reed K: Amitriptyline versus placebo in postherpetic neuralgia. *Neurology* **32**: 671–673, 1982.

Williams ACdeC: Measures of function and psychology. In *The Textbook of Pain*, 4th edn (Eds PD Wall and R Melzack), pp 427–444, Churchill Livingstone: Edinburgh, UK, 1999.

Williams ACdeC, Nicholas MK, Richardson PH, Pither CE, Justins DM, Chamberlain JH, Harding VR, Ralphs JA, Jones SC, Dieudonne I, Featherstone JD, Hodgson DR, Ridout KL and Shannon EM: Evaluation of a cognitive behavioural program for rehabilitating patients with chronic pain. *Br J Gen Practice* **43**: 513–518, 1993.

Williams ACdeC, Richardson PH, Nicholas MK, Justins DM, Morley S, Diamond A, Linton S, Vlaeyen J, Nilges P, Eccleston C: The effects of cognitive-behavioural therapy in chronic pain. Letters to the Editor. *Pain* **65**: 82–83, 1996a.

Williams ACdeC, Richardson PH, Nicholas MK, Pither CE, Harding VR, Ridout KL, Ralphs JA, Richardson IH, Justins DM and Chamberlain JH: Inpatient vs outpatient pain management: results of a randomised controlled trial. *Pain* **66**: 13–22, 1996b.

Williams ACdeC, Nicholas MK, Richardson PH, Pither CE and Fernandes J: Generalizing from a controlled trial: the effects of patient preference versus randomization on the outcome of inpatient versus outpatient chronic pain management. *Pain* **83**: 57–65, 1999.

Williams DA and Thorn BE: An empirical assessment of pain beliefs. *Pain* **36**: 351–358, 1989.

Wright JH, Thase ME, Beck AT and Ludgate JW: *Cognitive Therapy with Inpatients: Developing a Cognitive Milieu.* Guilford Press: New York, 1993.

Zeltner L, Altman A, Cohen D, leBaron S, Munuksela E and Schechter N: Report of the subcommittee on the management of pain associated with procedures in children with cancer. *Pediatrics* **86**: 826–831, 1990.

Zigmond AS and Snaith RP: The Hospital Anxiety and Depression Scale. *Acta Scandinavica* **76**: 361–370, 1983.

6

Psychological and Psychiatric Practice in Oncology Populations

Andrew Baum
University of Pittsburgh, Pennsylvania, USA
Diane Thompson
Western Psychiatric Institute, Magee-Women's Hospital and University of Pittsburgh, Pennsylvania, USA
Susan Stollings, John P. Garofalo and Ellen Redinbaugh
University of Pittsburgh, Pennsylvania, USA

INTRODUCTION

Increasingly, behavioral research and theory are becoming an integral part of the care and treatment of cancer patients. Evidence continues to suggest that behavioral and psychological factors contribute to cancer morbidity and are key factors in prevention efforts. At the same time, quality of life issues for patients and their families have become more prominent. It now seems likely that well-being, mental health, and other psychosocial factors affect disease course, response to medical treatment, and survival. Behavioral involvement in cancer care, research, and patient management has become more common as a result and has led to new and larger roles for psychologists and psychiatrists in oncology settings. This chapter considers some aspects of these emerging roles, with emphasis on the complementary roles each can play and how behavioral medicine may best be integrated with evolving medical treatments and models of patient care. Palliative care programs are described as examples of the effective and successful integration of a range of disciplines in care of cancer patients.

Before considering these issues, it is useful to consider briefly the bases of behavioral intervention in cancer care. As we will describe later, this involvement extends across prevention, early detection, treatment, and palliation-related issues. The rationale for this is essentially that behavioral factors explain some or much of

Psychology and Psychiatry: Integrating Medical Practice.
Edited by J. Milgrom and G. D. Burrows © 2001 John Wiley & Sons, Ltd.

the variance in these areas and that recognition of their influence enhances overall care and patient welfare. We know that behavior is centrally involved in people's risk for cancer; in particular, tobacco use, sun exposure, diet, exercise, and alcohol or drug exposures can dramatically alter a person's risk for cancer (e.g. Baum & Cohen 1998). More recently, data have begun to suggest that psychosocial issues also affect disease course and response to cancer treatment (e.g. Andersen et al 1994; Helgeson & Cohen 1996; Spiegel et al 1989). There are clearly many sources of stress and strain associated with cancer diagnosis, treatment, and survival, beginning with the trauma of cancer discovery and diagnosis and continuing throughout treatment and post-treatment transitions. This stress can affect physiological systems, mood, and behavior in ways that can affect disease processes and illness-related behavior (e.g. Baum & Posluszny 1999). Cancer-related stressors can increase a patient's risk for mental health problems as well (e.g. Jenkins et al 1991). Psychiatric complications that are not detected, treated, or prevented can cause complications and compromised treatment and may result in higher medical costs and poorer patient outcomes.

The next section describes some major aspects of psychologists' increasing involvement in cancer care. This activity reflects an overall shift in models of pathogenesis and treatment of chronic diseases associated with the emergence of behavioral medicine. We then turn to parallel involvement by psychiatrists and the complementary benefits associated with psychological and psychiatric engagement. Finally, we consider issues related to integrating these models of care and the role of behavioral care in multidisciplinary or interdisciplinary cancer-care teams. More specific specialization, such as that reflected in palliative care, offers an important example of the need for and benefits of integration of behavioral medicine with prevailing models of care.

PSYCHOLOGICAL EVALUATION AND TREATMENT OF CANCER PATIENTS

Application of psychological treatment in the care of cancer patients is complex and varies dramatically across stage of illness, patient characteristics, and the phase of discovery or treatment of the disease. Issues raised when cancer is diagnosed are very different from those associated with survival or with disease recurrence. Systematic investigation of patient needs, distress, and provider interventions has not evaluated these different contexts, but clinical experience strongly suggests that different approaches should be taken. In particular, early, pre-emptive interventions that seek to prevent development of major psychological problems are warranted when cancer is suspected or found. These early interventions, generally delivered before major problems may be anticipated, seek to enhance coping and provide support necessary for appropriate adaptation.

Diagnosis and Early Intervention

The diagnosis of cancer presents the patient with extraordinary circumstances that exceed the demands commonly encountered in his or her daily life. Fear, stress, and uncertainty are quickly aroused because of the severe life threat associated with cancer diagnoses (Stanton & Snider 1993). Many patients report having adjustment problems and feelings of depression, anxiety, and isolation. In some instances, a patient may experience feelings of guilt when past behaviors are highly associated with cancer (e.g. tobacco use, sun exposure). Some distress and difficulty achieving adaptation appear nearly universal and are expected among recently diagnosed patients. For some this distress may not be manageable, impairing adjustment. Adjustment problems may persist for years or develop into debilitating psychological disorders. Even when medical screening or biopsy yields negative results, patients may experience difficulty coping with feelings of uncertainty about their medical status and can become overly preoccupied with their health (Baum et al 1997)

There are several reasons to provide early psychosocial intervention to people who have been undergoing diagnostic testing or who have been recently diagnosed with cancer. First, it should assist the patient in coping more effectively with the acute onset of cancer-related psychosocial distress. Interventions offered at this point in the disease experience are often designed to equip patients with skills that will permit more effective coping with the stressful demands of the surgery and/or adjuvant treatment. Early intervention and reinforcement of more effective coping can also reduce some of the detrimental effects that stress can have on health behaviors. Patients who are diagnosed with cancer are likely to experience an array of strong emotions and coping strategies, and face stressors that may tax coping skills as well as compromise judgment. As a result, poor health behaviors, adherence problems, and delays in the initiation of treatment may increase. These factors may collectively compromise medical treatment and lead to more negative outcomes. Early intervention can better prepare cancer patients for future psychological sequelae and minimize the likelihood of future mood disturbance and other psychiatric morbidity (i.e. sexual dysfunction, unemployment, job discrimination, changes in body-image, etc.).

Psychosocial interventions are not all the same and can be shaped to address specific stressors or characteristics of a patient's situation. For example, site of disease is important because it dictates prognosis and affects the nature of possible impairment. Men with testicular cancer demonstrate a 90% survival rate, while there are poorer survival rates among women diagnosed with advanced ovarian cancer or men and women found to have advanced colon cancer. Differences in mortality rates across disease site may lead to qualitatively and quantitatively different sources of worry and coping responses among cancer patients. In addition, treatment-related issues (i.e. treatment modality, duration of treatment) also vary across site. Many cancers require surgical intervention and the location and nature of the disease dictate the extent, severity or likely disfiguring effects associated with surgery. Whether adjuvant radiation or chemotherapy is indicated, how severe treatment side-effects are and how often or how long treatments are needed are also important variables associated with site. Often the weighing of pros and cons in selecting a treatment represents a major source of distress for cancer patients and programs providing decision-making support are warranted. Because distress may hamper judgment and behavior it is important that interventions assist cancer patients with coping and problem-solving when making decisions regarding treatment selection.

Prognosis also depends on the stage of disease at diagnosis. Early detection and treatment is generally the best predictor of survival. Because evidence suggests that the needs and issues of cancer patients change during the cancer experience, some treatment plans may be more appropriate than others at different stages of disease. These interventions are developed and fashioned to address the salient issues of each stage as well as any presenting adjustment difficulties experienced by patients. However, interventions include some components that are inherently valuable regardless of stage of disease (e.g. Andersen 1992). Emotional support, information regarding the disease and its treatment, coping strategies, and relaxation training appear to be valuable across disease stage.

As an example, consider the fact that issues regarding death and dying become more prominent in later stages of disease and represent a major concern for both the patient and family. While interventions for early-stage cancer patients emphasize preparation for and prevention against cancer-related distress, patients with advanced disease frequently report a significant level of depression and anxiety as well as needs to work through existential issues. A number of studies have found that patients with advanced disease report more distress than patients with early-stage disease (Degner & Sloan 1995). Systematic investigation has found that intervention at later stages benefits the patient (e.g. Spiegel et al 1989). At the same time, data suggest that the same approaches that appear to work among late-stage patients are not necessarily effective with early-stage patients (e.g. Helgeson et al 2000).

Patient gender and age are also important because disease and treatment can affect gender identity and sexual functioning. For example, men diagnosed with testicular cancer experience a significant level of concern regarding future fertility and sexual functioning (Arai et al 1996). These issues may assume different meanings among older and younger men. Similarly, women diagnosed with ovarian cancer report distress regarding fertility functioning, and concerns about post-treatment sexuality characterize many cancers. Self-esteem issues, intertwined with body-image, are also a major problem area for women diagnosed with breast cancer (Rowland 1997). In addition, some cancer treatments can induce "premature" menopause, eliminating reproductive options and introducing new problems for the patient and her family.

INDIVIDUAL PSYCHOTHERAPY AND MENTAL HEALTH

When pre-emptive approaches to patient management do not prevent more serious disturbances, more traditional approaches are necessary. The psychological toll of cancer and its treatment often includes poor adjustment to the disease, expressed as depressed mood and an impoverished view of the patient's self and future. There is general agreement that mental health treatment can alleviate cancer-related psychological distress and improve overall quality of life for cancer patients (Andersen 1997).

A traditional mental health approach is warranted when the cancer patient presents with major psychopathology or maladaptive personality traits, especially when they interfere with case management of the patient. A past psychiatric history increases the likelihood of poorer adjustment to cancer (Stanton 1997). However, there is some debate about how common psychopathology is in a cancer patient population. Derogatis and colleagues (1983) conducted one of the first studies of the rate of psychopathology among cancer patients, reporting that approximately 50% of cancer patients carry a psychiatric disorder. The majority of the diagnoses were adjustment disorders (68%), followed by affective disorders (13%), organic mental disorders (8%), and anxiety disorders (4%). More recently, reports have suggested that psychopathology is not a modal response among cancer patients. For example, Van't Spijker et al (1997) found more depression among cancer patients but did not find differences in anxiety or distress between cancer patients and the general population. When major psychopathology does present, interventions are generally more symptom-oriented and based on providing immediate relief. In these instances, a traditional mental health approach usually replaces more preventive behavioral medicine approaches.

Mental health interventions can be particularly helpful when a patient uses denial as a coping strategy to the point that physical health is endangered. One of the major issues encountered in medical settings is use of denial or avoidance coping. Greer (1992) described three different ways that cancer patients may use denial, including complete denial, denial of the implications of the cancer diagnosis, and denial of affect. The frequency of this coping strategy is likely due to the reduction of psychological distress associated with its use. However, this is often a transient effect and when denial breaks down or people must finally confront the event, distress may be heightened (Collins et al 1983). Denial and avoidance can also frustrate health providers who become concerned that patients are not fully processing information provided by the treatment team, prompting them to refer the patient for psycho-social services. In instances in which denial is extreme, crisis intervention may be required.

Adjuvant psychological therapy (APT) represents one of the most common approaches used to treat cancer-related psychological disorders (Greer & Moorey 1997). APT has been described as a brief, problem-focused, cognitive-behavioral form of therapy. This approach is generally directed towards current problems lasting approximately six sessions, and often tries to involve the spouse or the partner of the patient. The goal of therapy is to help the patient focus on the personal meaning of the disease and the manner in which he or she copes with having cancer. Clinical trials have found this form of therapy to be particularly effective in reducing psychological distress for the patient (Greer & Moorey 1997). In one trial, patients receiving APT had significantly higher scores on fighting spirit and lower scores on measures of helplessness and anxiety than did control subjects who received no therapy (Greer et al 1992).

PREVENTION

Primary Prevention

Prevention is another important objective for behavioral medicine and mental health efforts. Primary prevention programs are tailored towards risk factors for disease. For example, smoking-cessation programs are frequently used to prevent the onset of cancers that are particularly vulnerable to the carcinogenic effects of smoking (e.g. lung cancer). This level of prevention is very effective in reducing the risk of disease onset for the general population as well as reducing the risk of disease recurrence among disease-free cancer patients. However, cessation of addictive or habitual behaviors is difficult and success rates are not very high.

Although addressing maladaptive health behaviors may reduce cancer morbidity, evidence suggests that some people are more at risk to develop cancer than are others. A primary example includes people with a heritable, family risk. During the past three decades, technology has led to the development of a number of screening procedures for detecting cancer. Recent advances such as the identification of the BRCA1 and BRCA2, two breast–ovarian cancer susceptibility genes, has enhanced our ability to identify individuals at risk for developing cancer. The value of this form of screening is predicated on the idea that identification of people at risk will lead to and encourage health-promoting behaviors to reduce the likelihood of cancer onset and/or better surveillance and early detection of disease. Appropriate surveillance (e.g. mammography, biopsy) can lead to early detection and better prognosis. The important roles for psychologists in risk identification programs and risk modification are readily apparent, see for example Baum et al (1997).

Prevention-Education of Health-Care Providers

A large part of prevention is education (Ivey 1980), with an important first step of educating medical practitioners about cancer risk factors. A recent study found that approximately one-third of physicians questioned were not aware that early detection was a significant strategy to reduce oral cancer deaths (Voelker 1996). Similarly, a study of a group of nurse practitioners found that approximately 78% were unaware that most breast cancers occur after age 60 and roughly half cited erroneous beliefs about risk factors that have not actually been linked to cancer (Tessaro et al 1996). Thus, making clinicians aware of risk factors and emphasizing the importance of conducting routine screening examinations is particularly important in cancer prevention (Voelker 1996). At the same time, increasing the frequency of routine inquiries about patients' preventive or surveillance behaviors should help (Wechsler et al 1983).

Another form of education is to conduct training for health-care providers in cancer prevention strategies. Such training could include facilitating conversations with patients about their health habits and advising patients of ways to improve those habits. A group of nurse practitioners in one study reported that they had little or no training in smoking cessation or discussing diet as a risk factor (Tessaro et al 1996). In another study, it was reported that physicians' lack of comfort discussing and facilitating treatment for alcohol problems kept them from inquiring about drinking behaviors in their patients (Israel et al 1996). When given a nonintrusive method for screening patients, however, 81% agreed to use that method (Israel et al 1996). Often, discussions about patients' alcohol use do not occur routinely (Pearson & Terry 1994), nor do discussions about diet and cancer (Soltesz et al 1995). Although lack of time is cited as one factor (Soltesz et al 1995), Wechsler et al (1983) noted that physicians and other medical staff may believe that they are not prepared to intervene to modify patients' behaviors or may not feel that their interventions will be helpful.

Secondary and tertiary prevention are more concerned with detecting disease in its earliest stages and preventing progression of already established disease. With varying rates across disease, early detection is associated with improved prognosis and a higher curative rate, and psychosocial research has focused particularly on the mechanisms that impede screening behavior (e.g. breast self-examination, mammography, routine physical examinations). Lerman et al (1991) reported that women with moderate levels of distress were more likely to practice breast self-examinations than women with either high or low levels of distress, suggesting that the optimal condition for adherence may require the experience of some distress. Further research is needed to develop interventions that will help to reduce overwhelming levels of distress that inhibit screening behavior. Research is also needed to address those who have a false sense of security that they are immune to disease.

PSYCHOLOGISTS' ROLES ON A MULTIDISCIPLINARY TEAM

Psychologists make many contributions in the oncology setting, addressing psycho-social issues that could affect medical treatment, working with other team members on developing patient care programs and evaluating these programs, addressing treatment compliance issues, supporting staff, and planning discharge recommenda-tions (Hunter et al 1997). Other duties include education, consulting on patient issues, conducting therapy as needed, and conducting research (Kagan et al 1988). At times, neuropsychologists provide cognitive and diagnostic assessment as well (Massie & Holland 1987). Educational issues can be particularly important and may include teaching the rest of the team about when and how to make referrals for psychological treatment and about advances in psychological treatment such as new relaxation or pain management techniques (Kagan et al 1988). This is important because mental health services are frequently under-used by physicians, often because of a lack of familiarity about the benefits of such services or because of stigma attached to mental health issues (Gobar et al 1987).

The psychologist typically has a substantial clinical role on these teams. Although the majority of cancer patients do not have or develop serious psychopathology, some psychological problems may appear and interventions at several points in the diagnostic and treatment process are important. If preventive interventions are not applied or fail to enhance adjustment, mental health consultations are more likely. Common reasons for referring medical patients for mental health services include affective disorders and suicidality, anxiety, adjustment problems, and behavior management issues (Feldmann 1987). The psychologist on a medical team can play a large role in evaluating patients with these problems and conducting time-limited individual or group therapy or behavioral medicine interventions such as stress management, pain management, smoking cessation, or biofeedback (Kagan et al 1988). Psychological intervention sometimes includes the family and may focus on coping with change in family structure or addressing grief issues. Finally, the psychologist can also make psychiatric referrals if warranted.

Having a mental health professional on a medical treatment team also allows for more timely and informal discussions about patient issues and can help remove the stigma associated with psychotherapy (Shapiro & Kornfeld 1987). It is important that the psychologist be present and available on the oncology unit to facilitate such discussions (Massie & Holland 1987). More formal consideration of all aspects of the patient's care can occur in multidisciplinary treatment team meetings (Masera et al 1998). The psychologist can also become involved in grand rounds or teaching rounds for medical students (Belar 1989; Massie & Holland 1987). Helping medical students become more aware of psychosocial aspects of the oncology patient can be done didactically or through a group discussion format, and can help the student feel greater comfort in working with seriously ill patients (Wise 1977).

STAFF SUPPORT

Psychologists are often called on to provide staff support, often with other members of their team. Education and advice about psychological techniques for managing patient behavior are helpful, but for a variety of reasons patients may not behave as recommended or desirable, due to poor communication between physician and patient, patients' lack of trust of their physician, or past experiences on the part of the patient and/or physician (DiMatteo 1997). A psychologist can be helpful in such situations by helping to identify the reasons for nonadherence. A consultation with a mental health practitioner is also appropriate for patients who are angry with the physician, fearful of treatment, who have psychological issues that stand in the way of medical treatment, or who are not responding (Beckman 1997).

A further form of staff support is working collaboratively with staff on specific issues of patient care, such as using psychological treatments for chemotherapy-related nausea or cancer pain (Massie & Holland 1987). Another example is working with patients who have relationship difficulties. Since cancer-related morbidity and quality of life may be affected by social support, physicians may need to assess the amount of support patients are receiving from significant others in their lives (Peteet & Greenberg 1995). If significant relationships are conflicted, the physician may be called upon to take action. Psychologists can support physicians in negotiating this with the patient and assist as needed, either through educating the physician on working with the patient or by seeing the patient and/or couple in therapy (Peteet & Greenberg 1995).

Increasingly, psychologists on multidisciplinary or interdisciplinary teams are called on to provide emotional support to other members and to help them deal with personally disturbing issues or events. At the same time, validation and discussion of their concerns and intuitions regarding patient care can sustain job satisfaction and job performance on the team. Psychologists can offer support to the medical team dealing with grief or stress issues (Kagan et al 1988; Stoter 1997). Such peer support can be helpful in preventing burnout by fostering a safe environment where feelings can be shared (Colon 1996; Eisendrath 1981). If staff members are stressed, a strained atmosphere may result and patients may not be cared for as carefully or empathetically as usual (Stoter 1997). Burnout on the oncology unit can come from several sources, including death and dying, bioethical issues, staff isolation, poor communications or management or identification with patients (Lederberg 1990; Ramirez et al 1995; Davidson & Foster 1995). Symptoms may include exhaustion, decreased empathy for patients, and a sense of decreased productivity (Ramirez et al 1995). Psychologist team members who recognize early signs of burnout can intervene to facilitate coping often by formal or informal peer group discussions or participation in patient treatment team meetings (Fawzy et al 1983). These discussions can be useful in solving practical or ethical issues and in helping the staff find meaning in patients' suffering (Lederberg 1990). Instrumental support can also be arranged through multidisciplinary meetings (Davidson & Foster 1995). Such interventions become important when one considers that the burnout rate for medical staff in oncology settings ranges from 47 to 66% (Colon 1996).

PSYCHIATRIC CARE OF CANCER PATIENTS

Psychiatric management of cancer patients typically involves some form of inpatient or outpatient intervention for patients who are experiencing significant distress. It overlaps considerably with screening and pre-emptive mental health interventions, and assumes several forms, including traditional consultation-liaison psychiatry, commonly consulted for inpatient adjustment problems.

Consultation-Liaison Psychiatry

The consultation-liaison psychiatrist addresses the interface of psychological and medical issues experienced by oncology patients, counseling the patient and working with the oncology team so that they may better understand the patient, family and their own feelings about a particular patient. Recommended treatments may include pharmacotherapy as well as psychotherapy. The psychiatrist's specialized knowledge of drug interactions and side-effects makes an essential contribution to the care and the well-being of the patient, as does overall control of distress and establishing better patient and family adjustment to the situation.

Psychiatric consultations are typically requested in both outpatient clinics and in the hospital. Outpatient evaluations are usually for patients who experience increasing symptoms of anxiety or depression which have become disabling and detrimental to their quality of life. On the other hand, an inpatient consult often follows an acute change in mental status. This frequently involves a delirium, psychosis or onset of severe depression.

CASE STUDY

Mrs S was a 40-year-old married women diagnosed with breast cancer. She had no significant past medical or psychiatry history but could be considered at high risk for adjustment problems due to the breast cancer. She had undergone a lumpectomy and had tolerated the surgery well. After two weeks of adjuvant therapy with the anti-estrogen drug tamoxifen, she called her oncologist in significant distress. The sudden onset of crying spells, lack of energy, hopelessness and otherwise unexplainable suicidal ideation was initially linked to the tamoxifen (the initiation of tamoxifen may include depressive symptoms). The oncologist discontinued the tamoxifen and the patient improved within two weeks. Although her mood had improved, the patient became fearful that the cancer would return if she did not continue with the medication. The oncologist agreed to another trial with tamoxifen. Shortly after re-starting the tamoxifen, Mrs S experienced a recurrence of depressive symptoms. At that time a psychiatrist was consulted.

On evaluation, Mrs S appeared anxious and exhibited persistent wringing of her hands through most of the interview. She was pleasant and cooperative and no neurological symptoms were apparent. She described her mood as being very anxious and she was upset about feeling so "down". She reported a depressed mood with sleep and appetite disturbances, hopelessness, no energy, significant guilt about not being able to care for her children and vague thoughts about "ending it all". Her affect was congruent with these thoughts. She denied active suicidal ideation but sometimes "wished it was over". There was no evidence of delusions or perceptual disturbances such as hallucinations. She recognized that the depression and anxiety appeared abruptly and necessitated further treatment.

TABLE 6.1   Recommended Treatment for Mrs S

1. Implement a safety plan: Active planning with the patient established a hierarchy of options and contacts Mrs S could utilize should she experience a worsening of her symptoms or have further suicidal ideation.
2. Check thyroid-stimulating hormone: An underactive or overactive thyroid can present with symptoms of depression or anxiety. Thyroid abnormalities may result from chemotherapy or radiation.
3. Begin antidepressant medication: In this case a family history revealed that the patient's father had become depressed following a myocardial infarction and fully recovered from depressive symptoms after being placed on sertraline (Zoloft), a selective serotonin re-uptake inhibitor. If one member of a family has a good response to an antidepressant, the success of a similar response in another family member is increased.
4. Consider further organic work-up: If the symptoms persisted or worsened despite intervention, further studies would be merited, such as a CAT scan of the head and/or other laboratory data.
5. Drug interactions: The patient was not on any other medications and there are no known adverse effects associated with the use of sertraline and tamoxifen. However, it is important for the patient and treatment team to be aware of other potential interactions and to consult with the psychiatrist should they have any concerns in the future.

Several recommendations for treating this patient were made (see Table 6.1), including additional screens for organic causes, pharmacotherapy, and implementation of a safety plan. The potential benefits and side-effects of antidepressant therapy were discussed with Mrs S. She began a course of sertraline (Zoloft) and bi-monthly therapy sessions. After two weeks, improvement was marked and she was able to continue tamoxifen therapy.

This case illustrates some of the complexities of mental health intervention with cancer patients. First, as with other medical patients experiencing distress, there are aspects of cancer treatment that can cause or contribute to symptoms of depression, anxiety, or distress. In this case tamoxifen, an effective chemoprevention agent, was implicated in the agitated depressive symptoms characterizing the patient. Some treatments may cause fatigue or other symptoms of anxiety or depression, and drug interactions are also likely. Second, the relative paucity of effective cancer treatments means that one cannot simply discontinue a treatment due to troublesome symptoms. In this case fears about recurrence of breast cancer may have been as debilitating as the initial symptoms associated with tamoxifen. The need to take into account the possibility of such complex causal interconnections makes psychiatric care of cancer patients difficult.

Evaluation of Mental Status

As suggested above, psychiatric evaluations are important because they address multiple potential etiologies of psychopathology and consider several different aspects of mental status. A number of criteria can be evaluated. Some of these are readily assessed, including a patient's appearance, including his or her hygiene, grooming, or abnormal movements. Mood should be assessed as well, including feelings associated with statements like, "I feel hopeless, why should I go on?" Here the patient may describe sleep and appetite disturbances, low energy, lack of interest (anhedonia), guilt or panic. Evaluation of affect describes the degree to which the patient's presentation is congruent with mood; for example; the patient may be tearful, irritable, or inappropriately euphoric.

Speech should also be assessed, including how slowly or rapidly the patient is talking. The patient may be talking very loudly and may be difficult to interrupt (pressured speech), or the volume may be very soft and seem to lack all energy. Perceptions, hallucinations, and thought content should be evaluated and tests for degree of alertness and orientation are frequently useful. One can ask the patient to introduce himself, describe where he or she is, and so on. A more formal exam can be useful where the patient is asked a standard battery of questions, engages in activities such as drawing and follows complex commands.

The mental status exam develops a differential diagnosis in conjunction with the history of present illness, past psychiatric history, family history and other collateral information. A depressed oncology patient may get the same medication whether the symptoms are primarily psychiatric or due to a medical condition. However, it is often helpful for the patient and family to understand the potential causes, different triggers that worsen or improve symptoms, and estimated length of treatment. For example, if a woman with breast cancer had a depressive episode during her initial diagnosis and later has a recurrence of the breast cancer, it is likely that she will again experience depressive symptoms (Helgeson et al 2000). For such a patient, early assessment and consideration of prophylactic treatment can be beneficial.

Whenever depressive symptoms are assessed, the issue of lethality should be discussed. There is an unfortunate misconstruction that asking about suicide might "put the idea into a patient's head". In the case of a suicidal patient, the thought is already there. Addressing the issue does not suggest suicide to the patient but allows for detection of a potentially serious condition. An actively suicidal patient with a distinct plan may be hospitalized. However, there may be less restrictive alternatives; together with the psychiatrist or other behavioral health professionals they may agree to outpatient treatment with an appropriate back-up plan. At such times psychiatric intervention can range from a detailed assessment to a brief telephone consultation and outpatient follow-up.

Psychiatric Emergencies

The most frequent psychiatric emergencies that the oncology team may encounter include suicidal or homicidal ideation/aggression, delirium, psychosis, and neuroleptic malignant syndrome. Suicidal ideation varies in degrees of treatment urgency based on additional risk factors. A patient with a specific plan (e.g. overdose on pain medications) is at considerable risk and one who has a more detailed plan (counting out the pills) is at still higher risk. Other risk factors include feeling hopeless, prior attempts, male gender, pain, and age over 45 for males or over 55 for females. The diagnosis of a potentially lethal medical illness is also a factor. Half of the men with cancer who commit suicide do so within the first year of diagnosis and 70% of all female oncology patients who commit suicide have a diagnosis of gynecologic or breast cancer (Kaplan et al 1994). When treating a suicidal patient, the case should be discussed with a mental health expert. Treatment options range from frequent outpatient appointments with a specific safety plan to voluntary or involuntary hospitalization for the actively suicidal patient.

Homicidal ideation or violent behavior reflects the patient's intent to injure or kill someone. Although it is less common than suicidal ideation in this population, the clinician has a legal obligation to address this dangerous situation immediately. An example would be an actively psychotic patient who has auditory command hallucinations to kill a particular individual. Mental health support is imperative, and issues involving patient safety and safety of the potential victim must rapidly be addressed.

Delirium is a waxing and waning of consciousness due to an organic disturbance. It is an unfortunate but frequent complication in the medically compromised patient, particularly post-operative patients and the chronically ill. Delirium causes confusion, agitation, hallucinations, paranoia, disorganization and sleep disturbances. Many terminally ill cancer patients exhibit symptoms of delirium (Massie et al 1983) and although delirium resulting from a drug reaction or infection may quickly resolve, delirium associated with a chronic illness such as cancer has a poor prognosis. In a study of delirium that merited a psychiatric consult, 25% of the patients died within six months of initial assessment (Trzepacz et al 1985).

Delirium usually has a rapid onset but it is unlikely that a patient will be able to alert the treatment team of subjective mental status changes. In cases where the delirium progresses over several hours or days, warning signs may include complaints about vivid nightmares, unusual concerns about medications or staff, mild paranoia and periods where the patient drifts from states of confusion to baseline alertness. This return to baseline can often lull family and staff into thinking that the episode has passed. Unfortunately this symptom defines delirium, and though quick examination may lead one to believe the patient is "cured", a longer, more detailed evaluation may unmask the delirium.

Treatment includes correcting organic causes when possible. Patients with delirium due to metastatic brain tumor or medication that cannot be discontinued require management focused on ensuring the patient's safety. For example, a steroid-induced delirium may be managed with antipsychotics when discontinuation of the steroid would further compromise the patient. Several antipsychotic medications are commonly used to treat the agitation, confusion and hallucinations associated with delirium. Haloperidol can be administered by mouth, injection or intravenously while benzodiazepines should be avoided as they can increase confusion and agitation. Close supervision should occur in a low stimulation environment.

The psychotic patient, whether due to delirium or a primary psychiatric disorder, presents a particular challenge to the treatment team. Illogical, disorganized thinking, paranoia and internal stimulation characterize psychosis. Antipsychotic medications are frequently helpful and psychiatric involvement is necessary. For example, Mrs A, a 42-year-old married woman who had had a hysterectomy for uterine cancer, was brought to the hospital because she was "scaring the children". For the past two days she had been mumbling to herself, rhyming nonsensical words and complaining that her real problem was low blood levels of vitamin C, not uterine cancer. In the emergency room she became combative. After a consultation with a psychiatrist an antipsychotic was administered intramuscularly. The patient, while still suspicious, allowed the treatment team to conduct a physical examination and collect blood and urine. Laboratory data revealed a urinary tract infection. After 36 hours of antibiotic therapy, the delirium cleared. The patient was maintained on an oral antipsychotic during that time. Her agitation and confusion diminished in parallel to resolution of the infection.

While rarely encountered in the oncology patient, neuroleptic malignant syndrome (NMS) is a true emergency. Defined by the triad of autonomic instability (fever, high blood pressure, increased heart rate, sweating), muscle rigidity and confusion, it is a potentially fatal reaction to antipsychotic medication. Emergency medical treatment involves stabilization of blood pressure and temperature. The antipsychotic is discontinued and the patient is placed on intravenous fluids to ensure adequate hydration. Medication management may include use of the muscle relaxant dantrolene and the dopamine agonist bromocriptine. Kidney function must be closely monitored due to potential nephrotoxicity from elevated creatinine levels.

PSYCHOPHARMACOLOGIC MANAGEMENT OF DISTRESS

Antidepressant medication, antipsychotics and stimulants are effective in alleviating distress in the oncology patient. The three most common groups of antidepressants are tricyclics, monoamine oxidase inhibitors and serotonin re-uptake inhibitors. Each group has unique side-effects. The serotonin or combination serotonin/ norepinephrine medications convey fewer high-risk effects than do other medications.

Tricyclics have long been the "gold standard" and are effective for symptoms of depression and anxiety. They have also been used to treat neurological pain. Although they are more commonly prescribed for neuropathic and chronic pain syndromes than for the oncology patient, the analgesic effects may be particularly useful. Untoward side-effects include cardiac arrhythmias, hypotension, weight gain and sedation. While cardiac arrhythmias are rare, the risk may increase in those already medically compromised (Glassman et al 1998).

Monoamine oxidase inhibitors (MAOIs) are also useful in treatment of anxiety and depression. However, the potential for a hypertensive crisis makes them less attractive in the patient taking multiple medications. When a MAOI is combined with certain tyramine-containing foods, beverages or medications, the resulting rapid increase in blood pressure can be lethal (Davidson et al 1984). This is particularly relevant to the oncology patient as a MAOI combined with pain medication, especially meperidine (Demerol), can precipitate such a crisis. As the chemotherapeutic agent procarbazine has MAOI characteristics, similar precautions must be taken. A patient on procarbazine should not be placed on an antidepressant without careful evaluation and close observation due to the hypertensive risk.

Serotonin re-uptake inhibitors (SSRIs) and the dual acting serotonin/norepinephrine antidepressants offer comparable efficacy without the cardiac risk. They are effective in both depression and anxiety. Common side-effects include nausea, headache, activation and sleep disturbance, typically subsiding after several days. As with the other antidepressants, drug interactions can occur. However, the risk is significantly less than with the MAOIs. This class of antidepressants provides the clinician with a variety of medications that are well tolerated, and efficacious. The serotonin/norepinephrine combination antidepressants such as mirtazapine (Remeron) and venlafaxine (Effexor) may be particularly effective for augmentation of pain control without some of the more hazardous cardiac side-effects associated with the tricyclic medications (Stimmel et al 1997).

Antipsychotics, especially those that can be administered in intramuscular and intravenous forms, are frequently used for the delirious hospitalized oncology patient. The consultation-liaison psychiatrist should work with the treatment team so that a safe and rapidly effective medication is promptly administered. High doses of haloperidol may be administered intravenously with minimal cardiac or extrapyramidal side-effects (Tesar et al 1985; Lerner et al 1979). Low-potency agents such as chlorpromazine have considerable risk of causing extrapyramidal side-effects. Parkinsonian movements, dystonias (sustained muscle contractions) and akathesias (intolerable subjective restlessness) usually occur early. Careful monitoring and rapid treatment are necessary.

Stimulants offer another choice for the depressed patient. They are not recommended in confused or agitated patients as they can exacerbate delirium. Stimulants can be used to treat three prominent problems in the oncology patient: depression, oversedation secondary to narcotics, and pain. The anti-depressant effects of stimulants are well documented, and they are efficacious and well tolerated in the medically ill. In one large report of patients that included diagnoses of laryngeal/ tracheal cancer, lung cancer, prostate and renal cancer, 82% of the patients showed improvement, most within the first two days of treatment (Masand et al 1991). The anti-sedative effect may be very beneficial for the patient on high doses of pain medications. This is especially meaningful for the patient who is not able to visit with family and friends due to excessive daytime sedation. Lastly, stimulants augment pain medications. While not a primary analgesic, stimulants appear to enhance narcotic pain control without intensifying sedation.

There are a variety of medications that are used to treat the multiple psychiatric illnesses that may be encountered while treating the cancer patient. The psychiatrist is able to make the diagnosis and initiate pharmacotherapy that then leads to clinically observable improvement. Use of the appropriate medication with a knowledge of potential drug interactions can improve the mental status of the patient, lessen family and staff distress, and allow the treatment team to pursue ongoing medical issues more effectively.

WORKING WITH ALLIED HEALTH PROFESSIONALS

The oncology patient with a psychiatric disorder does not suffer in isolation. These patients are often viewed as "difficult" by the treatment team. They may not want to get out of bed, may miss appointments, or may forget to take medications. In the case of psychosis or delirium, they may become agitated, combative, try to leave their hospital room or pull out catheters. A clear understanding of the psychiatric illness and assurance that the behavioral health team is closely involved in the case can greatly reduce the apprehension of the treatment team. Not only does the psychiatrist educate the team about a specific psychiatric illness and its manifestations but they also address the countertransference or feelings the treatment team experiences with regard to the "difficult" patient or towards the terminal patient to whom they have become attached. For example, a 40-year-old woman with breast cancer was hospitalized with a new seizure disorder. A psychiatrist was consulted after negative results from a full organic work-up. The psychiatric evaluation suggested a conversion disorder, a psychiatric condition that cannot be accounted for by another medical disorder. The conversion disorder patient does not intentionally produce his or her physical symptoms, and typically has little insight as to the cause. Ordinarily these disorders are associated with a stressful event, although the patient may not be able to recall the event.

In this particular case, the patient's mother had recently died of breast cancer that had metastasized to the brain. Once the treatment team began to understand that her "seizures" were a form of "controlling" a symptom the patient felt sure she would get, they were better able to deal with her situation. The staff was more receptive to learn about the patient's disorder and how they could respond to her more appropriately during these episodes.

ISSUES ASSOCIATED WITH PRACTICE IN AN ONCOLOGY SETTING

Psychologists and psychiatrists can and should be an integral part of multidisciplinary or interdisciplinary teams in oncology settings. In addition to the benefits for the patient, they can assist other members of the team in a variety of ways. Some of these include facilitating the integration of behavioral and medical approaches to health care, supporting the staff and medical team, and assisting primary physicians in cancer prevention activities. In short, "...a major advance has been our recent development of a greater appreciation of the value of interdisciplinary activity in patient management" (Lenhard et al 1995, pp 64–65). However, this integration of research, theory, and therapeutic approaches is not easy to achieve and should be considered in the context of several thorny issues.

Integrating the Medical and Behavioral Models

The traditional medical model assumes a disease perspective, as diagnosed illness leads to prescription of treatment and ultimately to a cure (Ivey 1980). It is fundamentally biological in nature; the physician analyzes physical signs, diagnoses a disease, and concentrates on treating the specific body part that is disordered (Barbour 1995). The patient as a whole becomes less important than the part of the patient that contains the disease. A limitation of the model is that it limits the scope of the problem such that other contributing issues are sometimes missed. The physician bears the responsibility for fixing the problem (Barbour 1995), and some modern approaches are more technology-centered than human centered (Webb 1996).

Traditional approaches to treating disease are limited in how they view the cause of a disease and the breadth of factors considered to support or maintain pathophysiology. While these models focus on biological courses of disease or dysfunction, behavioral models focus on the relationship between illness and behavioral or lifestyle factors, both in terms of disease prevention and coping with the aftermath of illness (Matarazzo 1980). This model takes a more holistic approach to the patient and integrates biological and psychological aspects of normal or disordered functioning (Pomerleau & Rodin 1986). Psychiatrists and psychologists view patients' behaviors in the face of disease as normal reactions to unusual circumstances. They attempt to build on the patients' strengths and help patients to conceptualize solutions from a developmental perspective (Kagan et al 1988). Empirically supported psychological or behavioral techniques are applied to medical issues (Pomerleau & Rodin 1986). The ultimate goal of this model is "...the promotion and maintenance of health, prevention and treatment of illness, and identification of etiologic and diagnostic correlates of health, illness, and related dysfunction..." (Pomerleau & Rodin 1986, p 485).

The medical and psychological models are probably best integrated by working collaboratively in clinical settings. One example is in the area of cancer pain management. Cancer pain clearly has a biological basis. It also has psychological sequelae that may exacerbate it, such as fear of unremitting pain that causes the patient to focus more on the pain and thus attend to it more often or experience it more severely. Integrated pain management should address both issues, through the development of multidisciplinary treatment protocols. Pharmacotherapy or medical intervention is usually the most effective initial treatment applied to reduce the pain, but use of behavioral methods may achieve comparable relief with fewer side-effects and at lower cost. Together, these approaches should achieve superior pain control at less cost and with fewer complications (e.g. Friedman et al 1995).

Ultimately, "Achieving health depends on . . . collaboration. The emphasis has shifted from the doctor fixing what has gone wrong to what the patient needs to do for himself or herself" (Barbour 1995, p 33). Each model makes its own unique contributions, and integrating the models provides patients with more comprehensive care that addresses the medical illness and its resulting sequelae. Adoption of a biopsychosocial model that integrates all aspects of patient care may be the preferred approach (Matarazzo 1980).

BEHAVIORAL MEDICINE INTERVENTIONS WITH PALLIATIVE CARE CANCER PATIENTS

Palliative care refers to medical care that has patient comfort and quality of life as its primary goal, typically involving patients with advanced cancer that no longer responds to curative treatments. "Hospice" and "palliative care" are often used interchangeably, but palliative care subsumes hospice in both a time context and a treatment context. Hospice care is usually used during the last six months of life, whereas palliative care can last for many months or years. Also, hospice services usually do not include palliative radiation or chemotherapy treatments aimed at reducing patient pain, but a palliative care model does.

Palliative care teams typically include medicine, psychology, psychiatry, social work, nursing, pastoral care, and pharmacology, and these teams can work in a hospital setting or in a home-care setting. Each discipline shares the goal of optimizing patient comfort, but each has its own objectives and approaches to achieving this goal. In providing patient care, the palliative care team relies on an interdisciplinary model where all disciplines enjoy equal status, and no single discipline spearheads all cases. Rather, the patient's presenting problem defines which team members will be most involved in providing care, and the combination of disciplines can change from one case to another. Therefore, the psychologist in palliative care can anticipate working with different disciplines, depending on the referral reason.

The importance of palliative care is reflected in the rapid medical advances and changes in the provision of health care services that characterize our time. Medical technology has extended the survival of advanced cancer patients, but these scientific advances frequently have a negative effect on patient quality of life. For example, palliative radiation and chemotherapy can have a deleterious effect on a patient's energy level, appetite, and mood. Furthermore, the current trend in health care is to decrease the length of hospital stays and provide more of the medical care in the home. Palliative care services are designed to train patients and families about quality-of-life issues, including symptom management, and psychology offers several areas of expertise that can facilitate the obtainment of patient comfort.

Common Problems and Interventions in Palliative Care

Pain is a common symptom of advanced cancer, and over 75% of patients referred to inpatient palliative care services had pain as one of their presenting problems (Ellershaw et al 1995; Weissman & Griffie 1994). The experience of pain has a negative effect on patient quality of life and can impair psychological well-being by inducing anxiety and depression as well as interfering with social interactions (Paice 1996). The palliative care team addresses the physical as well as the psychosocial aspects of patient cancer pain, seeking to minimize patient pain while optimizing patient mental status and alertness. Frequently, nursing assesses patient pain, including the patient's openness toward behavioral pain management techniques, and may begin to offer assistance. From the assessment, the palliative care team identifies a viable treatment protocol that includes a pain medication regimen and a behavioral pain management program implemented by the psychologist. The team monitors the success of the intervention and makes adjustments as needed to ensure optimal quality of life for the patient.

Managed care and escalating health costs have caused hospitals to discharge patients "quicker and sicker", and an increasing number of terminally ill cancer patients receive their medical care at home (Croft et al 1997). Although home health-care services reduce the overall patient health-care costs, when compared to traditional hospital care, home health care places more of the care burden on family members (Robinson & Pham 1996). Research on family caregivers of advanced cancer patients found that only 15% felt that they coped adequately with their caregiving role (Barg et al 1995). Inadequate coping has been consistently linked with psychological distress in family caregivers (Haley et al 1987; Pruchno & Resch 1989), and strain among family caregivers of cancer patients has been associated with more extensive physical and psychological problems during bereavement (Beery et al 1997; Kurtz et al 1997). Stress and coping interventions with caregivers of Alzheimer's patients have been successful (Lovett & Gallagher 1988), and preliminary studies with cancer caregivers suggest that psychoeducational interventions generalize to caregivers of the terminally ill (Ferrell et al 1995; Toseland et al 1995).

Palliative care is broadly focused, and the palliative care team treats the caregiver and family as well as the patient, identifying sources of caregiving stress (e.g. lack of knowledge regarding patient care, lack of community resources that provide respite/support, family conflict, etc.), and suggesting coping strategy interventions. Frequently, psychology intervenes in tandem with nursing and social work to facilitate the success of the intervention. For example, psychologists' expertise in human learning can enhance nursing's training the family in patient care, and psychologists' understanding of family systems can enhance social work's interventions aimed at decreasing family conflict by increasing support from the community.

The following case provides an example of how behavioral medicine addresses patient pain and depressive symptomatology in palliative care settings.

CASE HISTORY

Mr E was a 73-year-old white married male whose renal cancer had metastasized to his spine, femur, and lungs. He was admitted to the hospital with severe back pain, and his attending physician consulted the palliative care service to assist in (1) managing the patient's pain, and (2) discussing hospice/home care options. Palliative care assessment of the patient indicated the need for medicine, nursing, and behavioral medicine involvement for pain management and family discussions regarding home-care concerns.

The behavioral medicine interventions complemented nursing and medicine's treatment plans for Mr E. The palliative care physician developed a pharmacological treatment regimen for Mr E's pain and the palliative care nurse trained the patient and his wife on the use of pain medications. Behavioral medicine helped Mr E identify a relaxation exercise that fit his personal style (he frequently prayed the Rosary, so this activity was used for the intervention). The behavioral medicine psychologist reviewed the medical pain management regimen with Mr E and his wife and then trained the couple to use relaxation exercises (i.e. pray the Rosary) immediately after the patient takes medication for breakthrough pain.

It became apparent that Mr E and his wife could not talk about discharge plans/home care because such conversations made them painfully aware of his dying. The palliative care nurse and behavioral medicine psychologist worked in tandem with the couple on discharge planning. The psychologist assisted the couple in reframing hope: the couple could no longer hope for a cure, but they could identify their hopes for today. Bringing the couple into the "present" allowed them to establish concrete, obtainable goals (e.g. we want to watch a movie together, we want to have our children over for dinner, we want to watch one of our grandchild's Little League games) that promoted their togetherness as opposed to their separation by death. Subsequently, the palliative care nurse was able to approach Mr E and his wife about discharge plans and home-care needs.

Psychological Distress

The prevalence of major depression among terminally ill cancer patients ranges from 25 to 60%, but fewer than 5% of patients receive treatment for their depression (Breitbart et al 1995). Considering the findings that spouses' levels of psychological distress parallel those of the patients (Cassileth et al 1985; Ell et al 1988), one can easily see the need for the palliative care team to address psychological distress within the family system.

All team members become involved when a patient or spouse has clinically significant psychopathology, but psychology or psychiatry plays a central role in the evaluation and treatment of mental disorders. Medicine, psychiatry, and pharmacology provide expertise in the pharmacological treatment of these disorders in cancer patients, particularly when considering that some of the side-effects from advanced cancer (e.g. fatigue, sleep disturbance, neuropathic pain) respond well to certain types of antidepressants (Hill 1994). Social work addresses social resource deficits that frequently accompany depression, and pastoral care facilitates the continuance of hope via spirituality and religion. Nursing monitors the interaction between psychological distress and patient care issues in order to identify areas where the psychopathology interferes with adequate medical care (e.g. patient's depression creates noncompliance with the treatment plan, spouse's depression interferes with appropriate patient care).

Grief and Bereavement

The grieving process begins with the acceptance of a poor cancer prognosis, and for this reason patients and families will try to deny the lethality of the illness for as long as possible. Denial is further perpetuated by the family and patient's need to maintain hope that a cure will be found. Frequently, family members will suggest that, "if we don't have hope, what else do we have to hang onto?"; however, as the patient becomes sicker and exhibits profound functioning deficits, hope begins to wane, and the family system moves toward the grieving process.

When families recognize that curative therapy is no longer viable, they describe intolerable feelings such as, "the rug has been pulled out from under us", or "our world has been shattered". Their distress is further exacerbated by feeling grief for someone who is still alive and sitting right next to them! Assisting the patient and family with the grief process begins with the reframing of "hope"; although cure is unlikely, the patient and family can still hope for the day-to-day maintenance of the patient's quality of life. The social worker or psychologist facilitates a conversation with the family and patient about their short-term hopes.

Among these shorter-term goals, family and patients tend to want: (1) patient comfort, (2) maintenance of normal family patterns (e.g. if the family always shared Sunday dinner together, then continue that tradition), and (3) minimization of family members' caregiving burden. Palliative care teams specialize in managing patient symptoms (e.g. pain, hydration, shortness of breath) as well as helping families maintain a sense of continuity during the end-of-life process. The medical team members assist the family manage patient symptoms and the psychosocial team members help the family identify specific areas of functioning that will maintain continuity and minimize caregiver burden.

Most bereavement reactions fall within the normal range where the bereaved individual experiences sadness and loss but rarely feels hopeless, guilty, worthless or suicidal. In these cases, social work and pastoral care provide supportive counseling as well as access to community resources that will help the bereaved cope with their loss. Complicated or traumatic grief, on the other hand, occurs less frequently, but is associated with deleterious physical and psychological outcomes (Prigerson et al 1997). People experiencing complicated grief report intrusive thoughts about the deceased and pining for their loved one which can include searching or believing to see the deceased in a crowd of people. People with complicated grief tend to feel upset when confronted with reminders of their loved one, and the condition can last for over a year. Psychiatry and psychology contribute to management of complicated grief cases by incorporating techniques used in bereavement therapy as well as Post Traumatic Stress Disorder therapies.

Thirty years ago, terminally ill patients usually died in the hospital while family members passively watched physicians and nurses provide patient care. Now, the majority of cancer patients die at home under the care of their families. Although patients prefer to die at home, their medical care places a burden on the family that can in turn compromise caregiver and patient quality of life. Palliative care teams have developed in response to the changes in our health-care system, and the palliative care specialist plays an integral role in addressing psychosocial and behavioral symptom management issues. The success of behavioral and psychopharmacologic interventions relies heavily on the collaborative efforts of other team members, and it is through an interdisciplinary approach that the palliative care team helps families maintain patient quality of life and minimize caregiving strain.

CONCLUSIONS

The palliative care model described above is an excellent example of the benefits of newer medical environments and emphases that are characterized by integrated behavioral and medical care accomplished by interdisciplinary treatment teams. The activity of psychologists and psychiatrists in these settings is key to the success of these teams. Their success in extremely difficult situations offers considerable hope and promise for the care of cancer patients at all stages of their disease. Research strongly supports the notion that behaviors, emotional states, and other psychosocial processes are important factors in the etiology and progression of cancer and in patient and family quality of life. Successful integration of psychological and psychiatric approaches in a coherent behavioral medicine that addresses and anticipates adjustment problems while working in a multidisciplinary context will continue to advance our understanding of and care for cancer patients.

REFERENCES

Amunni G, Villanucci A, Tavella K, Veneziano AF, Boddi V, Susini T and Massi GB: The "age factor" in ovarian cancer. Clinical, therapeutic and prognostic aspects. *Minerva Medica* **89**(3): 65–75, 1998.

Andersen B: Psychological interventions for cancer patients to enhance the quality of life. *J Consult Clin Psychol* **60**: 542–568, 1992.

Andersen B: Breast Cancer: Biobehavioral aspects. In E.A Blechman and KD Brownell (Eds), *Behavioral Medicine and Women*. Guilford Press: New York, 1997.

Andersen BL, Kiecolt-Glaser JK and Glaser R: A biobehavioral model of cancer stress and disease course. *Am Psychologist* **49**: 389–404, 1994.

Arai Y, Kawakita M, Hida S, Terachi T, Okada Y and Yoshida O: Psychosocial aspects in long-term survivors of testicular cancer. *J Urol* **155**: 574–578, 1996.

Bal DG, Nixon DW, Foerster SB and Brownson RC: Cancer prevention. In GP Murphy, W Lawrence and RE Lenhard (Eds), *American Cancer Society Textbook of Clinical Oncology, Second Edition*. American Cancer Society: Washington, DC, 1995.

Barbour AB: *Caring for Patients*. Stanford University Press: Stanford, CA, 1995.

Barg FK, Pasacreta J and Freeman T: Development, implementation and evaluation of a cancer family caregiver education program. (Meeting Abstract). *Tenth National Conference on Chronic Disease Prevention and Control, December 1995*: Atlanta, GA, 1995.

Baum A and Cohen L: Successful behavioral interventions to prevent cancer—the example of skin cancer (Review). *Ann Rev Public Health* **19**: 319–333, 1998.

Baum A and Posluszny DM: Health psychology: mapping biobehavioral contributions to health and illness (Review). *Ann Rev Psychol* **50**: 137–163, 1999.

Baum A, Friedman AL and Zakowski SG: Stress and genetic testing for disease risk. *Health Psychol* **16**: 8–19, 1997.

Beckman HB: Difficult patients. In MD Feldman and JF Christensen (Eds), *Behavioral Medicine in Primary Care*. Appleton and Lange: Stamford, CT, 1997.

Beery LC, Prigerson HG, Bierhals AJ, Santucci LM, Newsom JT, Maciejewski PK, Rapp SR, Fasiczka A and Reynolds CF: Traumatic grief, depression and caregiving in elderly spouses of the terminally ill. *Omega* **35**: 261–279, 1997.

Belar CD: Opportunities for psychologists in health maintenance organizations: Implications for graduate education and training. *Professional Psychology: Research and Practice* **20**: 390–394, 1989.

Belar CD: Collaboration in capitated care: Challenges for psychology. *Professional Psychology: Research and Practice* **26**: 139–146, 1995.

Belar CD: Clinical health psychology: A specialty for the 21st century. *Health Psychol* **16**: 411–416, 1997.

Bender KJ: A dual-action antidepressant. *Psychiatric Times, Suppl*: 6–12, 1997.

Breitbart W, Bruera E, Chochinov H and Lynch M: Neuropsychiatric syndromes and psychological symptoms in patients with advanced cancer. *J Pain Symptom Management* **10**: 131–141, 1995.

Cassileth BR, Lusk EJ, Strouse TB, Miller DS, Brown LL and Cross PA: A psychological analysis of cancer patients and their next-of-kin. *Cancer* **55**: 72–76, 1985.

Collins DL, Baum A and Singer JE: Coping with chronic stress at Three Mile Island: psychological and biochemical evidence. *Health Psychology* **2**: 149–166, 1983.

Colon K: Running on empty. *Minnesota Medicine* **79**(4): 12–20, 1996.

Croft JB, Giles WH, Pollard RA, Caspar ML, Andra RF and Livengood JR: National trends in the initial hospitalization for heart failure. *J Am Geriat Soc* **45**: 270–275, 1997.

Davidson J, Zung W and Walker J: Practical aspects of MAO inhibitor therapy. *J Clin Psychiatry* **45**: 81–84, 1984.

Davidson KW and Foster Z: Social work with dying and bereaved clients: Helping the workers. *Social Work in Health Care* **21**(4): 1–16, 1995.

Degner LF and Sloan JA: Symptom distress in newly diagnosed ambulatory cancer patients and as a predictor of survival in lung cancer. *J Pain Symptom Management* **10**: 423–431, 1995.

Derogatis LR, Marrow GR, Fetting J, Penman D, Piasetsky S, Schmale AM, Henrichs M and Carnicke CL: The prevalence of psychiatric disorders among cancer patients. *JAMA* **249**: 751–757, 1983.

DiMatteo MR: Adherence. In MD Feldman and JF Christensen (Eds), *Behavioral Medicine in Primary Care*. Appleton and Lange: Stamford, CT, 1997.

Eisendrath SJ: Psychiatric liaison support groups for general hospital staffs. *Psychosomatics* **22**: 685–694, 1981.

Ell K, Nishimoto R, Mantell J and Hamovitch M: Longitudinal analysis of psychological adaptation among family members of patients with cancer. *J Psychosom Res* **32**: 429–438, 1988.

Ellershaw JE, Peats SJ and Boys LC: Assessing the effectiveness of a hospital palliative care team. *Palliative Med* **9**: 145–152, 1995.

Fawzy FI, Wellisch DK, Pasnau RO and Leibowitz B: Preventing nursing burnout: A challenge for liaison psychiatry. *Gen Hosp Psychiatry* **5**: 141–149, 1983.

Feldmann TB: Patterns of referral for psychiatric consultation at a VA medical center. *Hosp Commun Psychiatry* **38**: 525–527, 1987.

Ferrell BR, Grant M, Chan J, Ahn C and Ferrell BA: The impact of cancer pain education on family caregivers of elderly patients. *Oncology Nursing Forum* **22**: 1211–1218, 1995.

Friedman R, Sobel D, Myers P, Caudill M and Benson H: Behavioral medicine, clinical health psychology, and cost offset. *Health Psychol* **14**: 509–518, 1995.

Gerlach RW: Cancer prevention: what the physician can do. *Cleveland Clin J Med* **62**: 184–192, 1995.

Glassman AH, Rodriquez AI and Shapiro PA: The use of antidepressant drugs in patients with heart disease. *J Clin Psychiatry* **5**: Suppl. 16–21, 1998.

Gobar AH, Collins JL and Mathura CB: Utilization of a consultation liaison psychiatry service in a general hospital. *J Nat Med Assoc* **79**: 505–508, 1987.

Gordon NP, Rundall TG and Parker L: Type of health care coverage and the likelihood of being screened for cancer. *Med Care* **36**: 636–645, 1998.

Greer S: The management of denial in cancer patients. *Oncology* **6**(12): 33–36, 1992.

Greer S and Moorey S: Adjuvant psychological therapy for cancer patients. *Palliative Med* **11**: 240–244, 1997.

Greer S, Moorey S, Baruch JD, Watson M, Robertson BM, Mason A, Rowden L, Law MG and Bliss JM: Adjuvant psychological therapy for patients with cancer: a prospective randomized trial. *BMJ* **304**(6828): 675–680, 1992.

Haley WE, Levine EG, Brown SL and Bartolucci AA: Stress, appraisal, coping, and social support as predictors of adaptational outcome among dementi caregivers. *Psychol Aging* **2**: 323–330, 1987.

Helgeson VS and Cohen S. Social support and adjustment to cancer-reconciling descriptive, correlational, and intervention research (Review). *Health Psychol* **15**: 135–148, 1996.

Helgeson VS, Cohen S, Schulz R and Yasko J: Group support interventions for women with breast cancer: who benefits from what? *Health Psychology* **19**: 107–114, 2000.

Hill CS: Effective treatment of pain in the cancer patient. In GP Murphy, W Lawrence and RE Lenhard (Eds) *The American Cancer Society Textbook of Clinical Oncology*. American Cancer Society: Atlanta, GA, 1994.

Hunter SM, Larrieu JA, Ayad FM, O'Leary JP, Griffies WS, Deblanc CH and Martin LF: Roles of mental health professionals in multidisciplinary medically supervised treatment programs for obesity. *S Med J* **90**: 578–586, 1997.

Israel Y, Hollander O, Sanchez-Craig M, Booker S, Miller V, Gingrich R and Rankin JG: Screening for problem drinking and counseling by the primary care physician-nurse team. *Alcoholism Clin Exp Res* **20**: 1443–1450, 1996.

Ivey AE: Counseling psychology, the psychoeducation model and the future. In JM Whiteley (Ed), *The History of Counseling Psychology*, pp 196–204. Brooks/Cole Publishers: Monterey, CA, 1980.

Jenkins PL, May VE and Hughes LE: Psychological morbidity associated with local recurrence of breast cancer. *Int J Psychiatry Med* **21**: 149–155, 1991.

Kagan N, Armsworth MW, Altmaier EM, Dowd ET, Hansen JIC, Mills DH, Schlossberg N, Sprinthall NA, Tanney MF and Vasquez MJT: Professional practice of counseling psychology in various settings. *The Counseling Psychologist* **16**: 347–365, 1988.

Kaplan HI, Sadock BJ and Grebb JA: Psychiatric emergencies. In *Kaplan and Sadock's Synopsis of Psychiatry*, 7th edn, p 804. Williams & Wilkins: Baltimore, MD, 1994.

Kurtz ME, Kurtz JC, Given CW and Given B: Predictors of post bereavement depressive symptomatology among family caregivers of cancer patients. *Supp Care Cancer* **5**: 53–60, 1997.

Lederberg M: Psychological problems of staff and their management. In JC Holland and JH Rowland (Eds), *Handbook of Psychooncology*. Oxford University Press: New York, 1990.

Lemkau JP, Grady K and Carlson S: Maximizing the referral of older women for screening mammography. *Arch Fam Med* **5**: 174–178, 1996.

Lenhard RE, Lawrence W and McKenna RJ: General approach to the patient. In GP Murphy, W Lawrence and RE Lenhard (Eds), *American Cancer Society Textbook of Clinical Oncology, Second Edition*. American Cancer Society: Washington, DC, 1995.

Lerman C, Trock B, Rimer BK, Jepson C, Brody D and Boyce A: Psychological side effects of breast cancer screening. *Health Psychol* **10**: 259–267, 1991.

Lerner Y, Lwow E, Levitan A and Belmaker RH: Acute high dose parental haloperidol treatment of psychosis. *Am J Psychiatry* **136**: 1061–1064, 1979.

Lovett S and Gallagher D: Psychoeducational interventions for family caregivers: preliminary efficacy data. *Behav Ther* **19**: 321–330, 1988.

Masand P, Pickett P and Murray GB: Psychostimulants for secondary depression in medical illness. *Psychosomatics* **32**: 203–208, 1991.

Masera G, Spinetta JJ, Jankovic M, Ablin AR, Buchwall I, Dongen-Melman JV, Eden T, Epelman C, Green DM, Kosmidis HV, Yoheved S, Martins AG, Mor W, Oppenheim D, Petrilli AS, Schuler D, Topf R, Wilbur JR and Chesler MA: Guidelines for a therapeutic alliance between families and staff: A report of the SIOP working committee on psychosocial issues in pediatric oncology. *Med Pediatr Oncol* **30**: 183–186, 1998.

Massie MJ and Holland JC: Consultation and liaison issues in cancer care. *Psychiatr Med* **5**: 343–359, 1987.

Massie M, Holland J and Glass E: Delirium in terminally ill cancer patients. *Am J Psychiatry* **140**: 1048–1050, 1983.

Matarazzo JD: Behavioral health and behavioral medicine. *Am Psychol* **35**: 807–817, 1980.

Meyer TJ and Mark MM: Effects of psychosocial interventions with adult cancer patients: a meta-analysis of randomized experiments. *Health Psychol* **40**: 517–528, 1995.

Paice JA: Pain. In SL Groenwald, MH Hanson, M Goodman and CH Yarbro (Eds), *Cancer Symptoms and Management*. Jones and Bartlett Publishers: Boston, MD, 1996.

Pearson TA and Terry P: What to advise patients about drinking alcohol. *JAMA* **272**: 967–968, 1994.

Peteet J and Greenberg B: Marital crises in oncology patients. *Gen Hosp Psychiatry* **17**: 201–207, 1995.

Pomerleau OF and Rodin J: Behavioral medicine and health psychology. In SL Garfield and AE Bergin (Eds), *Handbook of Psychotherapy and Behavior Change*, pp 483–522. John Wiley & Sons: New York, 1986.

Prigerson HG, Bierhals AJ, Reynolds CF, Shear MK, Day N, Beery LC, Newsom JT and Jacobs S: Traumatic grief as a risk factor for mental and physical morbidity. *Am J Psychiatry* **154**: 616–623, 1997.

Pruchno RA and Resch N: Mental health of caregiving spouses: Coping as mediator, moderator, or main effect? *Psychol Aging* **4**: 454–463, 1989.

Ramirez AJ, Graham J, Richards MA, Cull A, Gregory WM, Leaning MS, Snashall DC and Timothy AR: Burnout and psychiatric disorder among cancer clinicians. *Br J Cancer* **71**: 1263–1269, 1995.

Rimer BK: Toward an improved behavioral medicine. *Ann Behav Med* **19**: 6–10, 1997.

Robinson BE and Pham H: Cost-effectiveness of hospice care. *Clin Geriat Med* **12**: 417–428, 1996.

Roche AM and Richard GP: Doctors' willingness to intervene in patients' drug and alcohol problems. *Soc Sci Med* **33**: 1053–1061, 1991.

Rowland JH: Breast cancer: Psychosocial aspects. In EA Blechman and KD Brownell (Eds), *Behavioral Medicine and Women*. Guilford Press: New York, 1997.

Shapiro PA and Kornfeld DS: Psychiatric aspects of head and neck surgery. *Consultation Liaison Psychiatry* **10**: 87–100, 1987.

Soltesz K, Johnson LW, Price JH and Telijohann SK: Perceptions and practices of family physicians regarding diet and cancer. *Am J Prevent Med* **11**: 197–204, 1995.

Spiegel D, Bloom JR, Kraemer HC and Gottheil E: Effect of psychosocial treatment on survival of patients with metastatic breast cancer. *Lancet* **ii** (8668): 888–891, 1989.

Stanton AL: Cancer: Behavioral and psychosocial aspects. In E.A Blechman and KD Brownell (Eds), *Behavioral Medicine and Women*. Guilford Press: New York, 1997.

Stanton AL and Snider PR: Coping with a breast cancer diagnosis: a prospective study. *Health Psychol* **12**: 16–23, 1993.

Stimmel GL, Sussman N and Wingard P: Mirtazapine safety and tolerability: analysis of the clinical trials database. *Primary Psychiatry* 82–90, 1997.

Stoter DJ: *Social Support in Health Care*. Blackwell Science Publishers: Malden, MA, 1997.

Tesar GE, Murray GB and Cassem NH: Use of high dose intravenous haloperidol in the treatment of agitated cardiac patients. *J Clin Psychopharmacol* **5**: 344–347, 1985.

Tessaro IA, Herman CJ, Shaw JE and Giese EA: Cancer prevention knowledge, attitudes, and clinical practice of nurse practitioners in local public health departments in North Carolina. *Cancer Nursing* **19**: 269–274, 1996.

Toseland RW, Blanchard CG and McCallion P: A problem-solving intervention for caregivers of cancer patients. *Soc Sci Med* **40**: 517–528, 1995.

Trzepacz PT, Teague GB and Lipowski ZJ: Delirium and other organic mental disorders in a general hospital. *Gen Hosp Psychiatry* **7**: 101–106, 1985.

Van Wersch A, Bonnema J, Prinsen B, Pruyn J, Wiggers T and Van Geel AN: Continuity of information in cancer care: evaluation of a logbook. *Patient Education and Counseling* **30**: 175–186, 1997.

Van't Spijker A, Trijsburg RW and Duivenvoorden HJ: Psychological sequelae of cancer diagnosis: a meta-analytical review of 58 studies after 1980. *Psychosom Med* **59**: 280–293, 1997.

Voelker R: New strategies to fight oral cancer. *JAMA* **276**: 1121, 1996.

Webb C: Caring, curing, coping: towards an integrated model. *J Adv Nursing* **23**: 960–968, 1996.

Wechsler H, Levine S, Idelson RK, Rohman M and Taylor JO: The physician's role in health promotion—a survey of primary-care practitioners. *N Engl J Med* **308**: 97–100, 1983.

Weissman D and Griffie J: The palliative care consultation service of the Medical College of Wisconsin. *J Pain Symptom Management* **9**: 474–479, 1994.

Wise TN: Training oncology fellows in psychological aspects of their specialty. *Cancer* **39**: 2584–2587, 1977.

Psychological Management of Chronic Illness and Disability

Paul Kennedy
Warneford Hospital, Oxford, England
Mal Hopwood
Austin & Repatriation Medical Centre, Heidelberg West, Australia

and

Jane Duff
Stoke Mandeville Hospital, Aylesbury, England

INTRODUCTION

In the move into the new millennium there will be many changes in the nature and structure of society; with these changes will also come changes in the illnesses and disabilities that are experienced. Chronic illnesses and disabilities will become more common experiences in the lives of many individuals. Living longer does not necessarily mean living better. At the beginning of the last century, infectious diseases dominated the health lives of individuals, but now there are many chronic health conditions that have a significant impact on individuals' physical, psychological and social functioning. Some of these conditions may be congenital, such as spina bifida, or acquired in adolescence, adulthood or old age. Some are discrete events, such as traumatic injury resulting in amputation, brain injury or spinal cord injury, or may be associated with a progressive deteriorating condition such as rheumatoid arthritis, multiple sclerosis or Parkinson's disease. The types of disabilities that these chronic conditions cause are varied and can include problems with locomotion and mobility, with reaching and stretching, with ability to perform personal care, or associated with continence, behavioural impairment, and/or cognitive deterioration.

Estimates of the prevalence of disability vary. Eisenberg et al (1993) estimated that there were 35 million Americans with some form of chronic illness or disability.

Psychology and Psychiatry: Integrating Medical Practice.
Edited by J. Milgrom and G. D. Burrows © 2001 John Wiley & Sons, Ltd.

The Office of Population Census and Surveys (OPCS 1988) estimates that there are over six million adults with one or more disabilities in the United Kingdom (out of a population of 58 million). In the United Kingdom, the prevalence of severe disability remains stable until the age of 60 and from then there is a considerable increase in the prevalence, severity and range. Eisenberg et al (1993) estimated that a typical American will spend twelve years of their life in a state of limited functioning because of both acute and chronic medical conditions. Brain injury and spinal cord injury, whilst accounting for a small percentage of those with disabilities, make up a significant proportion of those spending a long period of life with the condition. Because of the early onset (in young adult-hood) and decreased mortality, years of life living with the disability are considerable.

The Clinical Context of Rehabilitation and Disability

There are many definitions of rehabilitation. It is generally defined as a process of active change by which a person who has become disabled acquires the knowledge and skills needed for optimum physical, psychological and social functioning. Physical rehabilitation refers to the application of all measures aimed at reducing the impact of disabling and handicapping conditions and enabling the person with a disability to achieve maximal social integration. Interventions generally aim to improve the independence of the person and enhance their quality of life. Physical rehabilitation is a complex process which occurs across the acute and chronic phases of disease and disability and often occurs alongside complex issues which possess multiple co-morbidity. The focus of physical rehabilitation in the past 100 years has moved from a focus of dealing with the physical impairment, through functional disabilities, and now includes a more comprehensive concern for the person as a whole. Arokiasamy (1993) defines the essence of rehabilitation as a blending of caring with elements of science or technique. The World Health Organisation's (WHO 1980) taxonomy of Impairment, Disability and Handicap provides a framework for understanding the needs of disabled people. Other researchers have attempted to extend the capacity of this model's ability to predict outcome by including illness cognition variables (Johnson 1996) and social functioning and quality of life issues (Whiteneck et al 1992a, b).

When discussing the psychological management of chronic illness and disability, it is important to recognize that the experience of disability is not solely a condition of the individual. From the perspective of the disabled person, the negative experience of disability, such as architectural inaccessibility and social exclusion, are physical and social creations in a society geared by, and for, able-bodied people. Furthermore, in addition to these external physical and social factors, which influence the experience of disability, it is also important to understand that biological factors (such as functional impairments, pathology and disease) are predictors of poor quality of life.

Renal Failure, Spinal Cord Injuries and Traumatic Brain Injury

To examine psychological factors associated with adjustment, impact and treatment in chronic illness and disability, we have chosen three areas. The first examines emotional issues and adjustment concerns associated with renal failure. The second section examines psychological aspects and psychosocial interventions in the management of traumatic spinal injury, and the third examines the emotional and psychiatric sequelae, treatment and interventions for people with traumatic brain injury. These themes were chosen because of the range and diversity of disabilities associated with the conditions, and the years of life affected by them.

RENAL FAILURE

Physical Impact and Epidemiology

Acute renal failure (ARF) is an acute and usually irreversible deterioration in kidney function which develops over a period of days or weeks. The disorders giving rise to ARF are many, but commonly include a kidney stone or infection, and in the majority of patients normal or near-normal recovery of renal function can be expected. Recovery can be more limited in some medical conditions or if the patient is over 50 years old, and either short or long-term dialysis may be required (The Renal Association 1997). ARF becomes more common with age, the highest incidence is in 90-year-olds, but the largest absolute numbers occur in late middle age or early old age (The Renal Association 1997).

Chronic renal failure is a progressive and irreversible deterioration in kidney function. The most common causes are high blood pressure and diabetes, but chronic renal failure can be caused by any condition which destroys the normal function and structure of the kidney. In the UK, approximately 80 patients per million of the adult population commence dialysis each year, and in the USA the rate is approximately 200 patients per million (Khan 1998). Elderly patients are the fastest growing group of patients undergoing treatment for End State Renal Disease (ESRD) in many Western countries (Kutner 1994a). The management of chronic renal failure may require investigations to determine the nature of the disease and any reversible factors, measures to prevent further renal damage, and supportive measures such as dialysis or transplantation (Edwards et al 1995). Unless dialysis or transplantation is available, chronic renal failure will result in death.

The majority of patients with ESRD will be treated with some form of dialysis in the first instance, with transplantation only becoming a limited subsequent option. The technological advances in recent years have meant that dialysis is a viable option for a much greater number of patients, irrespective of age or presence of co-morbidity. There are two approaches to long-term dialysis: haemodialysis and continuous ambulatory peritoneal dialysis. Haemodialysis (HD) is primarily a hospital-based treatment, although some patients can be trained to carry out the treatment at home. A needle is placed into the blood stream for three to five hours, three times a week and patients are attached to a dialysis machine. Many patients receiving this treatment lead relatively normal and active lives, with survival in excess of 20 years being common (Edwards et al 1995). Continuous ambulatory peritoneal dialysis (CAPD) involves the insertion of a peritoneal catheter into the abdominal cavity, which is used for daily repeated instillation, and drainage of sterile dialysate. The treatment is self-administered and patients are free of a dialysis machine. Each treatment takes approximately one hour and is repeated three to six times each day. The potential benefits are of a more sustained control of uraemia, and a more liberal dietary and fluid intake regime. The patient is fully mobile during treatment and able to undertake normal daily activities. CAPD can be successfully used for in excess of 10 years without serious complications (Edwards et al 1995).

Transplantation offers the chance of restoring normal kidney function, and is at present the most economical, successful treatment for patients with ESRD (The Renal Association 1997). The supply of donor organs in the UK averages only 30 per million of population per year, for a demand of 48 per million of the population per year (The Renal Association 1997). Transplants are available from two sources, a cadaver or live donor (usually sibling or parent). Long-term immuno-suppressive therapy is required, which in itself carries an increased risk of infection. In spite of this risk, transplant offers the best option for complete rehabilitation.

Emotional Issues and Adjustment Concerns

Any chronic physical illness taxes an individual's ability to cope and demands a significant emotional adjustment. Renal failure places a significant psychological strain on the coping resources of the patient because of the number and variety of stressors arising from the strict and unremitting medical regime. Devins et al (1997) comment that "despite safe and effective long-term treatments, individuals with ESRD experience threat of death, loss of physical strength and stamina, economic hardships, dietary and fluid-intake limitations, and dependencies on medical technology and personnel" (p 529). Patients can feel they have lost control of their bodies through the dependence on dialysis for survival. There are often difficulties maintaining employment, and an individual's independence, self-concept and esteem can easily diminish. Body image is also constantly challenged by the disease progression. There may be weight gain, premature aging and changes in skin colour (Harries 1996). Patients commonly report a number of physical problems such as nausea and vomiting, and painful cramps during haemodialysis (Levine 1991, cited in Christensen et al 1995). Patients who use CAPD can feel self-conscious about the empty fluid bag, and the noises produced by the fluid, and have an uncomfortable feeling of fullness (Killingworth 1993).

The predominant psychiatric diagnoses are of anxiety and depression (Sensky 1993). However, estimates about the prevalence of psychiatric morbidity and psychological disturbance vary greatly. Smith et al (1985) comment that early research estimates of the prevalence of depression ranged from 0–100%. Reliable estimates are difficult to establish because of the variety of the definitions, criteria and measures used. For example, Smith et al (1985) found that 47% of patients having haemodialysis were depressed on the Beck Depression Inventory (BDI), 10% by the Multiple Affect Adjective Checklist, and 5% by DSM-III criteria. Sensky (1993) warns against the use of screening and case-finding instruments because it can lead to prevalence being over-estimated with any physical health population. Psychological adjustment in patients with renal failure can vary substantially over the course of treatment and adjustment of mood can be particularly complex because a number of somatic symptoms are strongly associated with depressed affect in dialysis. In addition, there are the difficulties interpreting the research because some studies use a single modality of treatment, and others mixed groups. Some studies assess patients shortly following diagnosis and treatment, and others do not record time since onset. Despite these difficulties, Sensky suggests a prevalence rate of about 30% for depression, when rigorous criteria are used. Estimates of suicidal ideation are high within both dialysis (Abram et al 1971) and transplantation populations (Washer et al 1983). Studies have estimated risk for dialysis patients to be 10 to 15 times that of the general population (Rodin 1994). It is difficult to obtain reliable figures for this population, particularly given the influence of non-adherence, but the general suggestion is that this is a higher-than-average risk group.

Non-adherence has major implications for the long-term outlook of the individual on dialysis or the viability of the transplant. Non-adherence is life-threatening and remains one of the most significant problems within this population. As was the case for the prevalence rates (cited above), reliable estimates of non-adherence are difficult to obtain because of the different definitions and assessment methods used. However, Brannon & Feist (1992) estimate that around 50% of patients with ESRD fail to adhere to their treatment. The impact of depression on non-adherence is difficult to establish. There is some evidence that depression is associated with poor outcome and a higher rate of mortality (Burton et al 1986; Farmer et al 1979). However, Sensky (1993), in a review of the literature, does not consider depression and psychiatric morbidity to affect adherence except in a few studies, and suggests that a crucial factor influencing some patients' choices about discontinuation of treatment is perception of prognosis (which may be very different from objective disease status). Adherence to dialysis has been researched more than adherence to transplantation, but generally those who demonstrate poor adherence after transplantation showed similar patterns whilst on dialysis. Research about what makes people adhere is inconclusive, but Brannon & Feist (1992) suggested that long and complex disease regimens, lack of social support, individual beliefs that behaviour cannot affect health, locus of control, poor communication between the individual and the practitioner, delays in obtaining an appointment and in the waiting room may be contributory factors. The role of coping strategies and perceived control on adherence is discussed in the intervention section.

Researchers have also tried to compare mood disturbance with different treatment modalities. Comparisons have been made between patients on home and hospital haemodialysis, CAPD and those who have received a transplant. Clinicians and researchers generally consider there to be a hierarchy of adjustment in relation to treatment modality, with dialysis in hospital being most problematic through to home dialysis, CAPD and transplantation. However, few well-matched studies exist to make comparisons valid or worthwhile. One of the few was a study by Sayag et al (1990, cited in Levenson & Glocheski 1991), which found no differences in psychological adjustment between those who had received a transplant and those on dialysis. In addition, few studies when looking at adjustments and mood consider the effects of transplant failure, which may result in a much worse outcome.

Family and Social Issues

The chronic and progressive nature of renal failure has a significant impact on the family as well as on the individual. Wright (1975, cited in Brock 1990) suggests that the uncertainty about the condition, degree of low predictability, and the ever present threat of death place a significant strain on the family, contributing to the development of stress. The routines of dialysis often become a way of life for all family members, particularly in those who dialyze at home, and family roles will often change irreversibly (Sensky 1993). High levels of anxiety and depression in spouses have been reported (House 1987), and communication about the condition or concerns can be problematic. The impact of denial in families is unclear, one study suggesting that denial predicts failure in families training to do home haemodialysis, and another the opposite (Sensky 1993).

Studies examining family and social issues have demonstrated the success of a variety of coping and adaptation responses. One of the main coping responses of both patients and families is information seeking (Brock 1990). There is evidence that adaptation is better in couples with flexible rather than fixed roles, and that intimacy and good support between partners are key factors in minimizing psychological distress (Sensky 1993). Chowanec & Binik (1982) suggested that the main effect of dialysis is to intensify the relationship and bring couples together and, as a consequence, increase the strain in difficult relationships. Palmer et al (1984, cited in Killingworth 1993) found that strain was particularly introduced if the patient and partner had different perspectives of the problem. Reported difficulties include a narrowing of the family's social world and a generalized feeling of helplessness (Brock 1990). Parkerson & Gutman (1997) examined the role of social support and stress in rural patients with ESRD requiring haemodialysis and those in dialysis units. For both groups, severity of illness was not related to mental health or perceived disablement. However, the patient's perception of their own health status and of the amount of stress within family members appeared to be principal factors associated with the development of symptoms of anxiety and depression in the patient. They suggested that living with family members was protective against the development of anxiety and depression, providing that the patient did not perceive the family to be under strain.

Acute, Rehabilitation and Community Needs

One of the most important factors in the acute management of renal failure concerns the decision to dialyze. MacKay & Moss (1997) comment that about 5–10% of patients in intensive care require dialysis for acute renal failure, but that in-hospital mortality is higher for these patients than those without renal failure. They provide good evidence-based detail about the efficacy of dialyzing and when such a treatment should be offered to those with acute renal failure and how to affect the outcome following hospitalization. Levin et al (1997) also refer to this high mortality rate (estimated by the National Institutes of Health, 1994, to be as high as 25%) during emergency dialysis, and comment on two formal predialysis programs designed to proactively manage the onset of dialysis. A number of detrimental effects of later referral are identified, such as longer hospital stay, increased complications, morbidity and mortality; and preventive strategies discussed. Early referral to a specialist multidisciplinary team or centre is recommended.

Vachon (1992, cited in King 1994) defined renal rehabilitation as including all activities that are "intended to restore or improve the functioning of people with ESRD". Rehabilitation involves the promotion of independent living; the first step involves accurate assessment of an individual's level of functioning, from which rehabilitation goals can be developed. In chronic renal failure, functioning reflects both ongoing therapy and disease status. An important feature of rehabilitation within this population is secondary prevention. Factors such as improved adequacy of delivered dialysis, vascular access and reducing complications related to concurrent disease all contribute positively to patient functioning and well-being (Kutner 1994b). Kutner argues that efforts be made to address the psychological and psychosocial aspects of rehabilitation, but that survival has been the main element of care, with formal rehabilitation planning and the development of programs receiving little attention.

A more recent development within renal centres has been the introduction of regular exercise as part of the rehabilitation process. A number of studies have commented on the beneficial effects of exercise upon long-term outcome. Kouidi et al (1997) demonstrated that the application of long-term exercise training reduced the incidence of depression and improved the quality of life in patients using HD. Colangelo et al (1997) comment on the benefits for the individual and rehabilitation staff, and Cade (1997) provides a personal account of the impact of regular exercise. Structured exercise has also been found to be beneficial for older patients. Kutner et al (1992) found that older ESRD patients showed significantly compromised physical function and health outlook compared to other physically unwell controls and suggest a number of ways of developing an exercise regime with this population.

Although there have been significant medical advances in the treatment of patients with renal failure, there has generally been a failure to address the psychological needs of patients: "few units have a framework for dealing with psychosocial issues, despite the fact that most patients will inevitably encounter difficulties" (Harries 1996 p124). For all patients, the provision of specialist information is important, but within a renal population it can have a significant impact on survival (Binik et al 1993) and on the management of uncertainty within their families (Brock 1990). Structured education programs are part of the multidisciplinary service available in specialist centres, and psychologists have an important part to play in the development of such a program, the provision of booklets or video tapes or in the facilitation of support groups. A factor to consider within rehabilitation planning is the significant cognitive changes that occur during and immediately following haemodialysis. Research has demonstrated reductions in attention and speed of decision-making during haemodialysis compared to immediately prior (Smith & Winslow 1990; Osberg et al 1982). Patients often prefer to engage in psychological support during dialysis time, and this tends to be the usual time for nursing and other staff to engage in teaching the patient about self-care. The benefit of teaching during haemodialysis needs examination.

Approaches to Assessment

As commented upon earlier, severe and persistent depression is not a prerequisite feature in adjusting to chronic renal failure and occurs independently of disease severity (Sensky 1993). However, symptoms of depression are common in circumstances which are difficult and threatening and may be part of a normative response within ESRD rather than a psychiatric disorder (see Rodin 1994 for a good discussion of this area). Accurate diagnosis of depression in ESRD can be difficult because of overlapping symptomatology. Sensky (1993) suggests relying on symptoms such as depressed mood, hopelessness, worthlessness, guilt and suicidal ideation rather than fatigue, appetite and sleep disturbance.

Although the literature reviewed did not consider depression to play a significant role within non-adherence, its occurrence has an impact upon an individual's subjective quality of life and requires clinical intervention. There is some evidence that depression influences the performance of the immune system, which in turn may affect the frequency of infections in dialysis and transplant patients, and there is also evidence that depressed patients are more likely to evidence poor self-care (Levenson & Glocheski 1991).

Rustomjee & Smith (1996) researched the role of the liaison-psychiatrist in Australia and commented that there was a high incidence of misdiagnosis of patients' difficulties by staff working within a renal unit. Patients were often considered to have a "coping problem" when a diagnosis of anxiety, depression or staffing problems would have more accurately described the difficulty. Recognition of organic brain syndromes by staff was also low, patients often being referred for depression, behavioural disturbance or predialysis assessment. They comment upon the need for the involvement of liaison-psychiatrists in the assessment of delirium and careful monitoring of medication. Questions often arise about whether problems are organic or functional. Approximately 5% of transplant patients will experience a psychotic episode during the post-operative period of transplantation (Sensky 1993), but acute alterations may also herald an organic cerebral disturbance (Famularo & Kimball 1983) and require active management.

Psychological or psychiatric consultation may also be required in the assessment and management of a disorientated, non-compliant patient in an acute setting, and the psychologist has a particular role in supplementing the clinical interview with the use of standardized questionnaires to measure initial functioning as well as outcome.

There are a number of potential measures of outcome in renal failure. Quality of life is frequently employed as a measure of functional outcome, but there are many others, such as survival, adequacy of dialysis, interdialytic weight gain and complications (Levenson & Glocheski 1991). Indeed, Sensky (1993) warns against the assumption made by much of the research that adjustment or quality of life accurately reflects the physical outcome of treatment. Quality of life in itself is inherently difficult both to define and to assess, and research findings are often contradictory. As for depression, a hierarchy of quality is often assumed, from haemodialysis through to transplantation (e.g. Evans et al 1985; Molzahn et al 1997). However, the general conclusion now is that such a view is too simplistic. A number of studies have demonstrated that even when functional outcome is severely limited, life satisfaction and quality of life need not be impaired. A combined study in two UK centres (Auer et al 1990, cited in Khan 1998) reported patients' life satisfaction to be comparable to the general population, despite commencement of HD and CAPD treatment and deterioration in mobility. Johnson et al (1982) found that transplant patients achieved higher degrees of physical and occupational rehabilitation than HD patients, but were approximately equal on measures of quality of life. The patient's ability to choose between different treatment modalities has also been shown to have an impact upon quality of life. Szabo et al (1997) demonstrated that when freedom of choice for HD was removed from patients undergoing CAPD, their ratings of adjustment, life satisfaction and total quality of life deteriorated.

Often measures of quality of life are nothing more than an assessment of life satisfaction or affective disturbance. Sensky (1993) and Kutner (1994b) discuss the role of generic and disease-specific tools within this population, although both stress the importance of the patient's own assessment of quality and satisfaction.

Treatment and Interventions

Much of the research about quality of life and adjustment is non-specific in its recommendations for intervention. However, a body of coping research is being developed which provides treatment recommendations. As commented previously, non-adherence is a significant threat in the treatment of patients with renal failure.

In their research on coping, Christensen et al (1995) identified that planful problem solving was associated with favourable adherence if used in response to stressors involving a relatively controllable aspect of HD. For stressors with less controllable aspects, coping efforts involving emotional self-control were associated with more favourable adherence. The seeking of informational social support in response to an uncontrollable situation was associated with poorer fluid intake adherence. Christensen et al suggest that it is beneficial to teach patients to implement emotion-focused strategies such as relaxation training or distraction in situations of uncontrollable stressful encounters, and problem-focused strategies (such as information request and problem-solving skills) in contexts in which greater personal control can be exercised. Klang et al (1996) examined the use of coping strategies amongst predialysis and dialysis patients. Their results demonstrated that a variety of coping strategies were used, such as maintaining control, hope and information seeking. However, differences were found between the two groups. The dialysis patients tended to use more confrontational and palliative strategies, whereas the predialysis patients used more emotion-focused strategies.

Much of the literature on psychological impact and adjustment refers to the intrusive nature of renal failure upon both the individual and their family. Devins (1994) developed an "illness intrusiveness" model to explain this process and made a number of specific treatment recommendations, such as the integration of ESRD and its treatment into the patient's existing activities and interests, perhaps through the use of behavioural contracting; the development of additional activities involving pleasure and mastery; and health/illness education. In a later study, Devins et al (1997) suggest that illness intrusiveness is a powerful moderating variable on coping and self-concept in renal failure.

A few studies have also examined the benefits of group interventions. Friend et al (1986) found that patients who participated in a dialysis support group lived longer than non-participant controls, even after controlling for psychosocial and physiological co-variables. Hener et al (1996) examined the benefits of a support group, cognitive-behavioural group, and control group of patients and their spouses. Both intervention groups were found to be beneficial and promoted adjustment in comparison to the control group.

SPINAL CORD INJURIES

A spinal cord injury is most often associated with a fracture or fractured dislocation of the vertebral spinal column. The extent of the physical effects of a spinal cord injury (SCI) will depend on two factors, first, the level of the spinal cord at which injury occurs and secondly, whether neurotransmission is completely severed at the level of the lesion or some pathways remain intact, allowing preservation of some function below the damaged area. Cervical (neck) injuries may result in tetraplegia (quadriplegia) and injuries at the thoracic, lumbar and sacral levels (i.e. upper, middle and lower back) may result in paraplegia. Higher cervical injuries can also lead to a dysfunction of the respiratory muscles, which may require long-term artificial ventilation.

Physical Impact and Epidemiology

Functional losses, depending on the level of injury, may include the loss of trunk, arm and leg movement, losses of the sensation of touch, pressure and position, and the ability independently to control bladder, bowel and sexual functions. Whilst some people may have incomplete injuries which may result in partial neurological impairment, as the spinal cord is part of the central nervous system, complete injuries are permanent. Go et al (1995), using figures from the American National SCI Database, found that the most common discharge neurological category was incomplete tetraplegia (31%) followed by complete paraplegia (26%), complete tetraplegia (22%), incomplete paraplegia (20%) and complete recovery (1%).

The most common cause of traumatic SCI in developed economies is motor vehicle accidents (estimated to be 50%), falls (25%), and 20% are a result of recreational sporting activities (Kennedy 1995; Stover & Fine 1986). Diving into the shallow end of the swimming pool is the most common cause of sporting injuries. In the USA a significant proportion of injuries are caused by acts of violence, such as stabbing (accounting for almost 17% of injuries). In developing economies, road traffic accidents are less frequent, with agricultural accidents and falls being more common occurrences.

It is estimated that the annual incidence of spinal cord injuries, not including those who die at the scene of an accident, is approximately 40 cases per million in the United States, and between 10 and 15 per million in Europe and Australasia. Blumer & Quine (1995) reviewed the international literature on prevalence and found that rates ranged from 11 to 112 per 100 000 of the population. It is estimated that there are between 180 000 and 200 000 persons in the USA with spinal cord injuries and 40 000 people in the UK. Life expectancies for persons with SCI continue to increase, and whilst mortality rates are higher in the first year after injury, the relative survival rate is 69%, but is lower in those with higher tetraplegia and ventilator dependency. Guttmann (1976) reported that 80% of people with SCI died in the first few weeks, highlighting how these figures represent a dramatic improvement in life expectancy.

Overall, 82% of people with spinal cord injuries are male (Go et al 1995; Kennedy 1995) and an SCI primarily affects young adults. Fifty-six per cent occur among persons in the 16 to 30 age group, with a mean age of between 30 and 35 and the most frequently occurring age of injury being 19.

Psychological Adjustment

A spinal cord injury is often a sudden, devastating event that precipitates major changes in an individual's physical, psychological and social domains. Earlier attempts at conceptualizing the adjustment process proposed a variety of stages that were often based on mourning models (Bracken & Shepard 1980; Hohmann 1975). Morris (1992) and Trieschmann (1988) reviewed the literature and found there was little evidence to support the underlying assumptions of these models and concluded that psychological disruption was not inevitable, nor necessarily helpful in fostering the adjustment process. However, there have been a number of studies which have explored those factors which were predictive of psychological adjustment. Frank & Elliott (1989) found that SCI persons with an internal locus of control were less likely to be depressed than those who had attributed control to external factors. Using the Multidimensional Health Locus of Control Scale (MHLCS) they further identified that those with an external locus of control who believed chance factors accounted for events, were more depressed than those who felt powerful others were responsible for control.

A consistent finding in the literature is that young persons generally adjust better to SCI than older persons (Judd et al 1991; Morris 1992). Woodrich & Patterson (1983), using the Acceptance of Disability Scale, found that women adjusted better than men to SCI. However, Fuhrer et al (1993) found greater levels of depressive symptomatology in 40 community-resident women with SCI than a sample of 100 men. One of the few consistent findings in the literature, which is sometimes counterintuitive, is that the level of SCI, and therefore the extent of paralysis, is not related to adjustment variables in terms of acceptance of disability, emotional reaction or coping (Kennedy et al 1995b; Morris 1992; Judd & Brown 1988; Woodrich & Patterson 1983).

It is often assumed that the passage of time since injury is associated with increased adjustment. Whiteneck et al (1992a) reviewed the mortality, morbidity, health, functional and psychosocial outcomes of 834 individuals with SCI and found that whilst there is some deterioration in functional status over time, 75% of those interviewed rated their current quality of life as either good or excellent on a five-point scale. Kennedy et al (1995a) carried out a retrospective review of those who had acquired their spinal cord injuries during childhood. They found there was no evidence that childhood onset was a significant factor predicting an increased level of psychological difficulty when compared to an adult-onset control group. Crisp (1992) highlighted the important role of social support in fostering positive adjustment.

Research evidence indicates that there is no one single psychological response to SCI, and that social demographic factors and illness variables are insufficient to account for the variations in adjustment. More recently, an increased focus of research has been on the cognitive, behavioural and emotional coping strategies used by individuals to manage the consequences of their acquired disability. Buckelew & Hanson (1992) measured coping in 57 persons with SCI during their acute rehabilitation and followed them up five years post discharge. They found that cognitive restructuring was associated with high levels of acceptance of disability, whereas wish fulfillment and fantasy strategies were associated with low levels. Reidy et al (1991) found that depression had a strong positive correlation with escape and avoidant coping strategies. Kennedy (1995) employed a longitudinal methodology to examine psychological impact and coping strategies using the COPE developed by Carver et al (1989) following traumatic onset of SCI. He found a remarkably consistent pattern of coping strategies over nine observational periods, the most commonly used strategies being acceptance, positive reinterpretation and growth, active coping, planning and social support. Multiple regression analysis found that there was an association between a variety of coping strategies such as acceptance, behavioural disengagement, alcohol and drug use ideation and levels of anxiety and depression. Coping strategies assessed at six weeks post injury were found to predict 67% of the variance in depression at one-year post discharge. The model generated in this analysis included the use of focusing on and venting emotions, low acceptance and low functional independence. These applications of various coping models highlight the individual's cognitive appraisal processes in understanding adjustment to SCI as a major progression from the stage models which were prevalent in the middle part of the twentieth century.

Emotional Reactions

Emotional reactions to SCI are typified by increased levels of depression and anxiety, but cannot be considered to be either universal or necessary for successful rehabilitation. Judd et al (1991) followed 71 SCI patients through the course of their rehabilitation, and using the Beck Depression Inventory (BDI), found that about 20% of patients met the criteria for a major depressive disorder. Frank et al (1987) used a clinical interview approach to assess the prevalence of depression in a group of 32 SCI patients and found that 38% were diagnosed as having major depression. Kennedy et al (1995b) examined a group of 41 patients six weeks post injury and compared them with a group of 30 respondents between four and seven years post injury and found no differences on measures of depression, hopelessness or anxiety. In line with other findings, 34% of the inpatient group and 37% of the post discharge group scored above 14 on the Beck Depression Inventory. Hancock et al (1993) implemented a longitudinal study exploring depression and anxiety, and compared a group of SCI persons with a matched able-bodied group. They found that 25% of the SCI group were anxious and depressed, compared with less than 5% of the control group.

Suicide is another consequence of SCI that has been examined. DeVivo et al (1991) found that 50 people of a sample of 9135 persons had committed suicide (accounting for 6.3% of deaths) which produced a Standard Mortality Ratio (SMR) of 4.9. They concluded that although suicide occurred more often in the SCI population than the general population, in an absolute sense it was a rare event.

Overall the research would suggest that whilst a significant number of people following SCI have increased levels of anxiety and depression (case levels are thought to be between 25 and 35%) and there is a general increase in emotions of stress, most people do not experience severe psychological difficulties. Most of the research appears to have concentrated on exploring individuals in the first few years post rehabilitation, but there is a growing number of longitudinal studies which include those by Krause (1997), Kennedy (1995) and Eisenberg & Saltz (1991) which suggest that many people make a positive adjustment and do not experience severe emotional or psychological problems post injury.

Family and Social Issues

A study of marital relationships in a cohort of 60 000 people with spinal cord injury by Dijkers et al (1995) found that new marriages were less stable than pre-injury marriages and that marriage failures were more common in the younger age group. Changes in marital status tended to be higher in the earlier years post injury, and over time there was an increase in both divorces and marriages. DeVivo et al (1995) explored outcomes of post-SCI marriages in 622 individuals. They found that men had divorce rates two times higher than women, that divorce rates were high among persons with a college education and lower for persons with lower-level injuries. Sexual dysfunction following SCI is a major issue and Sipski & Alexander (1992) in their review highlight that between 70% and 93% of males with complete upper motor neurone lesions retained reflex erections but none sustained psychogenic erections. Sipski et al (1995) report on the first laboratory-controlled analysis of female sexual response and elaborated on the nature of female reflex vasoconges-tion. Despite the physiological changes following injury, most women returned to sexual involvement within 12 months.

Krause (1992) examined pre-injury and post-injury employment rates in a diverse sample of persons with spinal cord injuries. In a study of 286 persons, 75% had worked at some time since injury, but only 12% of persons who were employed at the time of injury returned to the same job. People with lower injuries were more likely to return to their pre-injury jobs and employment rates were dramatically lower in the 51–60-year-old group. Castle (1994) in a British sample, found that 23% of a sample of 114 persons were unemployed and seeking work and 25% were unemployed and not seeking work. However, re-employment figures after SCI vary tremendously. Trieschmann (1988) reports a range of return to competitive employ-ment varying between 13% and 48%.

Psychological Interventions

The primary aim of any psychological or psychiatric intervention with spinal cord-injured people is to assist the individual in the management of emotional concerns, foster general coping and adaptation, maximize the individual's rehabilitation potential and minimize general psychological and social disruption. The American Association of Spinal Cord Injury Psychologists and Social Workers (AASCIPSW, 1992) suggests that the psychosocial rehabilitation process should involve a continuity of services from the onset of SCI, through comprehensive rehabilitation, to follow-up in the community. Typically, these interventions are carried out at an individual and group level, but also in consultation with health professionals working in various treatment and rehabilitation centres. In the acute phase, the intervention is aimed at encouraging a sense of safety within the individual, normalizing their emotional reactions and providing them with an opportunity to explore their concerns and anxieties. Providing patients and families with information about what to expect has been shown to alleviate anxiety, and in the early stages the family should be informed of the timescale and main features of the rehabilitation process.

TRAUMATIC BRAIN INJURY

Traumatic Brain Injury (TBI) constitutes one of the current major public health problems. This particularly relates to the legacy of disability and handicap necessitating ongoing rehabilitation and causing grief to patients and families and cost to the community. With their diverse range of clinical problems, patients with TBI clearly need an integrative biopsychosocial approach to management. Given high rates of adjustment difficulties, cognitive and behaviour disturbance, and overt psychiatric disorder, there is clearly a strong role for the psychiatrist and psychologist in the TBI rehabilitation process. However, much yet remains to be examined as to how these disciplines can most effectively and efficiently contribute.

Epidemiology

Studies of the epidemiology of TBI demonstrate a range of estimates of the incidence, but fairly consistent trends emerge as to the group of individuals most at risk. Reasons for the discrepancy in estimates of the incidence may include variable likelihood of initial presentation, particularly with milder TBI, differences in accuracy of detection, differences in classification and differences in the likelihood of reporting of TBI in different treatment settings.

These discrepancies can be seen in two estimates of the incidence of TBI in the USA. Berker (1996) estimated that 7–10 million new cases of TBI occur in the USA each year, with 500 000 of these patients being hospitalized. Silver et al (1997) estimated that there are only 1–2 million new cases per year, of whom only around 300 000 are hospitalized. This latter figure would give a population incidence of around 360–720 per 100 000 per annum, broadly similar to most international studies. In terms of mortality, Lindsay & Bone (1997) estimated that in the UK, TBI alone was responsible for nine deaths per 100 000 per annum. Given the young average age of individuals at the time of acquiring a TBI, this figure would indicate that TBI rivals, if not exceeds, cardiovascular disease and cancer as the leading cause of potential years of life lost.

A more consistent profile of the sociodemographic characteristics of individuals suffering TBI has emerged. Typically, patients are predominantly male (2–4:1), with an average age in the 20s to 30s. In a Canadian study, Wong et al (1993) described several further characteristics of TBI populations. In their study of admission to a Toronto rehabilitation program, they found a relatively high proportion of their population were manual labourers (26%), students (15%) or were unemployed prior to their injury (13%). Thirty-six per cent had a pre-existing history of alcohol abuse and 9% of drug use. Patients with a history of alcohol or drug abuse were over-represented in the 7% of the sample that had a history of previous brain injury. It is striking given the high rates of adjustment difficulties and more overt psychiatric disturbance post injury that there has been relatively little study of pre-injury psychological functioning.

Physical Impairments

It is often the physical manifestations of TBI that are best recognized in the community and are often mistakenly taken to represent the most significant mani-festation of brain injury. The presence or absence of ongoing physical defects following a TBI is influenced by the severity, nature and localization of the injury. Pre-injury characteristics such as previous injury or illness, and the presence or absence of effective and timely acute and rehabilitative care, affect the long-term outcome of TBI.

The most commonly reported physical sequelae of minor TBI is the group of symptoms that have come to be known as the post-concussional syndrome. Whilst the aetiology and validity of this syndrome remain unclear, as reviewed by Lishman (1988), there appears to be a consistency in the symptoms reported worldwide in the three to six months post mild TBI, typically including several of headache, dizziness, fatigue, anxiety, insomnia, noise sensitivity, light sensitivity, decreased concentration, irritability, depression and frequent complaints of memory impair-ment not verifiable on neuropsychological testing. Typically, although not uni-formly, the syndrome is self-limiting. Clearly, given the above symptom profile, there often exists a need for differentiation from untreated mood or anxiety dis-order.

Moderate and severe TBI are associated with a range of pathological changes in the brain. These may be focal, such as contusion or laceration at the site of impact, at the opposite pole (contrecoup) or at the hemispheric poles generally. Diffuse so-called shear injury is due to the rapid acceleration/deceleration and rotational forces involved in many cases of TBI and is often asymmetrically distributed throughout the deep white matter of both hemispheres, the corpus callosum and the brain stem. A diffuse injury may also be produced, or exacerbated, by post-immediate injury factors such as hypoxia or hypotension. Broadly, physical outcome following TBI is often divided into five main groups (Jennett & Bond 1975): death, persistent vegetative state, severe disability (conscious but disabled), moderately disabled

(disabled but independent) or good recovery where an essentially normal life is resumed.

A large body of research now exists looking at those factors that may be useful in the prediction of eventual outcome from the early stage of injury. Factors examined include the initial depth of unconsciousness, as measured by instruments such as the Glasgow Coma Scale (Jennett & Teasdale 1976), and the length of Post-Traumatic Amnesia (PTA). This was defined by Russell & Nathan (1946) as the period after a head injury when new information about ongoing events is not stored, thus representing a disturbance of episodic memory. This typically follows an interval of impaired consciousness and often represents the initial stage of recovery. It is also characterized by attentional disturbance and behavioural changes ranging from lethargy to gross agitation. Studies such as that of Ellenberg et al (1996) have consistently shown duration of PTA to be a modest but reliable predictor of outcome in at least the medium term. In general terms, PTA of less than one hour is taken of evidence of mild injury and of greater than one day of significant injury.

A range of physical sequelae can then arise as a result of TBI, depending upon the site and severity of lesions, and some may only become evident once PTA is complete. Deficits may include motor, sensory and language deficits in addition to major cognitive disturbance. Initial attempts at rehabilitation following TBI tend to focus heavily on physical sequelae and increasing attention to cognitive difficulties has only become a major component of TBI rehabilitation in the past 20 to 30 years. Motor problems are often relatively responsive to rehabilitation and it is these deficits that are often rated by patients with TBI as the most troublesome (Prigatano & Schacter 1991). In the same study it was demonstrated that patients with TBI are much less accurate in rating their cognitive deficits, which are often the most troublesome to their families and carers.

Much of the initial neuropsychological investigation and treatment for individuals with TBI focused on disturbance in general intellectual function, language and memory. Increasing interest has now focused on the executive deficits which often accompany behavioural and emotional problems following TBI and include poor attention, decreased ability to regulate and control activity, problems with conceptual and problem-solving behaviour, and problems in assessment of self-deficit (Lezak 1983; Stuss & Gow 1992).

Emotional Adjustment and Psychiatric Sequelae

It is somewhat surprising, given the enormity of the personal challenge involved, that relatively little is written about what constitutes normal adjustment following TBI. It is clear that a number of factors combine to make adjustment to what is often a series of devastating losses in the case of moderate and severe TBI extremely difficult. Many patients will have long periods of unconsciousness followed by PTA, and when they "awake" often appear initially puzzled by their deficits from an injury that they are often unable to recall. Frequently repeated descriptions of the injury's nature are often required before the patient can begin to form an ongoing "memory" of what happened to them. From this point they may begin the process of adjusting to their new life. Hampering their progress in this challenging task may be other isolating deficits such as expressive or receptive language disturbance and denial or inability to cope in other ways among family members or other close supports. Several studies have demonstrated that the number of actual supports available progressively declines over many years after the initial accident (Thomsen 1984).

The traumatic nature of the events leading to TBI would no doubt often meet the criteria for the kind of event likely to be associated with a risk of Post Traumatic Stress Disorder (PTSD) in patients without TBI (APA 1994). However, the possible existence of a PTSD-like syndrome in those patients with prolonged PTA who are unable to recall freely any of the events around the time of their original injury remains a controversial area. It is clearly true that if the criteria for PTSD as outlined in DSM-IV are interpreted stringently, patients with amnesia for their initial trauma will not be able to meet criteria for this disorder. However, some patients clearly do form intrusive pseudomemories of their original traumatic event, possibly constructed from information given to them following recovery from PTA. In an interesting design, Bryant & Harvey (1996) demonstrated that some of these pseudomemories may be associated with the same physiological parameters of arousal as "true" memories in a clinical population suffering from PTSD.

Mood disorders, predominantly depression, remain the most commonly diagnosed psychiatric disorder post TBI (Gaultieri & Cox 1991) and, according to those authors, are as common as mood disorder associated with other major neurological disorders. They estimate that the risk of affective disorder is increased five to 10 times post TBI, giving a lifetime prevalence of 30 to 60% for major depression. They comment that whilst there has been no period of peak incidence of mood disorder following TBI identified, it does appear common in the first two years post injury. Experience is that mood disorder can also occur many years post TBI, often coinciding with the development of greater insight and is regularly under-recognized and undertreated. Debate still exists as to whether there is an increased risk of Bipolar Disorder following TBI.

The incidence of psychosis is also clearly increased post TBI. Gaultieri & Cox (1991) review what they describe as a paucity of studies but concluded that they were consistent in showing the prevalence of psychosis following TBI to be 2–5% following mild to moderate injuries and 10% following severe TBI. It is clear that the cognitive and language functioning of the patient influence the expression of psychosis. Presentation may occur many years after injury.

Family and Social Issues

The presence of an individual with TBI within a family has repeatedly been shown to produce high levels of family strain, which does not necessarily correlate with the overt severity of their relative's TBI. Families are more likely to rate emotional changes in the patient as more difficult to manage than the physical burden. Over-use of denial as a defense against the loss and increased burden is one response seen and important to recognize for the treating team. Overall, whilst some families cope well, there are high rates of moderate to severe psychiatric disturbance in families of patients with TBI (Gleckman & Brill 1995). It is important to take into account the nature of pre-morbid family dynamics and relationships in any post-TBI assessment of families. The nature of the relationship with a particular relative will influence the nature of the process. For example, Brooks et al (1987) commented that several studies have shown that wives cope less well than mothers, who in some senses may revert to an earlier role. It is pertinent in working with families of patients with TBI to review the 20-year Scandinavian follow-up study of Thomsen (1992), who demonstrated a progressive decline in the number of individuals still living with their parents or spouse in the years following TBI, which was attributed to a combination of parental death, frailty or exhaustion in most cases.

Acute, Rehabilitation and Community Needs

There is clear and widespread acknowledgement that appropriate, specialized and timely acute medical and neurosurgical care are essential to minimize the morbidity and mortality associated with TBI. Less clear is the point at which rehabilitation should be initiated. Morgan et al (1998) looked at the global outcome in individuals whose rehabilitation was commenced less than seven days post injury (i.e. during acute care) versus those whose rehabilitation was commenced more than seven days post injury. They found that earlier commencement of rehabilitation was associated with a shorter length of admission and a better outcome in terms of cognition, perception and motor skills. Despite this and some other similar findings, early rehabilitation involvement is not universal clinical practice. Many countries provide acute inpatient hospital rehabilitation, although in some areas such as the USA, this may only be available to those patients with appropriate insurance or a compensatable injury. Major studies such as that by Cope & Hall (1982) clearly demonstrate that early rehabilitation intervention has benefits in terms of cost savings in medical resources, both during the rehabilitation phase and subsequently, and is highly likely to improve global outcome. It is of note, however, that there is less systematic study of which components within such a program are the most effective—clearly each program must be tailored to the individual patient's needs.

Treatment programs in the post-acute phase tend to diversify greatly, again consistent with the range of patient needs. Systematic study of post-acute rehabilitation is less available, one of the critical factors being difficulty in determining appropriate endpoints. For example, an over-focus on vocational outcomes may be inappropriate for the majority of patients realistically unable to return to work in a difficult labour market. Nevertheless, Cope (1995) concluded in a seminal review that there was evidence to support overall effectiveness of post-acute rehabilitation up to five to 10 years post injury, particularly when the focus is appropriately moved from discrete measures of impairment to global handicap.

Of particular interest to psychiatrists and psychologists is the work of Eames & Wood (1985a) who designed an intensive inpatient rehabilitation program with a strong focus on behavioural intervention for those patients with severe head injury and behavioural disorder. Their group were on average four years post injury and stayed in the unit for an average of over 12 months. Given the limited scope for spontaneous recovery at this time, patients were used as their own controls, and by the end of the program, two-thirds of this difficult patient group had substantial improvement in residential or placement options compared with prior to the program, with good reduction in global handicap.

Approaches to Assessment

Adequate assessment of the multiple dysfunction resulting from TBI is a demanding task. Typically, poor attention, often necessitating multiple meetings to complete assessment, and on occasions other cognitive or language disturbance, will hamper assessment. Further, because of the diverse range of associated disabilities, a multidisciplinary approach is required. Regrettably, the attention to psychological and psychiatric assessment has been more evident in some rehabilitation programs than others, no doubt partly related to the relatively low numbers of individuals from these disciplines that have developed expertise in these areas.

In the assessment of current mood, anxiety and psychotic symptoms, there remains no substitute for careful patient interviewing, establishment of rapport and acknowledgement that symptoms may present in atypical ways in individuals with TBI. For example, in an individual with severe TBI, depression may present with reduced verbal output, a slackening of achievement or motivation in rehabilitation activities, or regression to a functional level previously achieved during rehabilitation.

Given the key role of adequate psychological and neuropsychological assessment in formation of effective rehabilitation planning, it is unfortunate that relatively little is written about appropriate classification and assessment of psychological disturbance following TBI that is readily transferable across settings. Levin et al (1987) developed what is currently the most widely used instrument for the assessment of the behavioural sequelae following head injury, the Neurobehavioral Rating Scale (NRS). They developed this instrument from the Brief Psychiatric Rating Scale (BPRS) (Overall & Gorham 1962) after they found that instrument to be of limited value in the post-TBI population. This 27-item scale involves rating items on a seven-point likert scale that are grouped into four areas: cognition/energy; metacognition (roughly correlating to executive function); somatic/anxiety; and language. An alternative approach is that of Eames & Wood (1985b) who attempted to classify behaviour disorders after brain injury, which often fit poorly into traditional psychiatric classificatory systems such as DSM-IV (APA 1994). They classified such disorders into three main groups: active (includes aggressive, impulsive, disin-hibited and anti-social); passive (insightless, driveless and abulic); and syndromal (manipulative, manipulative and dissociative, ritualistic, cyclothymic, confabulating and paranoid). Whilst this largely descriptive approach has potential merit, this schema has possibly failed to translate to use in a wide variety of settings. It also bears only limited commonality with taxonomies well known to psychologists and psychiatrists not working routinely with patients with TBI.

Treatments and Interventions

A very diverse range of treatments has been described and trialled in patients with post-TBI deficits. Any selection of techniques must involve the close matching of therapist strengths and weaknesses together with those of the patient and their environment. What has become increasingly clear is an emphasis on handicap which is more appropriate than selective focus on individual impairments and that significant improvement in overall functioning can be obtained years after TBI without necessarily involving change on more fixed measures of impairment like neuropsychological testing.

Behaviourally based techniques obviously form a major part of individual treatment for patients with TBI, particularly those with major behavioural disturbance. McGlynn (1990), in reviewing this area, examined a range of widely used behavioural techniques including token economies, stress inoculation training, skills training, utilization techniques, self-instructional training, shaping, chaining, prompting, modelling and the use of "time out from positive reinforcement". As in other areas of post-TBI rehabilitation, there remains a paucity of well-controlled studies. McGlynn (1990) was able to demonstrate that patients with severe behavioural disturbance were able to learn new associations, develop new skills or significantly alter behaviour, and head-injured patients having problems with impulsive and inappropriate behaviour can learn that this behaviour may have negative consequences, and more acceptable behaviours positive outcomes. Clearly crucial to success of behaviourally based interventions in a rehabilitation setting are structured assessment, monitoring and consistency of all individuals involved in the management plan.

Cognitive training, aimed essentially at the direct remediation of specific cognitive functions, remains a more controversial area. Although widely and at times intensively practiced, these forms of individual and group therapy have not yet been consistently proven to produce benefits to generalized situations. Central to the debate is controversy as to what is being attempted—restoration of function in damaged systems, compensation using alternative systems, or substitution of intact functions (Prigatano, Glisky & Klonoff 1996). Typical techniques of cognitive rehabilitation involve the use of exercises and drills, mnemonic strategies, external aids or strategies aimed at acquisition of domain-specific knowledge (see Prigatano et al 1996 for further information).

Relatively less is written about interpersonal forms of psychotherapy, group or individual, in patients with TBI. Clinically, there is clearly a role in many cases for both individual and family assessment and therapy, appropriately tailored to the situation (Florian et al 1989). Central themes in individual therapy often relate to the losses, both real and of future potential, involved in TBI and explorations of the potential to explore themes of "love", "work" and "play" in alternative ways to what were previously envisaged (Prigatano 1988). Similar challenges face the family which was described by Perlesz et al (1992) as involving grieving, restructuring the family organization, developing a new identity and growing through the tragedy.

Many of these techniques will be commenced in the acute rehabilitation setting and hopefully assist the patient during the period of gradual re-integration into the community. The importance of stable therapeutic relationships during this period should not be underestimated. Patients with TBI attempting to restructure their lives are confronted over many years with progressive social, financial, legal and personal challenges. Psychiatry and psychology are disciplines which have been involved in identifying clinical needs and promoting appropriate assessment and interventions with these individuals with complex needs.

THE ROLE OF THE PSYCHOLOGIST AND PSYCHIATRIST IN INTERVENTION: AN EXAMPLE OF SCI UNITS

Psychology

Trieschmann (1988) defined rehabilitation as a life-long process and conceptualized it in behavioural terms. Kennedy & Hamilton (1999) report on the efficacy of a goal planning/behavioural rehabilitation program in improving general rehabilitation outcomes, which includes reduction in mobility needs and improvement in activities of daily living and an increase in activities resulting in community placement.

The cognitive behavioural approach to managing more significant emotional concerns is highly applicable in the management of psychological problems following SCI. Whilst symptoms of depression may emerge as part of a normal response, they can precipitate seriously distorted modes of thinking. During therapy, thoughts and beliefs about the consequences of the injury are explored, and once specific negative thinking patterns are identified and related core assumptions made explicit, these can be the focus of the intervention. Many people following spinal cord injury generate very negative and catastrophic predictions about their future. Providing them with access to more realistic and adaptive cognitions can challenge these. Often this therapy is provided on a one-to-one basis, but more recently group interventions have been found to be effective in reducing levels of depression (Craig et al 1998, and King & Kennedy 1999). King & Kennedy utilized a combination of problem-solving and cognitive reappraisal processes to reduce mood disturbance significantly in a cohort of newly injured spinal cord people.

The most effective group approaches usually embrace information giving with basic problem-solving skills and include the use of patient education manuals and access to peer counsellors.

There is also general consensus (Alexander 1991) that the P-LI-SS-IT (Permission, Limited Information, Specific Suggestions, Intensive Therapy) developed by Annon (1974) provides a useful framework for organizing sexual counselling in rehabilitation. This model has four levels of intervention, each increasing in sophistication, enabling counsellors to structure their program according to level of competence. People with more complex sexual difficulties may require more intensive therapy, based on strategies and techniques developed by Masters & Johnson (1970). Other techniques include biofeedback and relaxation training.

Once the patient is discharged from the inpatient rehabilitation facility, there is often the dilemma about providing support to those who have ongoing psychological needs. Smith et al (1997) examined the durability of cognitive bibliotherapy for mild to moderately depressed adults, by conducting a three-year follow-up investigation. Bibliotherapy is the use of selected printed materials to extend therapy services into the home and may be particularly suitable for those who have difficulty in obtaining community support or accessing community mental health facilities. In this study they used a variety of measures of depression, including the Beck Depression Inventory and the Hamilton Rating Scale for Depression, to demonstrate the positive therapeutic gains that appear to be maintained at three years. Smith et al (1997) supported the usefulness of cognitive bibliotherapy as an adjunct to traditional treatment of depression in the community.

Liaison Psychiatry

Many spinal injury units have access to liaison-psychiatry services. Judd & Brown (1988) described the contribution of the liaison-psychiatry service as part of the psychosocial team. The psychiatrist contributes to the management of the patient in rehabilitation by excluding organic factors associated with psychiatric illness and providing a variety of forms of psychotherapy that would include individual and group therapy, family therapy and pharmacotherapy. Psychiatrists also contribute to the overall assessment and rehabilitation process by highlighting those at risk for the development of depressive illness or adjustment difficulties. Judd & Burrows (1986) recognize that whilst antidepressant and antipsychotic medication may be used, the side-effects may be particularly troublesome for those with spinal cord injuries. For example, anticholinergic side-effects may interfere with reflex bladder functioning. The liaison-psychiatrist clearly has an insight into the interactions of a variety of pharmacological interventions. Judd & Burrows concluded that all patients with preexisting psychiatric disorders and patients with a history of suicidal behaviour necessitate early psychiatric assessment and intervention. The psychiatrist also contributes to the psychosocial team and the medical and rehabilitation team in pursuing a more holistic perspective of a patient, especially one with special needs.

CONCLUDING REMARKS

This chapter has provided an overview of the impact and adjustment of three chronic conditions. The medical management and rehabilitation of each of these conditions have developed, and a significant number of the population now live for many years with a chronic illness or disability. The challenge has therefore become one of facilitating adjustment and enabling people to maintain a good quality of life. Significant advances have been made in the psychological management of chronic conditions. However, there continues to be a need to develop the science and contribute to the evidence base of clinical interventions. Dissemination of findings in scientific and lay publications will help with the application of the science and foster ongoing service development. These, taken together, will improve health outcomes and the quality of life for people with chronic conditions and disabilities.

REFERENCES

Abram HS, Moore GL and Westervelt FB: Suicidal behavior in chronic dialysis patients. *Am J Psychiatry* **127**: 1199–1204, 1971.

Alexander CJ: Psychological assessment and treatment of sexual dysfunctions following spinal cord injury. *J Am Paraplegia Soc* **14**: 127–131, 1991.

AASCIPSW (American Association of Spinal Cord Injury Psychologists and Social Workers): *Standards (1992)*. AASCIPSW: Jackson Heights, NY, 1992.

APA (American Psychiatric Association): *Diagnostic and Statistical Manual of Mental Disorders. 4th Edition*. American Psychiatric Association: Washington, DC, 1994.

Annon JS: *The Behavioral Treatment of Sexual Problems (Vol 1)*. Enabling Systems: Honolulu, HI, 1974.

Arokiasamy CV: A theory for rehabilitation? *Rehab Educ* **7**: 77–98, 1993.

Auer J, Gokal R, Stout JP, Hillier V, Kinsey J, Simon G and Oliver D: The Oxford/Manchester study of dialysis patients. *Scand J Urol Nephrol* **131**: 31–37, 1990.

Berker E: Diagnosis, physiology, pathology and rehabilitation of traumatic brain injury. *Int J Neurosci* **85**: 195–220, 1996.

Binik YM, Devins GM, Barre PE, Buttmann RD, Hollomby DJ, Mandin H, Paul LC, Hons RB and Burgess ED: Live and learn: patient education delays the need to initiate renal replacement therapy in end-stage renal disease. *J Nerv Ment Disease* **181**: 371–376, 1993.

Blumer CE and Quine S: Prevalence of spinal cord injury: an international comparison (Review). *Neuroepidemiology* **14**: 258–268, 1995.

Bracken M and Shepard M: Coping and adaptation to acute spinal cord injury: a theoretical analysis. *Paraplegia* **18**: 74–85, 1980.

Brannon L and Feist J: *Health Psychology*. Wadsworth: New York, 1992.

Brock MJ: Uncertainty, information needs, and coping effectiveness of renal families. *ANNA J* **17**: 242–246, 1990.

Brooks N, Campsie L, Symington C, Beattie A and McKinlay W: The effects of severe head injury on patient and relatives within seven years of injury. *J Head Trauma Rehab* **2**(3): 1–13, 1987.

Bryant RA and Harvey AG: Psychiatric and psychological sequelae of TBI. In J Ponsford, P Snow and V Anderson (Eds), *International Perspectives in Traumatic Brain Injury*. Australian Academic Press: Brisbane, 1996.

Buckelew S and Hanson S: Coping and adjustment following spinal cord injury. *Spinal Cord Injury Psychosocial Process* **5**: 99–103, 1992.

Burton HJ, Kline SA, Lindsay RM and Heidenham AP: The relationship of depression to survival in chronic renal failure. *Psychosom Med* **48**: 261–268, 1986.

Cade P: How exercise can change "disability" to "ability" in the ESRD patient. *Nephrology News and Issues* **11**(8): 55–56, 1997.

Carver CS, Scheier MF and Weintraub JK: Assessing coping strategies: a theoretically based approach. *J Personal Soc Psychol* **56**: 267–283, 1989.

Castle R: An investigation into the employment and occupation of patients with a spinal cord injury. *Paraplegia* **32**: 182–187, 1994.

Chowanec GD and Binik YM: End-stage renal disease and the marital dyad: a literature review and critique. *Soc Sci Med* **16**: 126–131, 1982.

Christensen AJ, Benotsch EG, Wiebe JS and Lawton WJ: Coping with treatment-related stress: effects on patient adherence in haemodialysis. *J Consult Clin Psychol* **63**: 454–459, 1995.

Colangelo RM, Stillman MJ, Kessler-Fogil D and Kessler-Hartnett D: The role of exercise in rehabilitation for patients with end-stage renal disease. *Rehab Nursing* **22**: 288–292, 1997.

Cope DN: The effectiveness of traumatic brain injury rehabilitation: a review. *Brain Injury* **9**: 649–670, 1995.

Cope DN and Hall K: Head injury rehabilitation. Benefit of early intervention. *Arch Phys Med Rehab* **63**: 433–437, 1982.

Craig AR, Hancock K, Chang E and Dickson H: Immunizing against depression and anxiety after spinal cord injury. *Arch Phys Med Rehab* **79**: 375–377, 1998.

Crisp R: The long-term adjustment of 60 persons with spinal cord injury. *Australian Psychologist* **27**: 43–47, 1992.

Devins GM: Illness intrusiveness and the psychosocial impact of lifestyle disruptions in chronic life-threatening disease. *Adv Renal Replacement Ther* **1**: 251–263, 1994.

Devins GM, Beanlands H, Mandin H and Paul LC: Psychosocial impact of illness intrusiveness moderated by self-concept and age in end-stage renal failure. *Health Psychol* **16**: 529–538, 1997.

DeVivo MJ, Black KJ, Richards JS and Stover SL: Suicide following spinal cord injury. *Paraplegia* **29**: 620–627, 1991.

DeVivo MJ, Hawkins LN, Richards JS and Go BK: Outcomes of post-spinal cord injury marriages. *Arch Phys Med Rehab* **76**: 130–138, 1995.

Dijkers MP, Abela NB, Gans BM and Gordon WA: The aftermath of spinal cord injury. In SL Stover, JA DeLisa and GG Whiteneck (Eds), *Spinal Cord Injury: Clinical Outcomes from the Model Systems*, pp 185–211. Aspen: Baltimore, 1995.

Eames P and Wood R: Rehabilitation after severe brain injury: a special unit approach to behavioural disorders. *Int Rehab Med* **7**: 130–133, 1985a.

Eames P and Wood R: Rehabilitation after severe head injury. Their nature and causes and strategies for management. *J Head Trauma Rehab* **3**(3): 1–6, 1985b.

Edwards CRW, Bouchier IAD, Hasle HC and Chivers ER: *Davidson's Principles and Practice of Medicine*. Churchill Livingstone: New York, 1995.

Eisenberg MG and Saltz CC: Quality of life among aging spinal cord injured patients: long term rehabilitation outcomes. *Paraplegia* **29**: 514–520, 1991.

Eisenberg MG, Glueckauf RL and Zaretsky HH (Eds): *Medical Aspects of Disability: A Handbook for the Rehabilitation Professional*. Springer: New York, 1993.

Ellenberg JH, Levin HS and Saydjari C: Posttraumatic amnesia as a predictor of outcome after severe closed head injury. *Arch Neurol* **53**: 782–791, 1996.

Evans RW, Mannien DL, Garrison LP, Blagg CR, Gutman RA, Hull AR and Lowrie EG: The quality of life of patients with end-stage renal failure. *N Engl J Med* **312**: 553–559, 1985.

Famularo RA and Kimball CP: Liaison psychiatry considerations in renal hemodialysis patients with acute organic cerebral disorders. In NB Levy (Ed), *Psychonephrology 2: Psychological Problems in Kidney Failure and their Treatment*, pp 71–78. Plenum: New York, 1983.

Farmer RA and Kimball CP: Survival on home haemodialysis: its relationship with physical symptomatology, psychosocial background and psychiatric morbidity. *Psychol Med* **9**: 515–523, 1979.

Farmer CJ, Bewick M, Parsons V and Snowden SA: Survival on home haemodialysis: its relationship with physical symptomatology, psychosocial background and psychiatric morbidity. *Psychological Med* **9**: 515–523, 1979.

Florian V, Katz S and Lahau V: Impact of traumatic brain damage on family dynamics and functioning: a review. *Brain Injury* **3**: 219–223, 1989.

Frank RG and Elliott TR: Spinal cord injury and health locus of control beliefs. *Paraplegia* **27**: 250–256, 1989.

Frank RG, Umlauf RL, Wonderlich SA, Askanasi GS, Buckelew S and Elliott T: Difference in coping styles among persons with spinal cord injury: a cluster approach. *J Consult Clin Psychol* **55**: 727–731, 1987.

Friend R, Singletary Y, Mendell N and Nurse H: Group participation and survival among patients with end-stage renal disease. *Am J Pub Hlth* **76**: 670–672, 1986.

Fuhrer MJ, Garber SL, Rintala DH, Clearman R and Hart KA: Pressure ulcers in community resident persons with spinal cord injury: prevalence and risk factors. *Arch Phys Med Rehab* **74**: 1172–1177, 1993.

Gaultieri T and Cox DR: The delayed neurobehavioural sequelae of traumatic brain injury. *Brain Injury* **5**: 219–232, 1991.

Gleckman AD and Brill S: The impact of brain injury on family functioning: implications for subacute rehabilitation programmes. *Brain Injury* **9**: 385–393, 1995.

Go BK, DeVivo NJ and Richards JS: The epidemiology of spinal cord injury. In SL Stover, JA DeLisa and GG Whiteneck (Eds), *Spinal Cord Injury: Clinical Outcomes from the Model Systems*. Aspen: Baltimore, 1995.

Guttman L: *Spinal Cord Injuries: Comprehensive Management and Research (2nd Edition)*. Blackwell Scientific: Oxford, UK, 1976.

Hancock KM, Craig AR, Dickson HG, Chang E and Martin J: Anxiety and depression over the first year of spinal cord injury: a longitudinal study. *Paraplegia* **31**: 349–357, 1993.

Harries F: Psychosocial care in end-stage renal failure. *Professional Nurse* **12**: 124–126, 1996.

Hener T, Weisenberg M and Har-Even D: Supportive versus cognitive-behavioural intervention programs in achieving adjustment to home peritoneal dialysis. *J Consult Clin Psychol* **64**: 731–741, 1996.

Hohmann G: Psychological aspects of treatment and rehabilitation of the spinal cord injured person. *Clin Orthopaedics* **112**: 81–88, 1975.

House A: Psychosocial problems of patients on the renal unit and their relation to treatment outcome. *J Psychosom Res* **52**: 41–46, 1987.

Jennett B and Bond M: Assessment of outcome after severe brain damage. *Lancet* **i**: 1031–1034, 1975.

Jennett B and Teasdale G: Predicting outcome in individual patients after severe head injury. *Lancet* **i**: 1031–1034, 1976.

Johnson J, Weissman MM and Klerman GL: Service utilization and social morbidity associated with depressive symptoms in the community. *JAMA* **267**: 1478–1483, 1982.

Johnson M: Models of disability. *The Psychologist* **9**: 205–210, 1996.

Judd FK and Brown DJ: The psychosocial approach to rehabilitation of the spinal cord injured patient. *Paraplegia* **26**: 419–424, 1988.

Judd FK and Burrows GD: Liaison psychiatry in the Spinal Injuries Unit. *Paraplegia* **24**: 6–19, 1986.

Judd FK, Brown DJ and Burrows GD: Depression, disease and disability: application to patients with traumatic spinal cord injury. *Paraplegia* **29**: 91–96, 1991.

Kennedy P: Psychological aspects of spinal cord injury: behavioural approaches, emotion and impact in coping strategies. Volume 2, *D Phil Thesis*, University of Ulster, 1995.

Kennedy P and Hamilton L: The Needs Assessment Checklist: A clinical approach to measuring outcome. *Spinal Cord* **37**: 136–139, 1999.

Kennedy P, Gorsuch N and Marsh N: Childhood onset of spinal cord injury: self esteem and self perception. *Br J Clin Psychol* **34**: 581–588, 1995a.

Kennedy P, Lowe R, Grey N and Short E: Traumatic spinal cord injury and psychological impact: a cross-sectional analysis of coping strategies. *Br J Clin Psychol* **34**: 627–639, 1995b.

Khan IH: Comorbidity: the major challenge for survival and quality of life in end-stage renal disease. *Nephrology, Dialysis, Transplantation* **13**: 76–79, 1998.

Killingworth A: Psychosocial impact of end-stage renal failure. *Br J Nursing* **1**: 905–908, 1993.

King C and Kennedy P: Coping effectiveness training for people with spinal cord injury: preliminary results of a controlled trial. *Br J Clin Psychol* **38**: 5–14, 1999.

King K: Vocational rehabilitation in maintenance dialysis patients. *Renal Replacement Ther* **1**: 228–239, 1994.

Klang B, Bjørvell H and Cronqvist A: Patients with chronic renal failure and their ability to cope. *Scand J Caring Sci* **10**: 89–95, 1996.

Kouidi E, Iacovides A, Iordanidis P, Vassiliou S, Deligiannis A, Ierodiakonou C and Tourkantonis A: Exercise renal rehabilitation program: psychosocial effects. *Nephron* **77**: 152–158, 1997.

Krause JS: Employment after spinal cord injury. *Arch Phys Med Rehab* **73**: 163–169, 1992.

Krause JS: Adjustment after spinal cord injury: a 9-year longitudinal study. *Arch Phys Med Rehab* **78**: 651–657, 1997.

Kutner NG: Psychosocial issues in end-stage renal disease. *Aging Advances in Renal Replacement Therapy* **1**(3): 210–218, 1994a.

Kutner NG: Assessing end-stage renal disease patients' functioning and well-being: measurement approaches and implications for clinical practice. *Am J Kidney Dis* **24**: 321–333, 1994b.

Kutner NG, Cardenas DD and Bower JD: Rehabilitation, aging and chronic renal disease. *Am J Phys Med Rehab* **71**: 97–101, 1992.

Levenson JL and Glocheski S: Psychological factors affecting end-stage renal failure. *Psychosomatics* **32**: 382–389, 1991.

Levin A, Lewis M, Mortiboy P, Faber S, Hare I, Porter EC and Mendelssohn DC: Multidisciplinary predialysis programs: quantification and limitations of their impact on patient outcomes in two Canadian settings. *Am J Kidney Dis* **29**: 535–540, 1997.

Levin HS, High WM, Goethe KE et al: The Neurobehavioural Rating Scale: Assessment of the behavioural sequelae of head injury by the clinician. *J Neurol Neurosurg Psychiatry* **50**: 183–193, 1987.

Levine DZ: *Care of the Renal Patient*. WB. Saunders: Philadelphia, 1991.

Lezak MD: *Neuropsychological Assessment (2nd Edition)*. Oxford University Press: New York, 1983.

Lindsay KW and Bone I: *Neurology and Neurosurgery, Illustrated*. Churchill Livingstone: Edinburgh, 1997.

Lishman WA: Physiogenesis and psychogenesis in the "post-concussional syndrome". *Br J Psychiatry* **153**: 460–469, 1988.

MacKay K and Moss AH: To dialyze or not to dialyze: an ethical and evidence-based approach to the patient with acute renal failure in the intensive care unit. *Advances in Renal Replacement Therapy* **4**: 288–296, 1997.

Masters WH and Johnson VE: *Human Sexual Inadequacy*. Little, Brown & Company: Boston, 1970.

McGlynn SM: Behavioural approaches to neuropsychological rehabilitation. *Psychol Bull* **108**: 420–441, 1990.

Molzahn AE, Northcott HC and Dossetor JB: Quality of life of individuals with end-stage renal disease: perceptions of patients, nurses and physicians. *ANNA J* **24**: 325–333, 1997.

Morgan AS, Chapman P and Tokarski L: Improved care of the traumatic brain injury (Abstract). In: *Proceedings of the Eastern Association for Surgery of Trauma, 1st Annual Conference, Longboat Key, Florida, 1998.*

Morris J: Psychological and sociological aspects of patients with spinal cord injuries. In HL Frankel (Ed), *Handbook of Clinical Neurology: Spinal Cord Trauma*, pp 537–555. Elsevier: London, 1992.

National Institutes of Health Consensus Statement: Morbidity and mortality of dialysis. *Ann Intern Med* **121**: 62–70, 1994.

OPCS (Office of Population Censuses and Surveys): *The Prevalence of Disability Among Adults.* HMSO: London, 1988.

Osberg JW, Meares GJ, McKee DC and Burnett GB: Intellectual functioning in renal failure and chronic dialysis. *J Chronic Dis* **35**: 445–457, 1982.

Overall J and Gorham D: Brief Psychiatric Rating Scale. *Psychol Rep* **10**: 799–812, 1962.

Palmer SE, Canzona L and Wai L: Helping families respond effectively to chronic illness: home dialysis as a case example. In RH Moos (Ed), *Coping with Physical Illness 2: New Perspectives*, pp 283–294. Plenum: New York, 1984.

Parkerson GR and Gutman RA: Perceived mental health and disablement of primary care end-stage renal disease patients. *Int J Psychiatry* **27**: 33–45, 1997.

Perlesz A, Furlong M and McLachlan D: Family work and acquired brain damage. *ANZ Family Therapy* **13**(3): 145–153, 1992.

Prigatano GP: Work, love and play after brain injury: observations from the neuroscience art and literature keynote address. *Proceedings of the 13th Annual Brain Impairment Conference, 1988.*

Prigatano GP and Schacter DL (Eds): *Awareness of Deficit After Brain Injury.* Oxford University Press: New York, 1991.

Prigatano GP, Glisky EL and Klonoff PSD: Cognitive rehabilitation after traumatic brain injury. In PW Corrigan and SC Yudofsky (Eds), *Cognitive Rehabilitation for Neuropsychiatric Disorders.* American Psychiatric Press: Washington, 1996.

Reidy K, Caplan B and Shawaryn M: Coping strategies following spinal cord injury: accommodation to trauma and disability. Paper presented at the 68th Annual Meeting of the American Congress of Rehabilitation Medicine, Washington, DC, 1991.

Rodin G: Depression in patients with end-stage renal disease: psychopathology or normative response? *Advances in Renal Replacement Therapy* **1**(3): 219–227, 1994.

Russell WR and Nathan PW: Traumatic amnesia. *Brain* **69**: 280–300, 1946.

Rustomjee S and Smith GC: Consultation-liaison psychiatry to renal medicine: work with an inpatient unit. *ANZ J Psychiatry* **30**: 229–237, 1996.

Sayag R, Kaplan De-Nour A, Shapira Z, Kahan E and Boner G: Comparison of psychosocial adjustment of male nondiabetic kidney transplant and hospital haemodialysis patients. *Nephron* **54**: 214–218, 1990.

Sensky T: Psychosomatic aspects of end-stage renal failure. *Psychother Psychosom* **59**(2): 56–68, 1993.

Silver JM, Hales RE and Yudofsky SC: Neuropsychiatric aspects of traumatic brain injury. In SC Yudofsky and RE Hales (Eds), *The American Psychiatric Press Textbook of Neuropsychiatry, 3rd Edition.* American Psychiatric Press: Washington, DC, 1997.

Sipski ML and Alexander CJ: Sexual function and dysfunction after spinal cord injury. *Phys Med Rehab Clin N Am* **3**: 811–828, 1992.

Sipski ML, Alexander CJ and Rosen RC: Physiological parameters associated with psychogenic arousal in women with complete spinal cord injuries. *Arch Phys Med Rehab* **76**: 811–818, 1995.

Smith BC and Winslow EH: Cognitive changes in chronic renal patients during haemodialysis. *ANNA J* **17**(4): 283–286, 1990.

Smith MD, Hong BA and Robson AM: Diagnosis of depression in patients with end-stage renal disease. *Am J Med* **79**: 160–166, 1985.

Smith NM, Floyd MR, Scogin F and Jamison CS: A three-year follow-up of bibliotherapy for depression. *J Consult Clin Psychol* **65**: 324–327, 1997.

Stover S and Fine R: *Spinal Cord Injury: The Facts and Figures.* University of Alabama, Birmingham, AL, 1986.

Stuss DT and Gow CA: "Frontal Dysfunction" after traumatic brain injury. *Neuropsychiatry Neuropsychol Behav Neurol* **5**: 272–282, 1992.

Szabo E, Moody H, Hamilton T, Kovithavongs C and Kjellstrand C: Choice of treatment improves quality of life. *Arch Intern Med* **157**: 1352–1356, 1997.

The Renal Association: *Treatment of Adult Patients with Renal Failure: Recommended Standards and Audit Measure* (2nd Edition). Royal College of Physicians: London, 1997.

Thomsen IV: Late outcome of very severe blunt head trauma: a 10–15 year second follow-up. *J Neurol Neurosurg Psychiatry* **47**: 260–268, 1984.

Thomsen IV: Late psychosocial outcome in severe traumatic brain injury. Preliminary results of a third follow-up study after 20 years. *Scand J Rehab Med (Suppl)* **26**: 142–152, 1992.

Trieschmann RB: *Spinal Cord Injuries: Psychological, Social and Vocational Rehabilitation* (2nd Edition). Demos: New York, 1988.

Vachon RA: Rehabilitation: should we just give up? *Nephrology News and Issues* **6**: 25, 29, 30, 45, 1992.

Washer GF, Schroter GPJ, Starzi TE and Weil R: Causes of death after kidney transplantation. *JAMA* **250**: 49–54, 1983.

Whiteneck GG, Charlifue SW, Frankel HL, Fraser BM, Gardner BP, Gerhart M, Krishnan K, Menter RR, Nusibeh I, Short D and Silver J: Mortality, morbidity and psychosocial outcomes of persons spinal cord injured more than 20 years ago. *Paraplegia* **30**: 617–630, 1992a.

Whiteneck GG, Charlifue SW, Gerhart KA, Overholser JA and Richardson GN: Quantifying handicap: a new measure of long-term rehabilitation outcomes. *Arch Phys Med Rehab* **73**: 519–526, 1992b.

Wong PP, Darnan J, Schentag CT, Ip R and Keating M: Statistical profile of traumatic brain injury: a Canadian rehabilitation program. *Brain Injury* **7**: 283–294, 1993.

Woodrich F and Patterson J: Variables related to acceptance of disability in persons with spinal cord injuries. *J Rehab* **49**: 26–30, 1983.

World Health Organisation: *International Classification of Impairments, Disabilities and Handicaps.* WHO: Geneva, 1980.

Wright TM: Family therapy and the nephrology patient. *Dialysis and Transplantation* **4**: 61–82, 1975.

8

Substance Abuse and Dependence

Peter E. Nathan
Department of Psychology, University of Iowa, USA

and

Nick Paoletti
Department of Psychiatry, University of Melbourne and Austin & Repatriation Medical Centre, Melbourne, Australia

INTRODUCTION

The Substance-Related Disorders

Clinical psychologists and psychiatrists are routinely called upon to diagnose and treat acute and chronic substance-related disorders, some of them primary, others secondary to comorbid disorders, in both in- and outpatient settings. These disorders include alcohol-, amphetamine-, cannabis-, cocaine-, hallucinogen-, inhalant-, opioid-, phencyclidine-, sedative-hypnotic-, and anxiolytic-related abuse, dependence, intoxication, withdrawal, intoxication delirium, and withdrawal delirium. They also include substance-induced psychotic states, substance-induced mood disorders, substance-induced persisting dementia, and substance-induced persisting amnestic disorder. In practice, most of the patients seen by both psychiatrists and psychologists suffer from abuse or dependence, one or more additional substance-related disorders, and additional comorbid psychiatric conditions. The definitions of these disorders on which this chapter relies are provided by DSM-IV (American Psychiatric Association 1994).

The lifetime prevalence of substance-related disorder in the United States was recently estimated to be 18%; the yearly cost in health care and job loss was placed at $144 billion per year; on average, in the United States, 20% of general medical inpatients and 35% of general psychiatric inpatients were estimated to have comorbid substance use disorders (Galanter & Kleber 1994). Similar figures are probably characteristic of most other developed countries.

Psychology and Psychiatry: Integrating Medical Practice.
Edited by J. Milgrom and G. D. Burrows © 2001 John Wiley & Sons, Ltd.

Comorbid Conditions

Many patients diagnosed with substance abuse or dependence present with comorbid disorders, physical and/or psychiatric. In addition to the actual substance-related disorders and comorbid psychiatric conditions, moreover, a complex interplay with other psychiatric and physical conditions is the rule.

The Epidemiological Catchment Area (ECA) study of the National Institute of Mental Health (NIMH) by Regier et al (1990) reported a lifetime prevalence of addictive behaviors in mentally ill patients in five American cities of about 29% (OR = 2.7). On the other side of this coin, comorbidity for mental disorder was found to be 37% (OR = 2.3) in alcoholics and 53% (OR = 4.5) in persons addicted to other drugs. Ries (1993), Sheehan (1993), Decker & Ries (1993) and Poole & Brabbins (1997) all emphasize the complex association of psychiatric illness and substance abuse, the frequency with which clinicians often fail to recognize one or the other of the dual diagnoses (depending on the setting in which the patient is treated), and the complexity of treatment. Ries (1993) also stresses flexibility in treatment format, with serial, parallel and integrated treatment models (referring to psychiatric and addictive treatment settings) for different patients.

As well, clinicians assessing or treating substance abusers must not ignore the likelihood of comorbidity with physical disorders (for example, hepatitis), since the latter will play an important role in determining the setting(s) in which the patient is treated. Clearly, a drug unit with close links to psychiatric facilities and medical units has many advantages. "Mainstreaming" of psychiatric and drug services hopefully facilitates such close links. A fairly "seamless" interface among these various services can only prove advantageous.

Roles and Responsibilities

Although the clinical work of psychologists and psychiatrists with substance abusers with or without comorbidity has increasingly moved in the direction of overlap, some generalizations are still apt. By virtue of their medical training, psychiatrists continue to be responsible for somatic assessment and treatment, including laboratory tests and the use of psychopharmacological interventions when appropriate. Likewise, as a result of the intensive training in assessment they receive, clinical psychologists generally undertake personality assessment and use detailed interviews and questionnaires to elicit information about the nature, antecedents and consequences of the patient's substance abuse and comorbid psychopathology (Nathan 1996). Although psychologists are more likely than psychiatrists to have been trained to employ the behavioral and cognitive-behavioral treatments that have become interventions of choice for many disorders in recent years, increasingly, psychologists and psychiatrists can both undertake syndromal diagnosis and both can provide a range of psychosocial treatments.

DIAGNOSIS AND ASSESSMENT

While some substance abusers may present with an uncomplicated picture, especially in the early stages of the disorder and in primary care rather than in psychiatric settings, those presenting to specialist clinics are much more likely to have complicated presentations, which might include one or more of the following:

- a pattern of abuse which is persistent and resistant to previous treatment attempts, often in the face of major psychosocial problems
- comorbidity with one or more psychiatric conditions, such as depression, antisocial personality disorder, or psychosis
- comorbidity with one or more physical conditions
  - caused by the substance abuse: for example, Wernicke's encephalopathy or cirrhosis of the liver in alcoholics, or hepatitis C or endocarditis in intravenous drug users
  - leading to the substance abuse: for example, chronic pain incidental to, but complicating, the total clinical picture: for example, patients admitted for an unrelated medical problem who are discovered to have comorbid drug abuse
  - co-existing pregnancy, with consequent need for early intervention (on the addictive behaviour) to prevent complications to the fetus
- special considerations, such as:
  - drug abuse by health care workers, especially those with access to drugs, such as physicians, nurses and pharmacists, but also anyone who may experience a reduction of mental function or abnormal behavior as a result of the drug use in settings where they engage in therapy of others
  - specific issues relating to age groups (children, adolescents, elderly) or gender
  - issues in transcultural settings or minority groups

Assessment Protocol

A comprehensive assessment protocol might well include the following sequence:

1. A proper referral request, with specific questions from the source of the referral, providing the reasons for referral and as much as possible about the patient's medical and psychiatric profile and likely areas of difficulties.
2. A comprehensive history, including the following elements:
   - alcohol and drug history
   - psychosocial history
   - current positive and negative circumstances
   - clinical assessment of personality characteristics, including weaknesses and strengths
   - psychiatric history, as appropriate (the depth will vary from case to case)
   - medical history.

3. Mental state examination.
4. Physical examination.
5. Laboratory investigations.
6. An assessment of addiction severity and areas of problems relating to the addiction, using interviews, questionnaires and rating scales.
7. Structured and semi-structured interviews for psychiatric diagnosis (see below) may be used in certain settings to accompany the clinical assessment.
8. Motivational interviewing (Miller & Rollnick 1991), especially in early stages, can set the stage for a less ambivalent involvement by the patient (Jarvis et al 1995).

A thorough alcohol and drug consumption/use history is an essential first step in assessing the patient who may be abusing alcohol or drugs. While alcohol-dependent patients may deny the extent of their abuse of alcohol, drug addicts are often quite candid about their "hard" drug intake, although they usually understate their concurrent benzodiazepine use. This last point can be very important, as benzodiazepines and/or alcohol can become potentially lethal when used with methadone (or any narcotic, for that matter).

Some assessment of personality and a psychiatric screening history should be part of the initial assessment process. A more thorough psychiatric history should be obtained where comorbid psychopathology is obvious or suspected.

Syndromal Diagnosis

Most syndromal diagnoses of substance-related disorders are accomplished according to unstructured diagnostic interviews that adhere reasonably closely to DSM-IV or ICD-10 (WHO 1992) diagnostic criteria. However, structured interviews for DSM-III (Diagnostic Interview Schedule: DIS; Robins et al 1981) and for ICD-10 (Composite International Diagnostic Interview: CIDI; WHO 1993), as well as a semi-structured interview for DSM-IV (Structured Clinical Interview for DSM-IV: SCID; First et al 1995), represent more highly reproducible and, hence, more reliable formats for syndromal diagnosis, including the diagnosis of substance-related disorders. In practice, the structured interviews (the DIS and the CIDI) can be administered reliably by trained lay interviewers, while the SCID works best when administered by a trained mental health professional. Of course, integration of diagnostic findings into a comprehensive assessment package for treatment planning that includes extensive information on family, social, and medical history, laboratory findings, and substance use pattern requires the skills, training, and experience of a psychiatrist or psychologist.

Assessment Interviews, Questionnaires and Rating Scales

Once interviews yielding substance abuse/dependence diagnoses, associated substance-related diagnoses, diagnoses of comorbid psychopathology, and additional information on family, social, and medical history have been completed, additional assessment measures designed to provide information to plan effective treatment are often employed by psychiatrists and psychologists who work with substance abusers.

These measures provide data on pre- and post-treatment consumption or use patterns, including periods of abstinence following prior treatment. The resultant information helps predict treatment effectiveness; in general, the heavier a person's prior abusive consumption pattern and the longer he or she has abused alcohol or drugs, the less likely he or she will benefit from treatment (Finney & Monahan 1996). Moreover, knowing as much as possible about the patient's previous history of success or failure in substance abuse treatment helps predict treatment outcome and motivation for change, as well as identify treatments more likely to be effective.

Two of the most widely-used measures of substance abuse patterns were originally developed for alcohol abusers, namely the Quantity-Frequency-Variability Index (QFV; Cahalan et al 1969) and the Timeline Followback Procedure (TLFP; Sobell & Sobell 1992). The QFV Index, developed for the first national study of drinking practices in the United States, asks respondents to provide a summary self-report of their drinking over an average week. Although it has proven valuable in epidemiological studies in non-treatment populations, it has been used less often with populations of substance abusers, perhaps because these groups might not be as willing to provide accurate data on their alcohol use.

The TLFP also elicits self-reports of drinking over discrete time periods, ranging from a month to a year; unlike the QFV Index, the TLFP was developed for use with patient populations. With the help of a clinician experienced in its use, the patient reconstructs consumption patterns following prompts which anchor drinking to special days, like birthdays, anniversaries, holidays, visits with friends, and the like. These prompts facilitate accurate recall of drinking behavior over time. The TLFP is especially useful when data on binge and abstinence periods are called for during treatment planning.

The Comprehensive Drinker Profile (CDP; Marlatt & Miller 1987), a structured interview, provides detailed information on drinking history and substance abuse pattern; it also aims to identify high stress environmental and psychological situations associated in the past with drinking, as well as current and prior correlates of motivation to change drinking. The CDP is one of the most useful substance abuse assessment methods, both because it is comprehensive and because it focuses on information of clear value in treatment planning.

The Severity of Opiate Dependence Questionnaire (SODQ; Sutherland et al 1986) is a 21-item Likert-type questionnaire, simply filled by the patient. It is used to assess the severity of opiate addiction.

Another important focus of assessment of the substance abuser are the life problems associated with the abuse. Knowing the nature of a substance abuser's life problems makes it possible to gauge motivation for change (if the problems are major, motivation will likely be higher than if they are not) as well as to plan treatment (physical problems reduce the likelihood that treatments designed to address psychological or psychiatric consequences will work). The best-regarded measure of substance-induced life problems is the Alcohol Dependence Scale (ADS; Skinner & Horn 1984). Based on the alcohol dependence syndrome concept, on which the diagnosis of substance dependence was based in DSM-III-R (American Psychiatric Association 1987), the ADS was developed empirically from extensive clinical samples; it reflects such life problems associated with alcohol dependence as compulsive drink seeking, loss of behavioral control over alcohol use, and many of the physical and perceptual sequelae of alcohol withdrawal.

Similarly, the Opiate Treatment Index (OTI; Darke et al 1991) and the Addiction Severity Index (ASI; McLellan et al 1980a) are useful in the assessment of lifestyle problems associated with drug addiction, which can then be further explored, leading to the tailoring of better therapy. McLellan et al (1980a), in particular, have stressed several commonly found problem areas, that are not correlated with each other, or with severity of chemical abuse. The OTI also includes an HIV Risk-Taking Behaviour Scale (HRBS), which is useful in patient education in reducing risk of acquiring blood-borne viruses.

A further category of information most often tapped during the assessment of a substance abuser is information on antecedents to and consequences of the abuse. This information is essential to treatment planning, especially cognitive behavioral treatment. Effective treatment typically requires that alternative ways be found by which substance abusers can access a suitable range of reinforcers to replace those lost when substance use is given up.

Over the past decade, a large and still-growing body of literature on alcohol expectancies has accumulated. Alcohol expectancies are the expectations one has of the effects of alcohol on one's behavior. Expectancies can be assessed in children before drinking begins. They appear to interact with personality risk factors to predict drinking behavior, and seem to mediate the impact of other early risk factors, including family history of alcoholism, on subsequent alcohol consumption (Goldman et al 1991). The alcohol expectancies most predictive of heavy drinking by high school students (Smith et al 1995), college students (Wood et al 1996), and young males aged 21 to 25 (Deckel et al 1995) have also been identified. The two alcohol expectancy questionnaires in current widest use were developed by Brown and her colleagues (Brown et al 1980) and Leigh & Stacy (1993).

Finally, scales that may be used include those to assess withdrawal, such as the Opiate Withdrawal Questionnaire (OWQ; Gossop et al 1987) and its condensation, the Short Opiate Withdrawal Scale (SOWS). These are used to monitor severity of symptoms, during and after an acute withdrawal phase, and are useful in heightening therapist awareness to patient risk and discomfort.

Physical Examination and Laboratory Tests

The importance of a thorough physical examination of the substance abuser cannot be overestimated. While it is outside the scope of this chapter to cover this complex topic in detail, it is important to note here that, depending on the type of substance abused, there will be particular foci of examination, as well as laboratory tests and radiological examinations relating to the systems potentially affected.

Even though the following list is not exhaustive, it does highlight some of the most important points that may be sought in a physical examination.

- Alcohol-dependent patients may have significant pathology in virtually any body system and, accordingly, require very thorough examination. The neurological, gastrointestinal (including hepatic), and cardiovascular systems are often affected, but one must also consider nutritional/hematological and endocrine problems, as well as the possibility of infections and injuries.
- Intravenous drug users will have tell-tales signs on the skin, such as puncture marks (often hidden by tattoos and birth marks) and signs of venous irritation or tissue induration.
- The nasal mucosa will be thinned or ulcerated in persons who snort their drug.
- Pupils will be constricted in narcotic users and dilated during narcotic withdrawal or in users of hallucinogens. These changes will not be seen in isolation, but will be accompanied by other signs of toxicity or withdrawal: for example, pupillary dilatation in narcotic withdrawal may be accompanied by piloerection ("goose bumps"), cramps and diarrhea.
- "Toxidromes" are rarely seen in their severe forms in the clinic, being more commonly seen in hospital emergency rooms. In their severe forms, they can be difficult to differentiate from each other: a sweating, semi-conscious patient, with high blood pressure, irregular heart rate, faltering respiration and an incipient seizure can have any one of several toxidromes, and it can be a real clinical challenge to make a precise diagnosis on clinical grounds alone. However, for those who work in clinics, early recognition of an impending state of toxicity is essential. Observational acumen and simply taken measurements, such as blood pressure and pulse and respiratory rates and rhythms, can prevent disasters. Slurred speech or reduced sensorium can indicate the need to perform a physical examination at a routine clinic review.

Laboratory testing should include at least urinary drug screening, full blood examination, liver function tests and screening for hepatitis. Depending on the results of these basic tests, other tests may become indicated (for example, following up an anemic pattern due to malnutrition with tests for a more precise diagnosis, such as iron deficiency). In addition, depending on the clinical picture that unfolds from the history and physical and mental examination, additional laboratory tests may also be ordered. HIV testing may be indicated, according to risk, but one must remember the necessity for pre- and post-test counseling when ordering such a test.

Urine drug screening, especially when used randomly, can be very useful in improving abstinence rates and retention in treatment programs (McCarthy & Borders 1985). A useful method is to have true randomization, using computer generated random tables, with a minimum testing rate, but also additional testing based on clinical suspicion. Urine for screening should be collected under supervision: a common trick used by some patients in methadone maintenance programs is to bring someone else's drug-free urine, to which a trace of methadone has been added, in a container kept close to the body for convincingly warm temperature felt through the clinic's official container, into which it is poured. Trust issues clearly come into play when random testing programs are in place, so the testing should be done in an atmosphere of openness, to minimize the likelihood that the procedure will become a challenging game.

Appropriate storage is essential if the urine is not going to be tested immediately. Laboratories use automated immunoassays for screening, to keep costs low. Presumptive identification is then followed up with more sophisticated techniques, such as chromatography and spectroscopic methods (Honour 1996). These more complex techniques, apart from confirming the presence of a class of drugs, for example, opioids, can also differentiate different compounds, such as morphine or codeine. Both a knowledge of pharmacological properties, such as the half-life of a drug, and of clinical facts, such as amount and time of ingestion, is essential to any conclusions drawn from testing.

Roles and Responsibilities

The role of the psychologist or psychiatrist is to administer (as appropriate) and interpret these diverse interviews, instruments, questionnaires, and tests, then interpret them and plan treatment accordingly. Many psychologists and psychiatrists find that sharing their assessments with their patients works well. Being informed of the extent of their abuse problem sometimes enhances patients' motivation to change their alcohol or drug use pattern; it also casts them in the role of collaborator in the planning and execution of their own treatment, another inducement to take responsibility for subsequent change efforts.

In practice, close collaboration between psychologist and physician is essential during assessment. The responsibility of the psychologist, generally, is to administer and interpret paper-and-pencil tests and questionnaires, while that of the physician is to order and interpret the results of laboratory tests. Both professional groups are involved nowadays in the diagnostic process. Comprehensive planning for treatment requires comprehensive knowledge of a broad range of assessment information, so psychiatrists and psychologists have a responsibility to ensure that they work closely together during this period in the best interests of their patients.

TREATMENT

Introduction and Aims of Treatment

O'Brien & McLellan (1996) point out that some clinicians continue to view treatment of the substance-related disorders as unrewarding because of unrealistic expectations of total and permanent cure. However, working in this area can be quite rewarding if one views treatment success as one or more of the following:

- Attenuation of the pattern of abuse, with total abstinence being only one of several possible positive outcomes
- Reduction of social consequences, such as:
  - reduction of crime
  - reduction of traffic accidents during intoxication
  - reduction of violence towards family and others
- Change in the abuse pattern so that it occurs less often and is less "driven" by craving
  - the need to engage in crime to obtain money for drugs may disappear
  - this more "elective" use may mean not sharing needles
- From the latter would follow a reduction in the spread of blood-borne viral diseases, such as hepatitis and HIV, which would be a major public health advance
- Improved mental health and reduction of comorbidity
- An improvement in personal functioning that may mean:
  - a return to at least part-time work
  - reduction of poverty through better management of money
  - enhancement of personal self-esteem
  - improvement of societal behavior
  - increase in frequency of behaviors other than drug-seeking
  - improved family life, including better care of children (an often forgotten group of sufferers in this context).

O'Brien & McLellan (1996) also note that both physicians and the general public tend to perceive the addictions "as...acute conditions such as a broken leg or pneumococcal pneumonia" (p 237). As a result, when the acute care procedure of detoxification is not followed by appropriate treatment follow-up and leads to the virtually inevitable relapse, "the treatment is regarded as a failure" (p 237). By contrast, these authors see addiction as a chronic disorder like hypertension, diabetes and asthma, stressing that, "as for the treatment of addiction, treatments for these chronic medical disorders heavily depend on behavioral change and medication compliance to achieve their potential effectiveness" (p 239).

McLellan et al (1980a) stress the importance of analyzing both severity and particular areas of problems in individual addicts. Their validated Addiction Severity Index is designed to "analyze the total addiction profile into its component treatment problems, and to estimate reliably and validly the severity of each of these problems" (p 32). The same group (1980b) advocates tailoring a treatment program to each patient. O'Brien & McLellan (1996) cite several studies confirming the usefulness of such an approach, with compliance with the recommended treatment plan a major predictor of therapeutic success, and psychiatric comorbidity and psychosocial difficulties prime predictors of therapeutic failure.

Ideally, psychologists and psychiatrists, together with other members of the team, plan substance-abuse treatment, based on their convergent assessments of the patient. While the patient might be treated by psychosocial or pharmacological means alone, a combined drug/psychotherapy treatment regimen probably works best, especially when the patient suffers both from a substance-related disorder and a comorbid psychiatric condition that responds to pharmacological treatment. As well, involving the patient simultaneously in self-help treatment is thought by many to be an essential component of treatment for substance abuse, especially when one of the substances abused is alcohol.

Detoxification

"Detoxification programs provide supervised withdrawal from a drug of dependence so that the severity of withdrawal symptoms and serious medical complications are reduced to a minimum" (Mattick & Hall 1996, p 97). Another desirable outcome of alcohol and drug withdrawal is "to foster the patient's motivation to enter rehabilitation therapy" (Gallant 1994, p 68). However, Mattick & Hall (1996) warn against "forcing too close a connection between treatment and detoxification" (p 97), since this may discourage patients from even entering a detoxification program, let alone further treatment.

Since space does not permit an elaborate description of the various withdrawal syndromes, or of detailed treatment protocols, we must limit ourselves to some general principles. Descriptions of opioid withdrawal syndromes can be found, among other sources, in Gossop et al (1987), Farrell (1994) and Mattick & Hall (1996); alcohol withdrawal in Mattick & Hall (1996); benzodiazepine withdrawal syndrome in Petursson (1994); and stimulant withdrawal in Lago & Kosten (1994). Hallucinogens probably do not cause a "true withdrawal syndrome" (Halikas 1993, p 697). West & Gossop (1994) provide an overview comparing withdrawal symptoms. Mattick & Hall (1996) broadly review the literature, concluding that alcohol withdrawal is a potentially lethal condition, whereas opioid withdrawal is uncomfortable to the point of being "immiserating" (p 98), but is rarely life-threatening.

Along with the use of benzodiazepines to control withdrawal symptoms (if indicated), alcohol withdrawal should be accompanied by prophylactic thiamine replacement to prevent Wernicke's encephalopathy (Mattick & Hall 1996). A clinical pointer for acute situations is always to inject thiamine before introducing carbohydrates in intravenous drips. This avoids Wernicke's encephalopathy being precipitated, as the last reservoir of thiamine may be drained when the Krebs' cycle is activated. Benzodiazepine withdrawal can sometimes result in seizures and psychotic reactions (Petursson 1994). This may also happen with withdrawal from the other CNS depressants, therefore withdrawal should be graded. It is always important to establish how much a patient is really using, to prevent overdosage and underdosage during withdrawal. Lago & Kosten (1994) review the literature on stimulant withdrawal and find contradictions about the presence of the classically described triadic sequence of "crash", "withdrawal" and "extinction". In any case, stimulant abstinence would not appear to produce as marked an effect as those produced by alcohol, opioids and sedatives.

Whether assisted withdrawal takes place in inpatient or outpatient settings depends on a variety of factors, some of which are outlined below.

The Likelihood of Medical Complications

Mattick & Hall (1996) conclude that alcohol withdrawal may need an inpatient setting, under medical supervision, especially "in those at greatest risk of life-threatening delirium tremens or seizures" (p 98) or where psychiatric or medical disorders may "complicate management" (p 98). However, they stress that "many people with mild-to-moderate withdrawal can be detoxified safely, successfully, and much more cheaply at home under the supervision of a visiting nurse to administer anxiolytic drugs, with medical practitioners providing necessary medical support" (p 98).

The Experience of the Treatment Provider

Obviously, experience is an essential requirement for home withdrawal of an alcoholic.

The Rate of Success

While opioid withdrawal, in most cases, could be conducted safely at home, Mattick & Hall's review (1996) suggests that inpatient settings not only tend to be favored by opioid addicts, but they have a higher rate of completion of the process. We refer here to patients who are detoxifying, as distinct from those entering a methadone program. Pettinati et al (1993) review the issues in inpatient versus outpatient studies and point out the methodological pitfalls in most previous studies. In particular, the exclusion from comparative studies of patients requiring inpatient treatment skews their results. In their study of inpatient versus outpatient detoxification from alcohol, they use a patient-treatment matching method, rather than random assignment, to prevent exclusion of those patients who required inpatient care. Preliminary analysis showed that outpatients were four times as likely to be early treatment failures ($\chi^2 = 41.2$, df $= 1$, $p < 0.01$). The same study showed that psychiatric illness and/or poor social supports were poor prognostic indicators for outpatient therapy; such subjects do better as inpatients.

The Motivation Behind Entering a Detoxification Program

Mattick & Hall (1996) alert us to motivations like entering a program to obtain drugs cheaply.

An Extreme Situation Requiring Inpatient Care of Any Addict Would Be a "Toxidrome"

These would normally be handled in emergency rooms or intensive care or other special units. A patient at risk of death from respiratory depression from opioids and/or benzodiazepines, for example, will need emergency use of antagonists, like naloxone for opioids and flumazenil for benzodiazepines, to displace the drug from its brain receptors and precipitate rapid withdrawal, which, obviously, will need close clinical monitoring.

Psychosocial Treatments

The psychosocial treatments for substance abuse briefly described below have been empirically supported. In each case, well-designed empirical research on the outcome provides assurance that the treatment is one of the most effective available for the condition in question (Nathan 1998).

The efficacy and effectiveness of psychosocial treatments for alcoholism were recently explored in two extensive studies: the United States National Institute on Alcohol Abuse and Alcoholism (NIAAA) study (Project MATCH Research Group 1993, 1997) and a United States Veterans Administration (VA) study (Ouimette et al 1997). Project MATCH (Project MATCH Research Group 1997) included two independent, parallel randomized clinical trials (RCTs). A total of 1726 alcohol-dependent outpatients (952 in one RCT, 774 in the other) were randomly assigned to one of three 12-week, manual-guided, individually delivered treatments, Cognitive Behavioral Coping Skills Therapy (CBT), Motivational Enhancement Therapy (MET), and Twelve-Step Facilitation Therapy (TST). Three separate, detailed treatment manuals were written, published, and provided to each therapist participating in the study (Kadden et al 1992; Miller et al 1992; Nowinski et al 1992). Clients were followed for a year; primary outcome measures were per cent days abstinent and drinks per drinking day during the one-year post-treatment period. The three treatments were described in a recent report on Project MATCH (1997) as follows:

> CBT was based on social learning theory and viewed drinking behavior as functionally related to major problems in an individual's life, with emphasis placed on overcoming skills deficits and increasing the ability to cope with situations that commonly precipitate relapse. TST was grounded in the concept of alcoholism as a spiritual and medical

> disease with stated objectives of fostering acceptance of the disease of alcoholism, developing a commitment to participate in AA and beginning to work through the 12 steps... MET was based on principles of motivational psychology and focused on producing internally motivated change. This treatment was not designed to guide the client, step by step, through recovery, but instead employed motivational strategies to mobilize the individual's own resources. (Project MATCH Research Group 1997, p 13)

The basic assumption underlying the Project MATCH study and its series of "matching hypotheses" was that substance abusers who are appropriately matched to treatments will experience better outcomes than those who are unmatched or mismatched. Surprisingly, however, given the widespread acceptance among clinicians of this assumption, only one of the matches was borne out. A secondary finding in terms of the basic purposes of Project MATCH, but of greater interest to the readers of this paper, was that significant and sustained improvements in drinking outcomes were achieved from baseline to one-year post-treatment by study subjects in all three treatment regimens. In other words, there was no difference in outcomes by type of treatment: the three treatments were comparable in efficacy.

The Veterans Administration study (Ouimette et al 1997) tested the comparative effectiveness of twelve-step and cognitive-behavioral (C-B) models of substance abuse treatment in 3018 detoxified inpatients from substance abuse treatment programs located at 15 United States Department of Veterans Affairs Medical Centers. Programs had a 21- to 28-day desired length of stay, used individual and group therapy, and were multidisciplinary in staffing. The two treatments were structured as follows:

> Twelve-step programs emphasized treatment activities such as 12-step meetings in the community and hospital, and psychotherapy groups covering topics such as working the steps, the *Big Book*, and writing an autobiography. Treatment targeted the patient's acceptance of an alcoholic-addict identity, acknowledgment of a loss of control-powerlessness over the abused substance, and adherence to abstinence as a treatment goal... C-B programs required participation in relapse prevention groups, cognitive skills training, behavioral skills training, abstinence skills training, and small C-B therapy groups. The goals of C-B treatment were to teach more adaptive ways of coping, to enhance the patient's sense of self-efficacy to cope with high-risk relapse-inducing situations, and to modify the patient's expectations of the abused substances' effects such that they were more realistic and appropriate. (Ouimette et al 1997, p 232)

Twelve-step patients in this study were somewhat more likely to be abstinent at the one-year follow-up; twelve-step, C-B, and combined twelve-step–C-B treatment programs were equally effective in reducing substance use and improving most other areas of functioning. The finding of equal effectiveness was consistent over several treatment subgroups, including patients attending the "purest" twelve-step and C-B treatment programs, and patients who had received the "full dose" of treatment. Moreover, patients with substance abuse diagnoses alone, those with comorbid psychiatric diagnoses, and those who had not entered treatment on their own volition all showed similar improvement at one-year follow-up, regardless of type of treatment received.

We conclude that psychologists and psychiatrists who have not yet been trained in the three treatment modalities empirically supported in these studies ought to seek this training. They currently represent the psychosocial treatments of choice for alcohol dependence.

Pharmacological Treatments—General Issues

Pharmacological treatments of drug-addicted patients are becoming more sophisticated, coincident with increased understanding of the neurochemical mechanisms involved in addiction, while PET and SPECT studies provide human data to support models previously based only on animal data. Nutt (1996) gives the following examples of how this understanding leads to better therapies or better understanding of empirically derived therapies:

- Endogenous opioids may be involved in the action of drugs other than opiates, such as alcohol and stimulants, thereby explaining the apparent efficacy of naltrexone in preventing relapse of alcoholism
- The decrease of noradrenergic neuron activity by opioids explains the efficacy of alpha-2 noradrenoreceptor agonists, clonidine and lofexidine, in the treatment of opioid withdrawal
- Increased calcium flux may contribute to neuronal death, which may be reduced by calcium channel antagonists, such as nitrendipine, which block some aspects of alcohol withdrawal.

Some of the established and emerging pharmacological treatments will now be considered.

Substitution Therapy (Agonists and Partial Agonists)

Methadone, the most widely known substitution treatment, has been described as "one of the best supported pharmacological treatments in all medical published research" (Seiverwright & Greenwood 1996, p 374). First described by Dole & Nyswander (1965), it is now widely used, with proven efficacy (Bertschy 1995; Sorensen 1996), whether patients enter treatment spontaneously or on referral by legal authorities (Brecht et al 1993). Methadone maintenance drastically reduces rates of HIV transmission (Metzger et al 1993) and criminal activity (Bell et al 1992). It is clearly cost-effective (Hubbard et al 1992).

The most effective dosage of methadone has been the subject of some controversy, especially as "client oriented" approaches, in which the patients have a larger say in the dose used and in whether complete abstinence is achieved, have tended to explore lower doses than the "blockade" doses of 80–120 mg per day originally used by Dole & Nyswander (1965). Studies such as those by Ball & Ross (1991) and

Caplehorn et al (1993) and a review by Lowinson et al (1992) support the efficacy of doses above 70–80 mg and the inefficacy of doses below 40–45 mg. Consensus now seems to be emerging on the value of tailoring dosage to patient, to ensure control, bearing in mind that lapse does not lead irrevocably to relapse (Johns 1994).

Other agents used for maintenance therapy of opiate addicts include Levo-alpha-acetylmethadol (LAAM) and Buprenorphine. LAAM, like methadone, is an opioid agonist, but has a much longer duration of action, allowing a three times a week rather than daily dosage (O'Brien 1996). One side-advantage is the elimination of weekend take-home doses, with the inherent risks of misuse and diversion. Buprenorphine, an opioid partial agonist, has also been shown to be effective in substitution therapy (Bickel et al 1988; Lewis 1985). Like LAAM, it has a long duration of action and additional advantages of reduced potential for toxicity, easier withdrawal and less interaction with other drugs (Seiverwright & Greenwood 1996). It may also have advantages in normalizing the endogenous opioid system and preparing the brain for naltrexone which, being an antagonist, has no addiction potential (Kosten et al 1992).

It is important to keep in mind that substitution therapy is not indefinite, but provides a period of time that allows the patient to gain control of the addiction, through better psychological control and skills.

Antagonists

Antagonists act by completely blocking receptors, so no further pharmacological activity on the receptors of interest can take place. Flumazenil (Hunkeler et al 1981) and naloxone (Senay 1994), in intravenous form, are useful in the reversal of benzodiazepine and opiate toxidromes, respectively. However, they can also induce acute withdrawal. In the case of naloxone, withdrawal symptoms can be managed with clonidine or lofexidine (Seiverwright & Greenwood 1996). In severe cases of withdrawal, general anesthetics, such as methohexitone, have been used by some (Loimer et al 1990). However, Farrell (1994) warns against using an expensive procedure with a risk of mortality (general anesthesia) for a condition (opiate withdrawal) which has negligible risk of death if unassisted.

Naltrexone is a longer-acting opiate antagonist than naloxone and, because it is more stable in the intestinal tract, can be given orally. It is useful as a relapse-preventing measure after detoxification (Seiverwright & Greenwood 1996), particularly in very motivated patients. Naltrexone has also been reported by Volpicelli et al (1992) to reduce craving and relapse into alcoholism.

Alpha-2 Adrenoreceptor Agonists

Clonidine (Gold et al 1978) and lofexidine (Washton et al 1983) are useful in alleviating narcotic withdrawal symptoms. Lofexidine is safe for outpatient use because it does not lower blood pressure (Seiverwright & Greenwood 1996).

Alcohol-Sensitizing Drugs

Disulfiram (Fuller et al 1986; Gerrein et al 1973), known more familiarly as Antabuse, has been widely used. It exerts its effect by serving as a psychological deterrent to using alcohol, the concurrent use of which will induce an unpleasant reaction (Gallant 1994). Pharmacologically, it works by blocking the metabolism of alcohol, thereby causing the accumulation of a noxious by-product, acetaldehyde (O'Brien 1997). This mechanism is also responsible for relatively low compliance (Fuller et al 1986), because it requires high motivation. Disulfiram works best under supervision (Azrin et al 1982; Sereny et al 1986). There are still clinicians who support its use (Gallant 1994), but Schuckit (1996, p 672) cautions that "additional large scale trials that incorporate behavioral and counselling techniques aimed specifically at enhancing the effect of disulfiram" are needed before its routine use can be recommended. Schuckit (1996) bases his caution on the presence of rare but serious side-effects (neuropathy, optic neuritis, blood dyscrasias and potentially lethal hepatotoxicity, not to mention severe depression, confusion and psychosis), and uncertain efficacy, in that the only large-scale trial is that by Fuller et al (1986).

GABA Agonists

Schuckit (1996) reviews several early trials of acamprosate (calcium acetylhomotaur-inate), a GABA agonist mostly used in Europe, which has shown promising early results in preventing alcoholism relapse.

Psychotropic Drugs

These drugs have important uses in many patients with psychiatric comorbidity, especially those with psychosis or major depression. Their use with substance abusers is similar to that in the treatment of the psychiatric condition alone, but with special issues relating to the alcohol or drug dependence:

- *Benzodiazepines* should be avoided for the treatment of anxiety, or prescribed with even more caution than normally, because of the almost certain chance of addiction. However, their short-term use in alcohol withdrawal is well estab-lished and essential to the prevention of a potentially lethal withdrawal syn-drome. Also, there will be patients with established addiction to these compounds, often in combination with other drugs, and they will need to be detoxified
- *Antipsychotic medications* do not present major problems, if used judiciously and in a manner that minimizes drug interactions
- The *antidepressants* are often used because of the high comorbidity of substance dependence and depression. Sierralta et al (1995) have shown various antide-

pressants (imipramine, clomipramine, maprotiline and zimelidine) to have anti-nociceptive activity in mice addicted to morphine. The newer antidepressants, particularly the SSRIs, apart from lower toxicity in overdose, are also finding use as "anticraving" medication (Seiverwright & Greenwood 1996). However, more studies, including pharmaco-epidemiological follow-up, are necessary to more fully understand drug interactions. Bertschy et al (1994) have reported cases of moderate to high (20–100%) increases in methadone levels after starting fluvox-amine, and also one case of opiate withdrawal syndrome after stopping fluvox-amine. Thus, "caution is needed when starting or stopping treatment with fluvoxamine in patients receiving maintenance treatment with methadone" (Bertschy et al 1994, p 42). Bertschy et al (1996) found a less marked interaction between fluoxetine and methadone, "unlikely to have clinical consequences" (p 570). Fluoxetine's long half-life has an additional advantage of maintaining therapeutic levels, as these patients, paradoxically, can be poorly compliant with prescribed medication.

Immunopharmacotherapy

This is an extremely interesting new area of development, although relatively remote at this time from clinical application. Active immunization has been used, only in rodent models so far, to block the psychostimulant action of cocaine (Fox et al 1996; Rocio et al 1995).

Roles and Responsibilities

Treatment roles and responsibilities may be related to professional roles, for ex-ample social milieu changes provided by social workers, cognitive behavioral ther-apy provided by psychologists and drug treatments provided by psychiatrists. However, combined drug-psychosocial treatment is often called for, especially when the substance abuser also suffers from a comorbid psychiatric disorder which is responsive to drug treatment. Hence, the closest possible cooperation between all members of the multidisciplinary team in the management of these patients is appropriate, if patients are to benefit from the empirically supported treatments-of-choice currently available.

SPECIAL ISSUES

Pregnancy

Raskin (1993) in reviewing the literature, states: "Alcohol, tobacco, and illicit drug addiction during pregnancy have been associated with low birth weight, prematur-ity, small-for-gestational-age babies, fetal alcohol syndrome, fetal loss, and obstetric complications, including placenta previa and abruptio placentae" (p 157). She also makes the point that "crack babies" have not only been covered widely by the popular media, but their "stereotypes...appear to influence our scientific judgment" (p 157). Thus she refers to the study of Koren et al (1989) which documents that papers showing adverse effects of fetal cocaine exposure were more likely to be accepted for scientific presentation than those which did not, even if the latter were methodologically superior. It would seem that systematic reviews of studies already done on risks of fetal drug exposure are badly needed, as well as further studies, such as retrospective cohort and case control studies, that would not present the ethical dilemmas that RCTs would have in this area.

For the clinician, until more evidence-based information is available, caution would appear to be of the essence:

- Firstly, as the malformation risks to the fetus in the first trimester are well established when the patient discovers she is pregnant, education about risks of fetal exposure to drugs, including alcohol and the often forgotten tobacco, should be part of the routine management of all patients in the drug clinic. This should include male partners, as a well-informed female patient may be no better off if she has a dominant male partner ignorant of or oblivious to this information
- It must be remembered that, apart from the mutagenic risks during organ formation in the first trimester, some substances, such as alcohol and tobacco, can continue to affect the fetus throughout pregnancy
- In those cases where it has been impossible to have the patient off all drugs throughout the pregnancy, the risks must be clearly understood by patient and partner. Also, cooperation with obstetric units specially staffed to deal with chemical dependence, which are appearing in some countries, improves monitoring of fetal structure and function, to maximize fetal health (where religion and the law are not obstacles, termination may need to be considered in some cases of malformation). The involvement of such specialized obstetric units also minimizes the impact of drugs on the birth process, such as suppression of the newborn's respirations by opioids and benzodiazepines
- Addiction in the newborn of such patients must not be forgotten, nor the effect of drugs passed through the milk.

Lanehart et al (1996) give encouraging preliminary evidence of the effectiveness of case management of women during pregnancy and the post-natal period.

Children and Adolescents

There are two issues to consider:

- Children of drug addicts are at risk. The literature on this issue is vast and will not be reviewed here. However, it is important to emphasize that health workers in this area need to be constantly vigilant of such risks in the infants, children and adolescents of drug-addicted patients

- Minors who are themselves patients present special issues that require special expertise. Yaster et al (1996) review the literature on the management of opioid and benzodiazepine dependence in this population, whilst Trad (1993) alerts us to the special, increasing, problem of the adolescent, drug-addicted mother.

The Elderly

Ghodse (1997) alerts us to the increasing problem of "harmful use" (United Nations International Drug Control Program 1997, pp 9–14) of drugs by the elderly. Ghodse (1997) highlights a number of issues and factors:

- Alcohol is the most abused substance in this group, particularly by those in pain or with sleep problems
- The increased use of prescribed psychotropic medications and over-the-counter preparations
- Changes in pharmacokinetics and reduced renal and hepatic function may lead to enhanced and prolonged drug effects, increasing the risk of dependence
- The aging of earlier generations of drug addicts means an increase in elderly recreational drug users; for example, Pascarelli (1981) reports an increasing proportion of methadone clinic attenders aged over 60 years.

Pain Patients

The use of opioids in controlling acute pain is well established (Shannon & Baranowski 1997), as it is in chronic cancer pain (Hanks & Justins 1992). However, the use of opioids in non-cancer, chronic pain remains controversial (Brena & Sanders 1991).

Shannon & Baranowski (1997) claim some differences between street addicts and pain patients, in opioid use:

- The former have euphoria, whereas the latter, especially cancer patients, often have dysphoria (Portenoy 1990)
- There is some evidence of pain patients not developing tolerance (Glynn & Mather 1982; Moulin 1996).

On this basis, Shannon & Baranowski (1997) recommend that, in the context of a multidisciplinary pain clinic, when all other reasonable attempts at analgesia have failed, having made a psychological assessment of addictive risk, opioids may be successfully used in the treatment of non-cancer chronic pain, using an "analgesic ladder", as proposed by Ahmedzai & Brook (1994) and advocated by the World

Health Organization for cancer pain, and with continual monitoring and downward dose adjustment whenever possible.

No doubt, this will remain a controversial issue. For those of us who work in consultation-liaison psychiatry and/or drug dependence, though, it is not uncommon to see patients who have become iatrogenically dependent on opioids, as a result of inappropriately enthusiastic and/or unmonitored use of opioids in chronic (for example, arthritis) or recurrent (for example, migraines) pain. The issues are then complex, as one needs to take into account pain management, not just achievement of the usual goals of abstinence or, at least, harm minimization, of the drug clinic. The setting in which these patients will be treated (drug clinic or pain clinic) needs to be evaluated case by case.

Cultural Issues

Closser & Blow (1993) emphasize the need to take into account issues of a social and economic nature when looking at rates of alcohol and drug abuse among various ethnic groups. They stress the importance of avoiding negative and unhelpful stereotypes. Brady (1995) highlights that negative stereotypes can also come from within the culture, and lead to singling out and rejection of those trying to escape some of these negative stereotypes. She gives the example of how some Australian aborigines who tried to escape alcoholism and save money have been branded within their immediate group as trying to be different, getting too "flash" or trying to be like white men.

Closser & Blow (1993) make reference to the paucity of research on efficacy and necessity for culturally specific programs. However, they do state that "every attempt should be made to incorporate culture-specific beliefs and concepts about healing and recovery into treatment programming" (p 205). Brady (1995) looks at innovative interventions by indigenous people in Australia and North America, in the field of treatment of addiction. Some of these treatment models incorporate mainstream ideas as well as indigenous healing techniques. Examples of this would be the adaptation of the North American Indian "sweat lodge" in the treatment of solvent abuse by adolescents and alcohol abuse by adults.

Substance Abuse by Physicians and Other Health Professionals

Brewster (1991) traced the source of wrongly quoted figures for increase in alcohol and other drug problems among physicians. Flaherty & Richman (1993) in their review of substance use and addiction among medical students, residents and physicians, were not able to corroborate the commonly held belief that these groups have higher use of substances. There may be methodological problems in studies in this area and more data need to be accumulated.

In the Flaherty & Richman (1993) review, an area of concern was that the drinking rates for women in these groups were found to approximate those of men by the end of medical school. The same authors also found that the most consistent predictive factor in alcoholism among physicians was the same as the general population, namely a family history of alcoholism. An important finding was that physicians as a group probably respond more favorably to alcohol and drug addiction programs than do members of the general population. This appeared to be directly or indirectly due to the dire consequences of continued use, including delicensure.

The issues relating to physicians and other health professionals being impaired by substance abuse are clearly of paramount importance, because of the potential risks to patients.

CONCLUDING REMARKS

Substance abusers are no longer denied attention by clinicians competent to diagnose and treat them. Instead, the assessment, diagnosis, and treatment of substance abuse has firmly entered mainstream mental health practice, and psychologists and psychiatrists in training are routinely taught these skills.

While some areas of assessment and treatment are more often pursued by psychologists than psychiatrists and vice versa, it is increasingly the case that cooperation between the disciplines so that substance-abusing patients enjoy the full armamentarium of assessment and treatment practices is the goal. This is certainly the approach to these disorders that we recommend. Perhaps it is in the care of the substance abuser that psychiatry and clinical psychology can best model the kind of cooperative attitude that effectively transcends old, outmoded competition, the better to serve our patients.

REFERENCES

Ahmedzai S and Brook D: Pain control in palliative care. *Hospital Update* **340**: 549–554, 1994.

American Psychiatric Association: *Diagnostic and Statistical Manual of Mental Disorders, Third Edition*. American Psychiatric Association: Washington, DC, 1980.

American Psychiatric Association: *Diagnostic and Statistical Manual of Mental Disorders, Third Edition, revised*. American Psychiatric Association: Washington, DC, 1987.

American Psychiatric Association: *Diagnostic and Statistical Manual of Mental Disorders, Fourth Edition*. American Psychiatric Association: Washington, DC, 1994.

Azrin NH, Sisson RW, Meyers R and Godley M: Alcoholism treatment by disulfiram and community reinforcement therapy. *J Behav Ther Exp Psychiatry* **13**: 105–112, 1982.

Ball JC and Ross A: *The Effectiveness of Methadone Maintenance Treatment*. Springer-Verlag: New York, 1991.

Bell J, Hall W and Byth K: Changes in criminal activity after entering methadone maintenance. *Br J Addiction* **87**: 251–258, 1992.

Bertschy G: Methadone maintenance treatment: an update. *Eur Arch Psychiatr Clin Neurosci* **245**: 114–124, 1995.

Bertschy G, Baumann P, Eap CB and Baettig D: Probable metabolic interaction between methadone and fluvoxamine in addict patients. *Ther Drug Monitoring* **16**: 42–45, 1994.

Bertschy G, Eap CB, Powell K and Baumann P: Fluoxetine addition to methadone in addicts: pharmacokinetic aspects. *Ther Drug Monitoring* **18**: 570–572, 1996.

Bickel WK, Stitzer ML, Bigelow GE et al: A clinical trial of buprenorphine: comparison with methadone in the detoxification of heroin addicts. *Clin Pharmacol Ther* **43**: 72–78, 1988.

Brady M: Culture in treatment, culture as treatment. A critical appraisal of developments in addiction programs for indigenous North Americans and Australians. *Soc Sci Med* **41**: 1487–1498, 1995.

Brecht M, Anglin MD and Wang J: Treatment effectiveness for legally coerced versus voluntary methadone maintenance clients. *Am J Drug Alcohol Abuse* **19**: 89–106, 1993.

Brena F and Sanders S: Opioids in non-malignant pain: questions in search of answers. *Clin J Pain* **7**: 342–345, 1991.

Brown SA, Goldman MS, Inn A and Anderson LR: Expectations of reinforcement from alcohol: Their domain and relation to drinking patterns. *J Consult Clin Psychol* **43**: 419–426, 1980.

Cahalan D, Cisin IH and Crossley HM: *American Drinking Practices: A National Study of Drinking Behaviour and Practices.* Rutgers Center of Alcohol Studies: New Brunswick, NJ, 1969.

Caplehorn JRM, Bell J, Kleinbaum DG and Gebvski VJ: Methadone dose and heroin use during maintenance treatment. *Addiction* **88**: 119–124, 1993.

Closser MH and Blow FC: Special populations. Women, ethnic minorities and the elderly. *Psychiatr Clin N Am* **16**: 199–209: 1993.

Darke S, Ward J, Hall W et al: *The Opiate Treatment Index (OTI) Manual. Technical Report Number 11.* National Drug and Alcohol Research Centre, University of New South Wales: Sydney, 1991.

Deckel AW, Hesselbrock V and Bauer L: Relationship between alcohol-related expectancies and anterior brain functioning in young men at risk for developing alcoholism. *Alcoholism: Clin Exp Res* **19**: 476–481, 1995.

Decker K and Ries R: Differential diagnosis and psychopharmacology of dual disorders. *Psych Clin N Am* **16**: 703–718, 1993.

Dole VP and Nyswander M: A medical treatment for diacetylmorphine (heroin) addiction. *JAMA* **193**: 80–84, 1965.

Farrell M: Opiate withdrawal. *Addiction* **89**: 1471–1475, 1994.

First MG, Spitzer RL, Gibbon M and Williams JBW: *Structured Clinical Interview for DSM-IV— Patient version (SCID-I/P, version 2.0).* Biometrics Department, New York State Psychiatric Institute: New York, 1995.

Flaherty JA and Richman JA: Substance use and addiction among medical students, residents and physicians. *Psychiatr Clin N Am* **16**: 189–197, 1993.

Fox BS, Kantar KM, Edwards MA et al: Efficacy of therapeutic cocaine vaccine in rodent models. *Nature Medicine* **2**: 1129–1132, 1996.

Fuller RK, Branchey L, Brightwell DR et al: Disulfiram treatment of alcoholism: a Veterans Administration cooperative study. *JAMA* **256**: 1449–1455, 1986.

Galanter M and Kleber HD: Preface. In M Galanter and HD Kleber (Eds), *Textbook of Substance Abuse*, pp xiii–xiv. American Psychiatric Press: Washington, DC, 1994.

Gallant D: Alcohol. In M Galanter and HD Kleber (Eds), *Textbook of Substance Abuse*, pp 67–89. American Psychiatric Press: Washington, DC 1994.

Gerrein JR, Rosenberg C and Manohar V: Disulfiram maintenance in outpatient treatment of alcoholism. *Arch Gen Psychiatry* **28**: 798–802, 1973.

Ghodse AH: Substance misuse by the elderly. *Br J Hosp Med* **58**: 451–453, 1997.

Glynn C and Mather L: Clinical pharmacokinetics applied to patients with intractable pain: studies with pethidine. *Pain* **13**: 237–246, 1982.

Gold MS, Redmond DE and Kleber HD: Clonidine in opiate withdrawal. *Lancet* **311**: 599–602, 1978.

Goldman MS, Brown SA, Christiansen BA and Smith GT: Alcoholism etiology and memory: broadening the scope of alcohol expectancy research. *Psychol Bull* **110**: 137–146, 1991.

Gossop M, Bradley B and Phillips GT: An investigation of withdrawal symptoms shown by opiate addicts during and subsequent to a 21 day in-patient methadone detoxification procedure. *Addictive Behaviours* **12**: 1–6, 1987.

Halikas JA: Treatment of drug abuse syndromes. *Psychiatr Clin N Am* **16**: 693–702, 1993.

Hanks G and Justins D: Cancer pain: management. *Lancet* **339**: 1031–1036, 1992.

Honour JW: Testing for drug abuse. *Lancet* **348**: 41–43, 1996.

Hubbard RL, Marsden ME, Rachal JV et al: *Drug Abuse Treatment: A National Study of Effectiveness.* University of North Carolina Press: Chapel Hill, NC, 1992.

Hunkeler W, Mohler H, Pieri L et al: Selective antagonists of benzodiazepines. *Nature* **290**: 515–516, 1981.

Jarvis T J, Tebbutt J and Mattick RP: *Treatment Approaches for Alcohol and Drug Dependence: An Introductory Guide.* John Wiley & Sons: Chichester, UK, 1995.

Johns A: Opiate treatments. *Addiction* **89**: 1551–1558, 1994.

Kadden R, Carroll KM, Donovan D, Cooney N, Monti P, Abrams D, Litt M and Hester R: *Cognitive-Behavioral Coping Skills Therapy Manual: A Clinical Research Guide for Therapists Treating Individuals with Alcohol Abuse and Dependence.* NIAAA Project MATCH Monograph, Vol. 3, DHHS Publication No. (ADM) 92–1895. Government Printing Office: Washington, DC, 1992.

Koren G, Graham K, Shear H et al: Bias against the null hypothesis: the reproductive hazards of cocaine. *Lancet* **ii**: 1440–1442, 1989.

Kosten TR, Morgan C and Kleber HD: Phase II clinical trials of buprenorphine: detoxification and induction onto naltrexone. In JD Blaine (Ed), *Buprenorphine: An Alternative Treatment for Opioid Dependence*, pp 101–119. NIDA: Rockville, MD, 1992.

Lago JA and Kosten TR: Stimulant withdrawal. *Addiction* **89**: 1477–1481, 1994.

Lanehart RE, Clark HB, Rollings GR et al: The impact of intensive case-managed intervention on substance-using pregnant and post-partum women. *J Subst Abuse* **8**: 487–495, 1996.

Leigh BC and Stacy AW: Alcohol outcome expectancies: Scale construction and prediction in higher-order confirmatory models. *Psychological Assessment* **5**: 216–229, 1993.

Lewis JW: Buprenorphine. *Drug Alc Dependence* **14**: 363–372, 1985.

Loimer N, Schmid R, Lenz et al: Acute blocking of naloxone-precipitated opiate withdrawal symptoms by methohexitone. *Br J Psychiatry* **157**: 748–752, 1990.

Lowinson JH, Marion IJ, Joseph H and Dole VP: Methadone maintenance. In JH Lowinson, P Ruiz, RB Millman and JG Langrod (Eds), *Substance Abuse—A Comprehensive Textbook*, 2nd Edition. Williams & Wilkins: London, 1992.

Marlatt GA and Miller WR: *Comprehensive Drinker Profile.* Psychological Assessment Resources Inc: Odessa, FL, 1987.

Mattick RP and Hall W: Are detoxification programmes effective? *Lancet* **347**: 97–100, 1996.

McCarthy IJ and Borders OI: Limit setting on drug abuse in methadone maintenance patients. *Am J Psychiatry* **142**: 1419–1423, 1985.

McLellan AT, Luborsky L, Woody GE and O'Brien CP: An improved diagnostic evaluation instrument for substance abuse patients: The Addiction Severity Index. *J Nerv Ment Dis* **168**: 26–33, 1980a.

McLellan AT, Druley KA, O'Brien CP and Kron R: Matching substance abuse patients to appropriate treatments: a conceptual and methodological approach. *Drug Alc Dependence* **5**: 189–193, 1980b.

Metzger DS, Woody GE, McLellan AT et al: Human immunodeficiency virus seroconversion among intravenous drug users in and out of treatment: an 18 month prospective follow-up. *J Acq Immun def Syn* **6**: 1049–1056, 1993.

Miller WR and Rollnick S: *Motivational Interviewing: Preparing People to Change Addictive Behaviour.* Guilford Press: New York, 1991.

Miller WR, Zweben A, DiClemente CC and Rychtarik RG: *Motivational Enhancement Therapy Manual: A Clinical Research Guide for Therapists Treating Individuals with Alcohol Abuse and Dependence.* NIAAA Project MATCH Monograph, Vol. 2, DHHS Publication No. (ADM) 92–1894. Government Printing Office: Washington, DC, 1992.

Moulin DE: Randomized trial of oral morphine for chronic non-cancer pain. *Lancet* **347**: 143–147, 1996.

Nathan PE: Assessing substance abusers. In LL Murphy and JC Impara (Eds), *Assessment of Substance Abuse*, pp xvii–xxix. The Buros Institute of Mental Measurements: Lincoln, NE, 1996.

Nathan PE: Practice guidelines: Not yet ideal. *Am Psychol* **53**: 290–299, 1998.

Nowinski J, Baker S and Carroll K: *Twelve Step Facilitation Therapy Manual: A Clinical Research Guide for Therapists Treating Individuals with Alcohol Abuse and Dependence.* NIAAA Project MATCH Monograph, Vol. 1, DHHS Publication No. (ADM) 92–1893. Government Printing Office: Washington, DC, 1992.

Nutt DJ: Addiction: brain mechanisms and their treatment implications. *Lancet* **347**: 31–36, 1996.

O'Brien CP: Recent developments in the pharmacotherapy of drug abuse. *J Consult Clin Psychol* **64**: 677–686, 1996.

O'Brien CP: A range of research-based pharmacotherapies for addiction. *Science* **278**: 66–70, 1997.

O'Brien CP and McLellan AT: Myths about the treatment of addiction. *Lancet* **347**: 237–240, 1996.

Ouimette PC, Finney JW and Moos RH: Twelve-step and cognitive-behavioural treatment for substance abuse: A comparison of treatment effectiveness. *J Consult Clin Psychol* **65**: 230–240, 1997.

Pascarelli EF: Drug abuse and the elderly. In JH Lowinson and P Ruiz (Eds), *Substance Abuse: Clinical Problems and Perspectives*, pp 752–757. Williams & Wilkins: Baltimore, 1981.

Pettinati HM, Meyers K, Jensen JM et al: Inpatient vs outpatient treatment for substance dependence revisited. *Psych Q* **64**: 173–182, 1993.

Petursson H: The benzodiazepine withdrawal syndrome. *Addiction* **89**: 1455–1459, 1994.

Poole R and Brabbins C: Substance misuse and psychosis. *Br J Hosp Med* **58**: 447–450, 1997.

Portenoy R: Chronic opioid therapy in nonmalignant pain. *J Pain Symptom Management* **5** (Suppl): 546–562, 1990.

Project MATCH Research Group: Project MATCH: Rationale and methods for a multisite clinical trial matching patients to alcoholism treatment. *Alcoholism: Clin Exp Res* **17**: 1130–1145, 1993.

Project MATCH Research Group: Matching alcoholism treatments to client heterogeneity: Project MATCH post-treatment drinking outcomes. *J Stud Alcohol* **58**: 7–29, 1997.

Raskin VD: Psychiatric aspects of substance use disorders in childbearing populations. *Psychiatr Clin N Am* **16**: 157–165, 1993.

Regier DA, Farmer ME et al: Comorbidity of mental disorders with alcohol and other drug abuse. *JAMA* **264**: 2511–2518, 1990.

Ries R: Clinical treatment matching models for dually diagnosed patients. *Psychiatr Clin N Am* **16**: 167–175, 1993.

Robins LN, Helzer JE, Croughan H and Ratcliff KS: National Institute of Mental Health Diagnostic Interview Schedule: Its history, characteristics, and validity. *Arch Gen Psychiatry* **38**: 381–389, 1981.

Rocio M, Carrera A, Ashley JA et al: Suppression of psychoactive effects of cocaine by active immunization. *Nature* **378**: 727–730, 1995.

Schuckit MA: Recent developments in the pharmacotherapy of alcohol dependence. *J Consult Clin Psychol* **64**: 669–676, 1996.

Seiverwright NA and Greenwood J: What is important in drug misuse treatment? *Lancet* **347**: 373–376, 1996.

Senay EC: Antagonists and partial agonists. In M Galanter and HD Kleber (Eds), *Textbook of Substance Abuse*, pp 223–236. American Psychiatric Press: Washington, DC, 1994.

Sereny G, Sharma V, Holt J et al: Mandatory supervised Antabuse therapy in an outpatient alcoholism program: a pilot study. *Alcoholism: Clin Exp Res* **10**: 290–292, 1986.

Shannon CN and Baranowski CT: Use of opioids in non cancer pain. *Br J Hosp Med* **58**: 459–463, 1997.

Sheehan MF: Dual diagnosis. *Psych Quarterly* **64**: 107–134, 1993.

Sierralta F, Pinardi G, Mendez M and Miranda HF: Interaction of opioids with antidepressant-induced antinociception. *Psychopharmacology* **122**: 374–378, 1995.

Skinner HA and Horn JL: *Alcohol Dependence Scale*. Addiction Research Foundation: Toronto, 1984.

Smith GT, Goldman MS, Greenbaum PE and Christiansen BA: Expectancy for social facilitation from drinking: The divergent paths of high-expectancy and low-expectancy adolescents. *J Abn Psychol* **104**: 32–40, 1995.

Sobell LC and Sobell MB: Timeline followback: A technique for assessing self-reported alcohol consumption. In R Litten and J Allen (Eds), *Measuring Alcohol Consumption*. Humana Press: Totowa, NJ, 1992.

Sorensen JL: Methadone treatment for opiate addicts. *BMJ* **313**: 245–246, 1996.

Sutherland G, Edwards G, Taylor C et al: The measurement of opiate dependence. *Br J Addiction* **81**: 485–494, 1986.

Trad PV: Substance abuse in adolescent mothers: strategies for diagnosis, treatment and prevention. *J Subst Abuse Treatment* **10**: 421–431, 1993.

United Nations International Drug Control Program: *World Drug Report*. Oxford University Press: Oxford, UK, 1997.

Volpicelli JR, Alterman AI, Hayashida M and O'Brien CP: Naltrexone in the treatment of alcohol dependence. *Arch Gen Psychiatry* **49**: 876–880, 1992.

Washton AM, Resnick RG and Geyer G: Opiate withdrawal using lofexidine: a clonidine analogue with fewer side effects. *J Clin Psychiatry* **44**: 335–337, 1983.

West R and Gossop M: Overview: A comparison of withdrawal symptoms from different drug classes. *Addiction* **89**: 1483–1489, 1994.

Wood MD, Sher KJ and Strathman A: Alcohol outcome expectancies and alcohol use and problems. *J Stud Alcoho* **57**: 283–288, 1996.

WHO (World Health Organization): *International Classification of Diseases, 10th Edition*. World Health Organization: Geneva, 1992.

WHO (World Health Organization): *Composite International Diagnostic Interview*. World Health Organization: Geneva, 1993.

Yaster M, Kost-Byerly S, Berde C and Billet C: The management of opioid and benzodiazepine dependence in infants, children and adolescents. *Pediatrics* **98**: 135–140, 1996.

9

Psychosocial Issues in the Management of Coronary Heart Disease

Stan Maes
Leiden University, The Netherlands
Thérèse van Elderen
Leiden University, The Netherlands

and

Lucio Sibilia
University La Sapienza, Rome, Italy

INTRODUCTION

Coronary heart diseases (CHD) are the leading cause of premature death in Western countries (WHO 1989). Although mortality rates due to CHD are declining (US Department of Health and Human Services 1994), the number of CHD patients in need of cardiac care is increasing because of higher survival rates. As a consequence of these developments, congestive heart failure is a leading cause of morbidity and mortality in industrialized societies, with a 6-year mortality rate of 80% for men and 65% for women (American Heart Association 1997). The mean age of onset and severity of cardiac problems are increasing, which leaves more individuals with disability, a decreased health-related quality of life, or both (Oldridge et al 1998).

This chapter is concerned with psychological and psychiatric issues in the management of CHD. More specifically, psychosocial consequences of CHD, psychosocial risk factors for CHD, objectives of cardiac rehabilitation, pharmacological issues, exercise-based rehabilitation programs, and health education and stress management programs are discussed, and recommendations for research, development and implementation of programs are formulated.

Psychology and Psychiatry: Integrating Medical Practice.
Edited by J. Milgrom and G. D. Burrows © 2001 John Wiley & Sons, Ltd.

PSYCHOSOCIAL CONSEQUENCES OF CORONARY HEART DISEASE

Experiencing a cardiac event or diagnosis of coronary heart disease is undoubtedly a traumatic event, since the disease poses a serious threat to an individual's current and future life perspectives. As some authors have put it: "the experience of a heart attack is typically sudden, frequently without forewarning, often dramatic, usually distressing, and almost always life-threatening" (Byrne & Johnson-Laird 1990, p 369).

As a consequence, learning to live with or adapt to CHD is not an easy task. This adaptation process can be characterized in terms of various stages. In an attempt to characterize stages of adaptation to chronic disease, Morse & Johnson (1991) developed the illness constellation model, which postulates four stages in the psychological development of an illness representation: (a) a stage of uncertainty, during which patients attempt to understand the meaning and severity of initial symptoms; (b) a stage of disruption, when it becomes obvious that the patient is affected by a serious disease (because of the disease state itself or communication of the diagnosis); during this stage the patient experiences a crisis, characterized by intense levels of stress and a high degree of dependence on professionals and/or relatives; (c) a stage which can be defined as a strive for recovery of the self, during which patients try to gain control over their illness with the help of their environment by using various forms of coping behaviour; and (d) a stage of restoration of well-being, in which the patient attains a new equilibrium within his or her environment by accepting the illness and its consequences. This model emphasizes that adaptation to chronic disease is largely dependent on the individual's evaluation of the stressor, the effectiveness of coping behaviour and the social support the patient receives in his or her attempts to gain control over the stressor. It also stresses that, despite the images of doom and the realities of disability accompanying a severe chronic condition, most patients adapt to chronic disease.

The Stage of Uncertainty

Many myocardial infarction (MI) patients experience an initial phase of uncertainty during their stay at the coronary care unit, sometimes accompanied by denial of the situation. This coping strategy may constitute a functional way of dealing with a life-threatening disease, since denial can protect patients from dangerous physiological arousal during their stay at the coronary care unit. Patients who exhibit relatively strong denial at this early stage have been found to spend fewer days in the CCU and to show fewer signs of cardiac dysfunction during hospitalization (Levine et al 1987). In addition, denial has been linked to favorable outcomes in patients with unstable angina pectoris (Levenson et al 1984).

The Stage of Disruption

Research has shown that patients suffering from CHD do report intense levels of stress in the disruption stage. The most characteristic stress reaction to a cardiac incident is undoubtedly anxiety, which tends to be initially very high, to drop after discharge from the coronary care unit, to rise again at discharge from the hospital and to return to normal levels about three to four months after discharge (Byrne & Johnson-Laird 1990). Anxiety can be seen from the perspective of the illness constellation model as a functional or normal reaction to an important life stressor, which activates the patient to take steps to gain control over his or her new circumstances. However, as Sykes (1994) has stated, high and prolonged levels of anxiety may inhibit adaptive change in the longer term. Fear of exercising may cause a patient to be inactive and as such may worsen his cardiac condition. In addition, the literature does not provide a consistent answer to the question of whether defensive coping strategies such as denial must be seen as beneficial during later phases of adaptation. While denial undoubtedly reduces anxiety and may thus enhance quality of life, such a response may interfere with life-style changes, such as smoking cessation, the adoption of healthy eating habits and exercise, which are advisable from a secondary prevention point of view. In the year following a cardiac event, strong deniers have been found to show less compliance with medical recommendations and to be rehospitalized more often than weak deniers (Levine et al 1987). Moreover, it has been found that avoidant coping strategies are positively related to quality of life directly after a cardiac event, but not at later measurement points; in contrast, approach coping strategies were found to be negatively related to quality of life variables when measured simultaneously, yet positively associated with quality of life assessed at subsequent measurement points (Van Elderen et al 1999). As a consequence, it is important to assess emotional states and coping strategies in cardiac patients over a longer period of time.

Assessment of Emotional States

This point is frequently overlooked, leading to a situation in which even a panic disorder may remain undiagnosed (Beitman et al 1993) in cardiac patients, despite the fact that such a disorder may reflect higher risk of recurrence of ischemic events through physiological worsening of the coronary disease (Katon 1990).

Depression is the second most important emotional state. It typically develops three to four days after admission, but is most prevalent during the first weeks after discharge from the hospital. Forrester et al (1992) concluded on the basis of several studies that a significant subset of CHD patients is vulnerable to serious depression after a cardiac event (e.g. Schleifer et al 1989), whereas high levels of depression have also been reported for a significant number of patients in the first five years after myocardial infarction or coronary bypass surgery (e.g. Follick et al 1988; Lange-luddecke et al 1989). Frasure-Smith et al (1993) have estimated that depressive symptoms arise in 20–30% of patients after the first myocardial infarction. In a recent study Brezinka et al (1998) found that about one-third of both male and female patients reported clinical levels of anxiety and depression (assessed with the SCL90) four and 12 months after a cardiac event. Using DSM-IV criteria, Gonzalez et al (1996) diagnosed 23% of 99 coronary inpatients as having had a major depressive episode. Prevalence of clinically relevant depression in patients with CHD is not only higher than in the general elderly population; its occurrence has an important prognostic significance, since these patients show higher mortality resulting from coronary events compared to cardiac patients who are free from depressive symptoms (Glassman & Shapiro 1998; Barefoot et al 1996).

These findings suggest that an important subgroup of CHD patients does not adapt to the incident within the expected time frame. Holahan et al (1995) found considerable variability in the level of depressive symptoms in cardiac patients; they also found that greater social support and use of active or approach coping strategies were associated with fewer depressive symptoms.

Adaptation, Coping Behavior and Social Support

Social support is thus also important in the adaptation process. A cardiac event is stressful not only for the patient, but also for the patient's spouse, children, friends and colleagues. And the way the patient's social environment adapts to the event in turn influences the patient's own adjustment. Research suggests that a good marital relationship supports recovery from CHD (Waltz et al 1988), and that having a partner is already an important source of social support, which may enhance effective emotion-focused (Sherbourne & Hays 1990) and/or problem-focused coping (Van Elderen et al 1994a). Nevertheless, the influence of the social context appears to be more complex. The Michigan Family Heart Study, which focused on couples coping with the husband's myocardial infarction (Coyne et al 1990), showed that coping with a myocardial infarction can be directed to at least three different functions: "coping with one's own distress (emotion-focused coping), attending to various instrumental tasks (problem-focused coping) and grappling with each other's presence and emotional needs (relationship-focused coping)" (Coyne & Fiske 1992, p 132). Relationship-focused coping is not necessarily congruent with emotion-focused and/or problem-focused coping. It is, in other words, not necessarily true that reducing one's own distress, or complying with medical advice, is effective in dealing with one's relationship, and vice versa. Coyne & Smith (1994) discovered that "protective buffering" by the wife (defined as conceding in response to disagreement and hiding of negative affect), but not overprotectiveness, was associated with higher levels of distress for the wife and greater self-efficacy for the patient. As a consequence it is important to assess emotional distress, coping and social support in both the patient and relevant others. While anxiety and depression are thus undoubtedly the most characteristic stress reactions to CHD, coping and social support are important mediators of adjustment.

Summarizing the findings of the above-mentioned studies, it can be concluded that the results support the illness constellation model, which states that many patients show effective adaptation over time to chronic disease conditions as a consequence of their coping behavior and social support. However, attention should be given at all phases of adaptation to psychiatric symptoms of depression, anxiety and panic disorders, and to emotional disorders and psychological symptoms not reaching the level of psychiatric clinical significance but impinging on quality of life and/or adherence to prescribed medical regimens; these symptoms include depressed mood, anxiety, insomnia, fatigue, denial or TABP components (hostility, anger, irritability, hyperactivity, etc.).

PSYCHOSOCIAL RISK FACTORS FOR CORONARY HEART DISEASE

From a biopsychosocial perspective, specific health behaviors and emotional disorders have been identified which increase the risk of coronary heart disease and contribute to its development. Among these, some are directly related to the traditional biomedical risk factors for CHD (e.g. hyperlipidemia and hypertension) and include smoking, excessive intake of salt or animal fat and lack of physical exercise. Others seem to be relatively independent of these risk factors, for instance hostility, anxiety, depression and type A behavior (an environmentally induced action–emotion complex or syndrome consisting of vigorous voice and psychomotor mannerisms, hard-driving and time-pressured job involvement, competitiveness, impatience and easily aroused anger and hostility). Although it is questionable whether type A behavior constitutes an independent risk factor, since recent studies have not replicated the earlier finding that it is a predictor of CHD (Dembroski et al 1985), components of type A behavior are still being considered in relation to the onset of coronary heart disease. Hostility was originally postulated to be the most coronary-prone dimension of type A behavior. In more recent studies the emphasis has shifted from hostility to the expression and suppression of anger. Anger refers to an unpleasant emotion ranging in intensity from irritation or annoyance to fury or rage. Anger has two components, angry affect and the perception of being subjected to illegitimate or unfair interference or harm (Lazarus 1991). On the one hand there is evidence for a relationship between the suppression or internalization of anger and health problems; on the other hand some studies suggest that it is the expression or externalization of anger that is related to the development of health problems (Van Elderen et al 1997). While the research findings with respect to hostility and anger are not unequivocal, there is more consistency in the research literature on anxiety and depression. There is evidence that anxiety is a prodrome of heart disease. It has been estimated that as many as 20% of the cases of sudden cardiac death are related to acute psychological stress (De Silva 1993). A prospective study demonstrated that the risk of fatal cardiac disease increases with the level of phobic anxiety, and that phobic anxiety was associated with a sixfold increase in incidence of sudden death. The fact that acute mental stress has been shown to be associated with a reduction in left ventricular function, regional wall motion abnormalities and coronary spasms in CHD patients suggests that anxiety may also be a risk factor for recurrence (Shapiro 1996). Finally, epidemiological studies have shown that depression is also associated with cardiovascular mortality. Booth-Kewley & Friedman (1987) showed on the basis of a meta-analysis of all studies published between 1945 and 1985 that the relative risk of coronary artery disease associated with depression is comparable to the risk associated with the classical biomedical risk factors. In addition, depression was shown to be related to recurrent MI and CHD mortality in CHD patients in more recent independent studies (Ladwig et al 1991; Frasure-Smith et al 1993).

Pathophysiological Effects of Emotional Disorders

There are many pathophysiological pathways linking emotional disorders to the various manifestations of CHD. A concise list should include both the acute and the chronic (sustained) effects of sympathetic activation (neurogenic and adrenergic) and the role of stress hormones, primarily cortisol, which in the long run are involved in dysfunction of the hypothalamic–pituitary–adrenal axis. Catecholamines impinge directly on heart activity (heart rate, rhythm, oxygen consumption, etc.), blood coagulation, platelets stickness (clotting), coronary activity, endothelium integrity, and last but not least, lipid metabolism (Sibilia 1993). Sympathetic disregulation also produces parasympathetic imbalance, resulting in reduction of heart rate variability and susceptibility to arrythmia.

Vital exhaustion, a disturbed emotional state characterized by unusual fatigue, a feeling of being dejected or defeated and increased irritability (Appels & Mulder 1989) also imparts a higher risk of angina pectoris and non-fatal myocardial infarction in cardiac patients who suffer from this "dystymic disorder".

As a consequence, in addition to life-style factors, clinical levels of hostility, anxiety, depression and vital exhaustion deserve increased attention within the framework of secondary prevention.

OBJECTIVES OF CARDIAC REHABILITATION

In 1993 the aim of cardiac rehabilitation was defined by the World Health Organization (WHO) as follows: "The rehabilitation of cardiac patients is the sum of activities required to influence favourably the underlying cause of the disease, as well as to ensure the patients, the best possible physical, mental and social conditions, so that they may, by their own efforts, preserve or resume when lost, as normal a place as possible in the life of the community" (p 5). Thus cardiac rehabilitation should facilitate the patient's return to his or her physical, psychological and social way of life before the cardiac event. That is, restoring everyday functioning (e.g. visiting a friend, driving a car, preparing meals, making household repairs, working in the garden, bicycling or making love) is the ultimate goal of rehabilitation. Furthermore, as the WHO definition states, secondary prevention should be added to the traditional goals of cardiac rehabilitation. Secondary prevention is the reduction of cardiovascular morbidity and mortality, including further incidents and complications, through pharmacological therapy, surgery and risk factor modification. This implies that the patient must be encouraged to return to his or her former way of life, with the exception of aspects of life-style (e.g. smoking) which promote hyperlipidemia, hypertension, diabetes, excessive weight and excessive stress.

As a consequence cardiac rehabilitation consists of medical advice, pharmacological therapy, physical exercise and psychosocial interventions.

PHARMACOLOGICAL ISSUES

An important problem in the psychological and psychiatric assessment of coronary patients, which should be always kept in mind, is that cardiovascular drugs are prone to have untoward (but sometimes favorable) psychotropic side-effects, so that the treatment itself may often have psychiatric implications. Cardiovascular drugs are the most commonly prescribed medication, especially in the elderly (Doucet et al 1996), a population in which drug responsiveness is usually altered for a variety of biological reasons. Moreover, many cardiovascular drugs, like digoxin, betablockers and calcium ion channel blockers, have a narrow therapeutic index. Psychologically relevant untoward side-effects include: neuropsychological impairment, lack of energy (fatigue), sleep disturbances, depression and loss of sexual desire. Using the Assessment of Symptoms and Psychological Effects in Cardiovascular Therapy (ASPECT) Scale, Jem (1990) found that subjective symptoms associated with cardiovascular drugs clustered into the following groups: cardiac symptoms, central nervous system or cognitive symptoms, fatigue, local/cutaneous symptoms, sleeping disturbances, and other symptoms.

It has been suggested that the frequency of side-effects (psychotropic or otherwise) of cardiovascular drugs should be reduced by limiting prescription of drugs associated with the most frequent and dangerous side-effects (Doucet et al 1996), limiting dosage to the lowest therapeutic levels, and giving initially low doses followed by gradual increases (Potempa & Roberts 1982). In any event, careful monitoring for side-effects, which is obviously advisable for acute patients, is also recommended in the elderly. Carbonin et al (1991) warn that there is virtually no useful information on the efficacy and safety of cardiovascular drugs in patients over 75 years of age.

Psychiatric treatment in cardiac patients must take into account the known cardiovascular effects of psychotropic drugs. Tricyclic antidepressant (TCA) drugs, which are the most common remedy prescribed for depressive states, but also bupropion, produce the same effects as class I antiarrhythmic drugs, because of their anti-cholinergic action. Such effects usually do not appear at normal therapeutic doses, but the severity of these effects necessitate careful monitoring for EKG abnormality. Like (or in addition to) the anti-arrhythmic drugs of class I, TCA are suspected to increase the risk of death for ventricular arrhythmias following myocardial infarction (Glassman & Roose 1994).

A new class of antidepressant drugs, the selective serotonin reuptake inhibitors (SSRI), such as fluoxetine, sertraline, and paroxetine, which are relatively free from such anti-cholinergic action, promise to provide better tools to counteract depressive states in cardiac patients, and are already considered the best choice for the treatment of depression in elderly patients. In fact, SSRI have a larger therapeutic index, yet are exempt from the many potentially serious adverse side-effects of TCA and other antidepressants (e.g. monoamine oxidase inhibitors (MAOI)), such as central nervous system and cardiovascular toxicity, orthostatic hypotension (due to alpha-adrenergic receptor blockage, with the associated subjective feelings of weakness and fatigue, and sedation; Preskom 1993). Conversely, benzodiazepines (the drugs most commonly prescribed as minor tranquillizers in a variety of anxiety states) show modest but positive cardiovascular side-effects, since they decrease heart workload by reducing the peripheral resistance or cardiac output (Gilman et al 1992). These connections at the pharmacological level demonstrate once again the close kinship between ischemic cardiovascular disorders and psychiatric conditions.

Tabrizi et al (1996) present a more extensive review of possible psychiatric side-effects of drugs commonly used for patients who have heart disease.

Although there is ample evidence of psychiatric side-effects of drugs commonly used for patients who have heart disease, the involvement of psychiatrists in cardiac rehabilitation services is relatively small compared to the involvement of other disciplines (Tabrizi et al 1996).

EXERCISE-BASED REHABILITATION PROGRAMS

In the past many CHD patients have been offered standard cardiac rehabilitation programs. Such a program generally starts after the initial or acute-care phase, when patients are transferred from the coronary care unit to a hospital ward. During this second stage in a regular hospital ward, in addition to pharmacological treatment, rehabilitation consists mainly of the provision of information to patients about their physical condition and its consequences for treatment and daily life, including life-style changes. In addition, the average patient receives a form of physical therapy in order to restore his or her physical condition. After about two weeks the patient is dismissed from the hospital and can than enrol in an exercise-based outpatient rehabilitation program. In most Western countries, patients who take part in such a program travel on average three times a week to and from the hospital in order to attend physical exercise sessions for a period of 8 to 16 weeks. This constitutes the third phase, after which the average patient is considered to be rehabilitated, implying that he or she should be able to resume normal daily activities (for example work, leisure activities and role in the family) as much as possible and should have adopted life-style changes that could prevent a future cardiac event. In several countries, groups organized by patient associations offer cardiac rehabilitation patients, in a fourth phase, the opportunity to join sports or exercise groups under the direct or indirect supervision of a health professional in their town or area. This fourth phase can last several years and is usually called the resocialization phase. For the small group of patients who do not recover as expected, most countries have a few rehabilitation clinics or departments where clinical rehabilitation is offered (Maes 1992).

It should be noted, however, that there are important differences between and within Western countries. At one extreme there are countries or health care centres within a country where forms of professional care other than pharmacological treatment, surgery and medical advice after discharge from the hospital are considered too expensive, not feasible or unnecessary. At the other extreme there are countries (e.g. Germany) and centres which offer a wide variety of interventions, including psychosocial interventions, in addition to standard medical care and exercise training, sometimes even in a clinical setting (Maes 1992).

Several meta-analyses have demonstrated positive effects of exercise-based rehabilitation programs on cardiac mortality. While Oldridge et al (1988) and O'Connor et al (1989) showed favorable effects of exercise training on cardiovascular and overall mortality in meta-analyses, which pooled the data of respectively 10 and 22 randomized trials, there is less evidence for effects on morbidity or psychosocial recovery. Randomized studies show that exercise programs have some effect on emotional distress, risk factors and health-related behaviors by the end of the programs, but these effects seem to disappear within a few months (Van Elderen 1991; Maes 1992). Moreover, since exercise-based interventions in most studies were combined with risk factor counseling, unique effects of both components could not be disentangled (Linden et al 1996; Oldridge et al 1989). Oldridge et al (1989) and O'Connor et al (1989) agree that further research is needed to isolate the distinct effects of various components of cardiac rehabilitation programs, such as exercise, health education, and psychosocial programs. Limitations in the effects of exercise-based rehabilitation programs and the extension of rehabilitation goals to include quality of life and secondary prevention have led to the development and evaluation of both health education and stress management programs.

EFFECTS OF HEALTH EDUCATION AND STRESS MANAGEMENT PROGRAMS

Psychosocial interventions have the potential to affect rehabilitation outcomes in two ways. Firstly, they may facilitate psychosocial recovery, including the return to everyday activities. Secondly, they may play an important role in secondary prevention, by improving compliance with medical advice concerning medication and life-style changes. In connection with these two objectives, two types of structured interventions have been well investigated. On the one hand, there are controlled studies of interventions which aim at improving quality of life via stress management. On the other hand, there are controlled studies of behavior modification and health education interventions, which are directed at life-style changes related to cardiac risk factors. Research by Langosch et al (1982) provides a good example of a study concentrating on the effects of stress management. Using a pre-test, post-test control group design, these authors compared three groups of CHD patients: a group receiving eight sessions of stress management training in addition to standard care, a group participating in eight sessions of relaxation training in addition to standard medical care, and a control group receiving standard medical care only. Both types of treatments focused on recognizing signs of tension and using coping techniques to reduce arousal. The stress management training included the following components: (1) emphasizing the harmful effects of pronounced achievement behavior on standard risk factors for CHD and on the impaired heart; (2) training in discrimination and modification of self-statements related to pronounced achievement and self-instructions inducing arousal, by means of thought-stopping and production of positive self-statements; (3) modifying non-assertive behavior, by means of thought-stopping and use of positive self-statements, role-playing and covert rehearsal; (4) discrimination training aimed at sensitization to signs of stress which can be alleviated by individual effort. Each session consisted of phases focused respectively on information, sensitization, discussion and training. Corresponding sections of a patient manual were given to the patients after each session. The relaxation training began with Jacobsonian muscular relaxation, proceeded to relaxation focusing on observation of breathing, followed by deep relaxation oriented towards two aspects ("heaviness" and "warmth") of autogenic training. After the last session the patients were given a scheme, describing the whole sequence and the areas in which relaxation could be applied (Langosch et al 1982, p 478). Both treatment procedures brought forth psychological improvements in assertiveness, social anxiety and components of achievement behavior. However, the effects of stress management training were superior to the effects of relaxation training in the sense that stress management subjects were more convinced than relaxation subjects that they were able to reduce stress through their own efforts. In other words, they had increased levels of perceived control, which seemed to be lacking in relaxation patients.

DeBusk and colleagues (1994) provide a good example of an effect study of a health education program focused on behavior modification related to risk factors. In this randomized clinical trial, CHD patients received either a health education intervention or standard medical care only during the first year after acute myocardial infarction. In the hospital, trained nurses implemented a case-managed approach to smoking cessation, exercise training and diet-drug therapy for hyperlipidemia. After discharge the intervention was conducted mainly via telephone and mail contacts with patients at home. All medically eligible patients received exercise training, all smokers received a smoking cessation intervention and all patients received dietary counseling, and, if needed, drug therapy aimed at lowering lipid levels. The health education intervention proved to have beneficial effects on smoking cessation, plasma LDL cholesterol levels and functional capacity.

These studies showed favorable results on outcome measures specifically related to the content of the programs in question, in agreement with the results in many review studies and meta-analyses (Dusseldorp et al 1999; Ketterer 1993; Linden et al 1996; Mullen et al 1992; Nunes et al 1987; Wenger et al 1995).

A number of narrative reviews and quantitative meta-analyses have assessed the effectiveness of stress management and health education programs. Ketterer (1993) compared behavioral therapies with pharmacological therapies and coronary artery bypass grafting in terms of their effects on risk for nonfatal myocardial infarction and cardiac death. The results observed so far suggest that behavioral therapies are superior to any form of medical therapy, with the possible exception of aspirin use in patients with unstable angina. In a meta-analysis of 18 controlled studies on the effects of treatments involving education, relaxation, cognitive therapy, imaging, behavior modification, emotional support and psychodynamic therapy, Nunes et al (1987) found that a combination of treatment techniques was most effective in reducing type A behavior and cardiac event recurrence. In addition, while one meta-analysis of 28 controlled trials (Mullen et al 1992) emphasized the effects of health education programs in cardiac rehabilitation, another meta-analysis of 23 controlled trials (Linden et al 1996) focused more on stress management programs. Although the two meta-analyses show an overlap of only three trials, both reviews included programs which combined stress management and health education. Favorable effects were observed by Mullen et al (1992) on mortality, systolic blood pressure, exercise and diet, but not on the recurrence of myocardial infarction and smoking. Linden et al (1996) found an overall reduction in mortality and nonfatal cardiac recurrence rates at short-term follow-up (two years or less), and lower mortality at long-term follow-up (between two and eight years). The review also showed positive effects on psychological distress and on systolic blood pressure and cholesterol, although only four trials reported results on these last two biomedical measures. A more recent meta-analysis (Dusseldorp et al 1999) examined 37 studies on the effects of a health education program, a stress management program or a combination of both types of programs. Attention was restricted to stress management and health education programs consisting of at least one face-to-face session. Substantial effects of health education and/or stress management programs were found, including: a 34% reduction in cardiac mortality and a 29% reduction in recurrence of myocardial infarction at two to 10 years follow-up, and significant beneficial effects on systolic blood pressure, total serum cholesterol, smoking behaviour, exercise and eating habits at six weeks to two years follow-up. No effects were found on coronary bypass grafting, incidence of angina pectoris, anxiety, or depression. There was one important moderating influence on the strength of program effects. Programs with success on proximal targets (systolic blood pressure, smoking behavior, exercise, and/or emotional distress) were more effective on distal targets (cardiac mortality and recurrence of myocardial infarction) than programs without success on proximal targets. This finding suggests that cardiac risk may be decreased through the reduction of excessive stress or improvement in health behaviors. This meta-analysis yielded no evidence of differential effectiveness of health education and stress management programs, however, which is a puzzling finding. One would expect health education programs to have effects on health- or disease-related variables and stress management to have effects on quality of life outcomes only. In fact, all three meta-analyses show a consistent pattern of positive effects on cardiac mortality and morbidity, risk factors for CHD and related behaviors, whereas only the meta-analyses of Linden et al (1996) showed favorable effects on psychological distress variables. The overall effects on mortality, morbidity, risk factors and health-related behaviors are probably due to the fact that so-called stress management programs focus directly and indirectly on life-style. Even in the program studied by Langosch and colleagues, which is considered to be a prototype of stress management programs, harmful effects of achievement behavior on standard risk factors for CHD are emphasized. Hence, there are virtually no programs which can be called pure stress management programs, and the same is true for health education programs. In fact, most intervention programs even officially claim to use a combined, concerted approach focusing on both health-related behaviors and stress management. The question remains, however, of why more substantial effects have not been found for emotional distress variables. In addition, an explanation is needed for the inconsistent results concerning emotional distress. Contrary to the positive effects on psychological distress reported by Linden et al (1996), the meta-analysis of Dusseldorp et al (1999) showed no favorable effects on anxiety and depression. The inclusion of two recent trials (Jones & West 1996; Frasure-Smith et al 1997) in the latter meta-analysis may have been responsible for this inconsistency in results. As both of these studies showed no significant effects on emotional distress and included very large numbers of patients, they had a considerable negative impact on the findings. Nevertheless, the absence of effects in these two studies and the overall absence of effects in the meta-analyses of Mullen et al (1992) and Dusseldorp et al (1999) requires further consideration. In response to the null findings of Jones & West (1996), Irving (1997) raised the question of why psychological interventions are ineffective. We disagree with his conclusion that the influence of psychological factors in precipitation of and recovery from myocardial infarction may have been overemphasized in earlier studies. As already mentioned in this article, there is accumulating evidence of the large impact of cardiac events on psychological functioning and of the role of anxiety and depression in both the onset and the progression of CHD. Lewin and colleagues (1997) have attributed the null findings of Frasure-Smith et al (1997) to the fact that the program was delivered by nurses untrained in psychological skills. And, even though the stress management programs examined by Jones & West (1996) were offered by clinical psychologists, it is questionable whether these clinical psychologists had sufficient experience with CHD patients, since a survey has shown that there are virtually no psychologists involved in cardiac rehabilitation in the United Kingdom (Maes 1992). A lack of training or experience with cardiac patients is a plausible explanation, since several studies evaluating interventions offered by experienced psychologists, psychiatrists, or specially trained nurses have shown positive effects on anxiety and depression (Burgess et al 1987; DeBusk et al 1994; Engblom et al 1992; Friedman et al 1986a; Langosch et al 1982).

RECOMMENDATIONS FOR RESEARCH, DEVELOPMENT AND IMPLEMENTATION OF PROGRAMS

The US Public Health Service definition of cardiac rehabilitation, used by the Cardiac Rehabilitation Guideline Panel, states that "cardiac rehabilitation services are comprehensive, long-term programs involving medical evaluation, prescribed exercise, cardiac risk factor modification, education and counselling" (p 3). The panel emphasized the added effectiveness of multifaceted cardiac rehabilitation services integrated in a comprehensive approach. If such an approach is adopted, there remains the issue of how to maximize beneficial effects. Within this framework there are two principal strategies available for the improvement of effects on emotional distress variables. The first is to improve the communication and psychological intervention skills of existing health care professionals, most of whom fail to realize that influencing emotional distress and health-related behaviors implies skills which go beyond the provision of information (Leventhal et al 1985). The second strategy is to add psychosocial professionals to rehabilitation teams. There is a trend in this direction in some European countries (e.g. The Netherlands, Austria, Italy), where there is a notable representation of psychologists and/or social workers in rehabilitation teams, but not in other countries (e.g. Denmark, Greece, Portugal, Sweden, Switzerland and the United Kingdom), where psychosocial care is lacking or is offered by other professionals, e.g. nurses. In contrast to the early days of cardiac rehabilitation, there now seem to be virtually no psychiatrists in cardiac rehabilitation teams in any European country (Maes 1992). As a consequence, despite the considerable literature on the effects of psychosocial interventions, systematic psychosocial interventions offered by qualified professionals seem to be the exception rather than the rule within cardiac rehabilitation settings in Europe.

Another issue concerns the fact that the overall effects of various health care programs for coronary heart patients have been evaluated in the past two decades. The underlying assumption in these evaluation studies is that patients with a given disorder constitute a homogeneous group. The moderate effects of the present programs may be attributable to the fact that standard programs are offered to all patients, even though some subgroups would profit more than others from these programs (Lipkin 1991). In 1990 the Dutch Rehabilitation Committee published the report "Cardiac rehabilitation tailor made, new ideas" (Baer et al 1990). This report stated that exercise-based cardiac rehabilitation was frequently offered to patients who hardly need it, while those who stood to benefit most (such as the elderly, the fearful, women, and patients living alone) were often overlooked. A patient-oriented approach was advocated, in which the patient is offered a rehabilitation program which addresses his or her specific needs. The underlying idea was that the majority of patients do not require an intensive or lengthy rehabilitation program. From this perspective, it is important to assess the patient's needs, or in other words to screen patients, so that they can be referred to an appropriate or "tailor made" form of care. To this end the Netherlands Heart Foundation Rehabilitation Committee has published new guidelines for cardiac rehabilitation (Part I, 1995; Part II, 1995/1996). In Part I of these guidelines, besides rehabilitation goals and subgoals with reference to quality of life and secondary prevention, screening questions and preliminary screening criteria are presented. Five core screening questions are formulated:

1. Is there an objective reduction in exercise tolerance (relative to the level required for work, domestic and leisure activities); and are there other locomotive restrictions detrimental to performance?
2. Is there a subjective reduction in exercise tolerance caused by fear of physical exertion (including sexual activity) or pronounced feelings of invalidity?
3. Is there a disturbance of or threat to emotional stability and is the patient dealing with his/her disease in a dysfunctional manner? In other words, to what degree is there a discrepancy between present and optimal psychological functioning?
4. Is there a disturbance of or threat to social performance, and what is the prognosis with respect to restoration of social roles (i.e. return to work/duties, leisure activities, role within the family/with important others); and how are the "quality" and "quantity" of the social network?
5. Are there behavioral risk factors subject to influence (e.g. smoking, diet (with regard to obesity and abnormal lipid levels), lack of exercise, nonadherence to therapy)?

Within the Dutch context, patients will be selected for cardiac rehabilitation programs based on these five screening questions. Rehabilitation subgoals are formulated based on the answers to these questions. The subgoals are subsequently translated into an individual rehabilitation program consisting of one or more modules, combined with individual coaching as necessary. Four group modules have been developed: two exercise modules, one short (FIT-short; 8–10 contact hours) and one long (FIT-long; 18–24 contact hours), both of which can be provided with or without use of an ergometer (Berkhuysen & Rispens 1995/1996); one information module (INFO-module; Van Elderen & Leenders 1995/1996), comprising four educational sessions; and a psycho-educational prevention module (PEP-module; Van Elderen & Echteld 1996; Van Elderen 1997), in which four or five sessions (including an intake session) are offered in the form of intensive workgroups. Various programs can be constructed by combining these modules. The modules, which are extensively described in Part II of the Guidelines, must be tailored to patient's and partner's individual needs.

In addition, the scientific literature does not provide sufficient evidence regarding differential effects of a variety of psychological interventions. Many authors recommend including psychosocial treatment components routinely in cardiac rehabilitation, but also stress the need to identify the specific, most effective types of psychosocial interventions via controlled studies (Dusseldorp et al 1999; Ketterer 1993; Lau et al 1992; Linden et al 1996; Miller et al 1990; Mullen et al 1992;

Wenger et al 1995). The question is thus not only: "Which types of patients profit from which kinds of programs?" but also: "What are the effective ingredients of successful programs?" In the meta-analysis by Mullen et al (1992), both content and procedural characteristics were studied. Outcomes were not found to be influenced by either type of communication channel, contact frequency, total contact hours, length of follow-up, or educational emphasis (didactic versus behavioral, although there was a trend in favor of behavioral interventions). In contrast, higher ratings on adherence to five educational principles were associated with larger effects. Mullen et al (1992) concluded that cardiac programs should use reinforcement, give feedback, offer opportunities for individualization, facilitate behavior change through skills and resources, and be relevant to patients' needs and abilities. However, Mullen & colleagues (1992) also concluded that "another apparent weakness of the interventions is that they were designed without explicit reference to a theoretical educational model. This appears to result in the omission of potentially significant techniques either from the intervention or from the writeup" (p 158).

The literature does not shed sufficient light on effective mechanisms or components of cardiac rehabilitation programs. In most evaluation studies, programs are described only vaguely, mostly without explicit reference to a theoretical model or to empirical findings pointing to specific causal relationships between a certain strategy or intervention and positive effects on outcome or intermediate indicators of success. There are some examples of very successful interventions, but these interventions combine a variety of different strategies, making it impossible to attribute beneficial effects to specific components or strategies.

Although the evidence for the efficacy of specific psychological methods or strategies is not clearly demonstrated, currently "best practice" psychological interventions are offered to cardiac patients. The following interventions or strategies are often included in psycho-educational cardiac rehabilitation services.

1. Relaxation training (Van Dixhoorn 1991; Friedman et al 1996b).
2. Health education concerning risk factors and life-styles (DeBusk 1994; Lindsay & Gaw 1997).
3. Cognitive restructuring focused on stress management and the modification of unhealthy life-styles (Bracke & Thoresen 1996; Lewin et al 1992; Langosch et al 1982; Van Elderen et al 1994b).
4. Self-control techniques (behavioral therapies) directed at the modification of unhealthy life-styles (Lewin et al 1992; Burell 1996).
5. Specific strategies for treatment of panic disorders, depressive symptoms, and anger problems (e.g. "the Hook procedure" (Powell 1996)).

In order to be able to demonstrate that these "best practice" psychological interventions are "evidenced-based" interventions, there is a need, however, for more theory-driven research focusing on the relationship between specific components of interventions and changes in intermediate and outcome indicators related directly both to specific subgoals of cardiac rehabilitation and to the needs of the individual patient. Perhaps we were too quick to conclude that strategies and procedures derived from traditional theoretical principles in clinical psychology could be applied without adaptation to the problems of chronic patients. Therefore, to gain insight into effective mechanisms, it would be worthwhile to study these mechanisms on a micro-level in qualitative research. Probably, the accumulation of case studies over time will give more insight into effective mechanisms for specific problems in specific patients.

CONCLUSION

Coronary heart diseases are the leading cause of premature death in Western countries and as such affect a very large portion of the population.

In the first section we described the most important psychosocial consequences of coronary heart disease. While many patients seem to adapt over time, anxiety and depression are prevalent at all stages of adaptation. In about one quarter to one third of the patients, clinical levels of anxiety and depression are reached at some stage, which may be a consequence of inadequate coping and social support.

In the second section, we turned our attention to psychosocial risk factors for coronary heart disease. There is growing evidence that vital exhaustion, hostility and anger, anxiety and especially depression may be associated with disease progression and/or cardiovascular mortality. The next sections were devoted to cardiac re-habilitation. First, the objectives of cardiac rehabilitation were clarified. Then psychological side-effects of cardiovascular drugs as well as cardiovascular effects of psychotropic drugs were discussed. Careful dosage of drugs and constant monitoring of these effects is strongly advised. In the following section the nature and effects of exercise-based rehabilitation programs were described. It was concluded that although beneficial effects of these programs on cardiovascular mortality have been demonstrated, there is less evidence for their effects on morbidity or psychosocial recovery. Finally, the effects of health education and stress management programs were discussed. It was noted that three independent meta-analyses show a consistent pattern of beneficial effects of such programs on cardiac mortality and morbidity, on risk factors for coronary heart disease and on health behaviors; effects on psychosocial outcomes are, however, inconsistent. This may be due to the fact that many programs were offered to all CHD patients rather than to patients who report high or clinical levels of anxiety or depression, and to a lack of experience or training on the part of health personnel in two recent large-scale studies yielding negative findings.

In the last section recommendations were given concerning future research, and concerning development and implementation of intervention programs. These recommendations include communication training for health professionals, increasing the number of psychosocial professionals (e.g. psychologists and psychiatrists) in cardiac rehabilitation teams, tailoring interventions to the patients' needs on the basis of screening, developing theory-based interventions and complementing quantitative research with qualitative research to gain insight into mechanisms of change.

REFERENCES

American Heart Association: *1997 Heart and Stroke Statistical Update*, 1997.

Appels A and Mulder P: Fatigue and heart disease: the association between vital exhaustion, and past, present, and future coronary heart disease. *J Psychosom Res* **33**: 727–738, 1989.

Baer FW, Cluitmans J, Elderen T van, Maes S, Rutten F, Soons P and Stiggelbout W: *Hartrevalidatie op maat, nieuwe visies (Cardiac rehabilitation tailor made, new ideas)*. Report of the Rehabilitation Committee of the Netherlands Heart Foundation. The Netherlands Heart Foundation: The Hague, 1990.

Barefoot JC, Helms MJ, Mark DB, Blumenthal JA, Calstt RM, Hamey H, O'Connor CM, Siegler JC and Williams RB: Depression and long-term mortality risk in patients with coronary artery disease. *Am J Cardiol* **78**: 613–617, 1996.

Beitman BD, Mukerji V, Russell JL and Grafting M: Panic disorder in cardiology patients: a review of the Missouri Panic/Cardiology Project. *J Psychiatr Res* **27**: 35–46, 1993.

Berkhuysen MA and Rispens P: Bewegingsmodules (Exercise-based rehabilitation). In *Revalidatie Commissie Nederlandse Vereniging voor Cardiologie en de Nederlandse Hartstichting, Richtlijnen Hartrevalidatie Deel II (Guidelines for Cardiac Rehabilitation Part II)*. The Netherlands Society of Cardiology and The Netherlands Heart Foundation: The Hague, 1995/1996.

Booth-Kewley S and Friedman HS: Psychological predictors of heart disease: A quantitive review. *Psychol Bull* **101**: 343–362, 1987.

Bracke PE and Thoresen CE: Reducing Type A behavior patterns: a structured-group approach. In R Allan and S Scheidt (Eds) *Heart and Mind*, pp 255–290. American Psychological Association: Washington, DC, 1996.

Brezinka V, Dusseldorp E and Maes S: Gender differences in psychosocial profile at entry into cardiac rehabilitation. *J Cardiopulmonary Rehabil* **18**: 445–449, 1998.

Burell G: Group psychotherapy in Project New Life: Treatment of coronary-prone behaviors for patients who have had coronary artery bypass graft surgery. In R Allan and S Scheidt (Eds) *Heart and Mind*, pp 291–310. American Psychological Association: Washington, DC, 1996.

Burgess AW, Lerner DJ, D'Agostino B, Vokonas PS, Hartman CR and Gaccione P: A randomized controlled trial of cardiac rehabilitation. *Soc Sci Med* **24**: 359–370, 1987.

Byrne RMJ and Johnson-Laird PN: Models and deductive reasoning. In KJ Gilhooly, MT Keane, R Logie and G Erdos (Eds) *Lines of Thinking: Reflections on the Psychology of Thought*, Vol 1. Wiley: Chichester, 1990.

Carbonin P, Bernabei R, Carosella L, Cocchi A, Menichelli P, Pahor M, Sgadari A and Zuccala G: Cardiovascular therapy problems in the elderly patient. *Cardiologia* **36**: 275–279, 1991.

Coyne JC and Fiske V: Couples coping with chronic and catastrophic illness. In TJ Akamatsu, JC Crowther, SC Hobfoll and MAP Stevens (Eds) *Family Health Psychology*, pp 129–149. Hemisphere: Washington, DC, 1992.

Coyne JC and Smith DAF: Couples coping with a myocardial infarction: contextual perspective on patient self-efficacy. *J Family Psychol* **8**: 43–54, 1994.

Coyne JC, Ellard JH and Smith DA: Unsupportive relationships, interdependence, and unhelpful exchanges. In IG Sarason, BR Sarason and G Perce (Eds) *Social Support: An Interactional View*, pp 129–149. Wiley: New York, 1990.

DeBusk RF, Miller NH, Superko R, Dennis CA, Thomas RJ, Lew HT, Berger WE, Heller RS, Rompf J, Gee D, Kraemer HC, Bandura A, Ghandour G, Clark M, Shah RV, Fischer

L and Taylor B: A case-management system for coronary risk factor modification after acute myocardial infarction. *Ann Intern Med* **120**: 721–729, 1994.

Dembroski TM, MacDougall JM, Williams RB, Haney TL and Blumenthal JA: Components of Type A, hostility, and anger—in relationship to angiographic findings. *Psychosom Med* **47**(3): 219–233, 1985.

De Silva RA: Cardiac arrhythmias and sudden cardiac death. In A Stoudemire and BS Fogel (Eds) *Medical-Psychiatric Practice*, Vol 2, p 199. American Psychiatric Press: Washington, DC, 1993.

Doucet J, Chassagne P, Trivalle C, Landrin I, Pauty MD, Kadri N, Menard JF and Bercoff E: Drug–drug interactions related to hospital admissions in older adults: a prospective study of 1000 patients. *J Am Geriatr Soc* **44**: 944–948, 1996.

Dusseldorp E, Van Elderen T, Maes S, Meulman J and Kraay V: A meta-analysis of psycho-educational programs for Coronary Heart Disease Patients. *Health Psychol* **18**: 506–519, 1999.

Engblom E, Hämäläinen H, Lind J, Mattlar CE, Ollila S, Kallio V, Inberg M and Knuts LR: Quality of life during rehabilitation after coronary artery bypass surgery. *Quality of Life Research* **1**: 167–175, 1992.

Follick MJ, Gorkin L, Smith TW, Capone RJ, Visco J and Stablein D: Quality of life post-myocardial infarction: Effects of a transtelephonic coronary intervention system. *Health Psychol* **7**: 169–182, 1988.

Forrester AW, Lipsey JR, Teitelbaum ML, DePaulo JR, Andrzejewski PL and Robinson RG: Depression following myocardial infarction. *Int J Psychosom Res* **22**: 33–46, 1992.

Frasure-Smith N, Lesperance, F and Talajic M: Depression following myocardial infraction. Impact on 6-month survival. *JAMA* **270**: 1819–1825, 1993.

Frasure-Smith N, Lesperance F, Prince R, Verrier P, Garber RA, Juneau M, Wolfson C and Bourassa MG: Randomised trial of home-based psychosocial nursing intervention for patients recovering from myocardial infarction. *Lancet* **350**: 473–479, 1997.

Friedman M and Rosenman RH: Type A Behavior and Your Heart. Knopf: New York, 1974.

Friedman M, Thoresen CE, Gill JJ, Ulmer D, Powell LH, Price VA, Brown B, Thompson L, Rabin DD, Breall WS, Bourg E, Levy R and Dixon T: Alteration of type A behavior and its effect on cardiac recurrences in post myocardial infarction patients: Summary results of the recurrent coronary prevention project. *Am Heart J* **112**: 653–665, 1986a.

Friedman M, Myers P, Krass S and Benson H: The relaxation response: Use with cardiac patients. In R Allan and S Scheidt (Eds) *Heart and Mind*, pp 363–384. American Psychological Association: Washington, DC, 1986b.

Gilman AG, Goodman LS, Ralf TW and Murad F (Eds) *The Pharmacological Basis of Therapeutics*. Macmillan: New York, 1992.

Glassman AH and Roose SP: Risks of antidepressants in the elderly: tricyclic antidepressants and arrhythmia-revising risks. *Gerontology* **40**: 15–20, 1994.

Glassman AH and Shapiro PA: Depression and the course of coronary artery disease. *Am J Psychiatry* **155**: 4–11, 1998.

Gonzalez MB, Snyderman TB, Colket JT, Arias RM, Jiang JW, O'Connor CM and Krishnan KR: Depression in patients with coronary artery disease. *Depression* **4**: 57–62, 1996.

Holahan CJ, Moos RH, Holahan CK and Brennan PL: Social support, coping, and depressive symptoms in a late-middle-aged sample of patients reporting cardiac illness. *Health Psychol* **14**: 152–163, 1995.

Irving JB: Psychosocial rehabilitation for patients recovering from acute myocardial infarction (Comment). *Lancet* **350**: 457, 1997.

Jem S: Questionnaire for the Assessment of Symptoms and Psychological Effects in Cardiovascular Therapy (the ASPECT Scale). *Scand J Prim Health Care* **1**: 31–32, 1990.

Jones DA and West RR: Psychological rehabilitation after myocardial infarction: multicentre randomised controlled trial. *BMJ* **313**: 1517–1521, 1996.

Katon MJ: Chest pain, cardiac disease, and panic disorder. *J Clin Psychiatry* **51**: 27–30, 1990.

Ketterer MW: Secondary prevention of ischemic heart disease. The case for aggressive behavioral monitoring and intervention. *Psychosomatics* **34**: 478–484, 1993.

Ladwig KH, Kieser M, Konig J, Breithardt G and Borggrefe M: Affective disorders and survival after acute infarction. Results from the post-infarction late potential study. *Eur Heart J* **12**: 959–964, 1991.

Langeluddecke P, Fulcher G, Baird D, Hughes C and Tennant C: A prospective evaluation of the psychosocial effects of coronary artery bypass surgery. *J Psychosom Res* **33**: 37–45, 1989.

Langosch W, Seer P, Brodner G, Kallinke D, Kulick B and Heim F: Behaviour therapy with coronary heart disease patients: Results of a comparative study. *J Psychosom Res* **26**: 475–484, 1982.

Lau J, Antman EM, Jimenez-Silva J, Kupelnick B, Mosteller F and Chalmers TC: Cumulative meta-analysis of therapeutic trials for myocardial infarction. *N Engl J Med* **327**: 248–254, 1992.

Lazarus RS: *Emotion and Adaptation*. Oxford University Press: New York, 1991.

Levenson JL, Kay R, Monteferrante J and Herman MV: Denial predicts favorable outcome in unstable angina pectoris. *Psychosom Med* **46**: 25–32, 1984.

Leventhal H, Prochaska TR and Hirschmann RS: Preventive health behaviour across the lifespan. In J Rosen and L Solomon (Eds) *Prevention in Health Psychology*, pp 191–235. NY University Press: New York, 1985.

Levine J, Warrenburg S, Kerns R, Schwartz G, Delaney R, Fontana A, Gradman A, Smith S, Allen S and Cascione R: The role of denial in recovery from coronary heart disease. *Psychosom Med* **49**: 109–117, 1987.

Lewin B, Robertson IH, Cay EL, Irving JB and Campbell M: Effects of self-help post-myocardial-infarction rehabilitation on psychological adjustment and use of health services. *Lancet* **339**: 1036–1040, 1992.

Lewin RJP, Thompson DR, Johnston DW and Mayou RA: Cardiac rehabilitation (letter). *Lancet* **350**: 1400, 1997.

Linden W, Stossel C and Maurice J: Psychosocial interventions for patients with coronary artery disease. *Arch Int Med* **156**: 745–752, 1996.

Lindsay GM and Gaw A: *Coronary Heart Disease Prevention: A Handbook for the Health Care Team*. Churchill Livingstone: New York, 1997.

Lipkin DP: Is cardiac rehabilitation necessary? *Br Heart J* **65**: 237–238, 1991.

Maes S: Psychosocial aspects of cardiac rehabilitation in Europe. *Br J Clin Psychol* **31**: 473–483, 1992.

Miller NH, Taylor CB, Davidson DM, Hill MN and Krantz DS: The efficacy of risk factor intervention and psychosocial aspects of cardiac rehabilitation. *J Cardiopulmon Rehab* **10**: 198–209, 1990.

Morse JM and Johnson JL: Towards a theory of illness: The illness constellation model. In JM Morse and JL Johnson (Eds) *The Illness Experience*, pp 315–342. Sage: London, 1991.

Mullen PD, Mains DA and Velez R: A meta-analysis of controlled trials of cardiac patient education. *Patient Education and Counseling* **19**: 143–162, 1992.

Netherlands Heart Foundation Rehabilitation Committee: Guidelines Cardiac Rehabilitation: Part 1, 1995, Part II, 1995/1996. The Netherlands Heart Foundation and the Netherlands Society of Cardiology: The Hague, 1995, 1995/1996.

Nunes EV, Frank KA and Kornfeld DS: Psychological treatment for the type A behavior pattern and for coronary heart disease: A meta-analysis of the literature. *Psychosom Med* **48**: 159–173, 1987.

O'Connor GT, Buring JE and Yusuf S: An overview of randomized trials of rehabilitation with exercise after myocardial infarction. *Circulation* **80**: 234–244, 1989.

Oldridge NB, Guyatt GH, Fischer ME and Rimm AA: Cardiac rehabilitation after myocardial infarction. Combined experience of randomized clinical trials. *JAMA* **260**: 945–950, 1988.

Oldridge NB, McCartney N, Hicks A and Jones NL: Improvement in maximal isokinetic cycle ergometry with cardiac rehabilitation. *Med Sci Sports Exercise* **21**: 308–312, 1989.

Oldridge NB, Gottlieb M, Guyatt GH, Jones N, Streiner D and Feeny D: Predictors of health-related quality of life with cardiac rehabilitation after acute myocardial infarction. *J Cardiopulmon Rehab* **18**: 95–103, 1998.

Potempa K and Roberts KV: Cardiovascular drugs and the older adult. *Nurs Clin N Am* **17**: 263–274, 1982.

Powell LH: The hook: a metaphor for gaining control of emotional reactivity. In R Allan and S Scheidt (Eds) *Heart and Mind*, pp 313–329. American Psychological Association: Washington, DC, 1996.

Preskom SH: Recent pharmacologic advances in antidepressant therapy for the elderly. *Am J Med* **94**(5A): 2–12, 1993.

Schleifer S, Macari-Hinson M, Coyle D, Slater W, Kahn M, Gorlin R and Zucker H: The nature and course of depression following myocardial infarction. *Arch Intern Med* **149**: 1785–1789, 1989.

Shapiro PA: Psychiatric aspects of cardiovascular disease. *Psychiatr Clin N Am* **19**: 613–629, 1996.

Sherbourne CD and Hays RD: Marital status, social support, and health transitions in chronic disease patients. *J Health Soc Behav* **31**: 328–343, 1990.

Sibilia L: Type A behavior and hostility in coronary heart diseases. In L Sibilia and S Borgo (Eds) *Health Psychology in Cardiovascular Health and Disease*, pp 77–89. Centro di Ricerca in Psicoterpia: Roma, 1993.

Sykes DH: Coping with a heart attack: psychological processes. *Irish J Psychol* **15**: 54–66, 1994.

Tabrizi K, Littman A, Williams Jr RB and Scheidt S: Psychopharmacology and cardiac disease. In R Allan and S Scheidt (Eds) *Heart and Mind*, pp 397–419. American Psychological Association: Washington, DC, 1996.

Van Dixhoorn J: Relaxation therapy in cardiac rehabilitation. *Doctoral dissertation*. Erasmus University: Rotterdam, 1991.

Van Elderen T: *Health Education in Cardiac Rehabilitation*. DSWO Press: Leiden, 1991.

Van Elderen T: Psycho educational prevention programme (Psychoeducatieve preventie module). *Hart Bulletin* **5**: 141–144, 1997.

Van Elderen T and Echteld M: Psycho-Educatieve Preventie Module. In *Revalidatie Commissie Nederlandse Vereniging voor Cardiologie en de Nederlandse Hartstichting, Richtlijnen Hartrevalidatie Deel II (Guidelines Cardiac Rehabilitation Part II)*. The Netherlands Heart Foundation and The Netherlands Society of Cardiology: The Hague, 1995/1996.

Van Elderen T and Leenders CM: Voorlichtingsmodule. In *Revalidatie Commissie Nederlandse Vereniging voor Cardiologie en de Nederlandse Hartstichting, Richtlijnen Hartrevalidatie Deel II (Guidelines for Cardiac Rehabilitation Part II)*. The Netherlands Heart Foundation and The Netherlands Society of Cardiology: The Hague, 1995/1996.

Van Elderen T, Maes S and Dusseldorp E: Coping with coronary heart disease: A longitudinal study. *J Psychosom Res* **47**: 175–183, 1999.

Van Elderen T, Maes S and Van den Broek Y: Effects of a health education program with telephone follow-up during cardiac rehabilitation. *Br J Clin Psychol* **33**: 367–378, 1994a.

Van Elderen T, Maes S, Seegers G, Kragten H and Relik-van Wely L: Effects of a post-hospitalization group health education program for patients with coronary heart disease. *Psychology and Health* **9**: 317–330, 1994b.

Van Elderen T, Maes S, Madalinska J and Komproe I: Coping, angst en vitale uitputting na een coronair incident. Een longitudinaal onderzoek. *Gedrag and Gezondheid* **24**: 207–214, 1996.

Van Elderen T, Maes S, Van der Kamp L and Komproe Y: The development of an anger expression and control scale. *Br J Health Psychol* **2**: 269–281, 1997.

Waltz M, Badura B, Pfaff H and Schott T: Marriage and the psychological consequences of a heart attack: a longitudinal study of adaption to chronic illness after 3 years. *Soc Sci Med* **27**: 149–158, 1988.

Wenger NK, Froelicher ES, Smith LK, Ades PA, Berra K, Blumenthal KA, Certo CME, Dattilo AM, Davis D, DeBusk RF, Drozda JP, Fletcher BJ, Franklin BA, Gaston H, Greenland P, McBride PE, McGregor CGA, Oldridge NB, Piscatella JC, Rogers FJ: In: *Cardiac Rehabilitation. Clinical Practice Guideline, 17.* US Department of Health and Human Services, Public Health Service, Agency for Health Care Policy and Research and the National Heart, Lung and Blood Institute. AHCPR Publication No 96–0672, Rockville MD, 1995.

US Department of Health and Human Services: Health, United States 1994. Public Health Service. DHHS Pub No (PHS) 95–1232, Hyattsville MD: 1995.

WHO (World Health Organization): *Statistic Annual.* World Health Organization: Geneva, 1989.

WHO (World Health Organization), Regional Office for Europe: Needs and action priorities in cardiac rehabilitation and secondary prevention in patients with CHD. World Health Organization: Copenhagen, 1993.

Psychiatry, Psychology and Health Promotion

Rhonda Galbally
Australian International Health Institute, University of Melbourne, Australia
Felicity Allen
Monash University, Melbourne, Australia

and

Chris Borthwick
Managing Editor, Health Promotion Journal of Australia

INTRODUCTION

That psychiatry and psychology can contribute to health promotion is now well recognized. Many areas, however, most notably models of addictive behaviour, are relatively underdeveloped and hinder progress in the field. This paper explores some of the problematic issues in current models of addiction, and explores briefly the benefits to health promotion of developing new approaches to deal with individual and social problems arising from substance use or abuse.

The major area of concern in this paper is cigarette smoking. Numerous efforts to reduce cigarette smoking have been tried, with mixed success. The deficiencies in these approaches are discussed and suggestions made for a more effective approach to social change in substance use.

HEALTH PROMOTION

Health promotion is defined as the process of enabling people to increase control over and improve their health; psychiatry is the area of medicine concerned with the treatment of mental illness and problems; psychology is the scientific study of the behaviour of humans and animals. These definitions are not so much mutually exclusive or even overlapping as lying at right angles to each other. Workers in

Psychology and Psychiatry: Integrating Medical Practice.
Edited by J. Milgrom and G. D. Burrows © 2001 John Wiley & Sons, Ltd.

any of the three fields could claim sole title to almost any of the areas each definition covers; in particular all three have a stake in questions of health-related behaviours, both positive and negative. It is sensible for the three disciplines to work together; however, if they are to co-operate, areas of responsibility must be assigned.

The field of health promotion, dealing as it usually does with behavioural change, has been identified as debatable ground. The development of health promotion as a separate cognate area with its own programs and policies has already led to realignments in the professional relationship of psychology and psychiatry.

Over recent years, clinical psychological services have diversified within the health sector, leading to a breakdown in the traditional nexus between clinical psychology and psychiatry, and to the emergence of the interdisciplinary field of behavioural medicine. From their earlier limited role as providers of psychometric assessments in educational and psychiatric hospital settings, clinical psychologists now provide a wide range of therapeutic services and research skills to general hospitals, universities, community health centres, and the private sector. This evolving trend has significant implications for the future structure and direction of clinical practices in clinical psychology, psychiatry and medicine (Touyz et al 1992).

This realignment may also be seen as an instance of the more practical analysis of Ross & Pam (1995). "Psychologists have made strategic end runs around psychiatry in the past two decades. Part of the strategy has been to use terms like behavioural medicine and to offer expertise in behavioural analysis and therapy, which psychiatrists tend to lack. These manoeuvres and counter-manoeuvres are all political in nature, on both sides" (Ross & Pam 1995, p 128).

The scientific study of human behaviour in any area is still in its infancy, particularly the study of health-related behaviours. Health promotion requires input from both psychology and psychiatry as well as from many other disciplines, including epidemiology, pharmacology, sociology, semiotics, ethics and politics. A major barrier to the advance of knowledge in this field is the absence of adequate theoretical development from health psychologists. When research in health psychology is theoretically based, and much of it is not, it usually relies either on the Theory of Planned Behaviour (Fishbein & Ajzen 1975), the Theory of Reasoned Action (Fishbein et al 1994) or the Health Belief Model (Rosenstock 1974). Tests of the predictions of these theories regularly show that they can explain only about 20% of the variation in human health behaviours, yet there has been no move to replace them. The utter unlikelihood of humans behaving rationally in any area, let alone where health is concerned, would seem to require no demonstration, yet health psychologists insist on acting as though it does.

An overview of the relevance of health promotion and prevention to health was provided in Chapter 2. In this chapter the example of nicotine dependence is used to emphasize the difficulties encountered in health promotion interventions, to illustrate the move from conceptualizing addiction as an individual problem suitable for treatment and to suggest alternatives that place the health problem in the context of the person, including both cultural and physical considerations.

NICOTINE DEPENDENCE

Cigarette smoking is the world's largest single preventable cause of death; just under half (45%) of all smokers will die of a tobacco-induced disorder. According to a tranche of research and internal company documents leaked to the American Congress from the Brown and Williamson Tobacco Corporation, smoking depends so directly on the absorption of and development of tolerance for and addiction to nicotine that tobacco companies are in the business of "selling nicotine" (Slade et al 1995). Since the mid-1950s, tobacco companies in Europe and America have devoted millions of dollars to research the effect of nicotine on the brain and to converting cigarettes into sophisticated "nicotine-delivery devices". This last is the basis for the American Food and Drug Administration (FDA) finally exerting control over the production, advertisement and distribution of cigarettes.

What have the professions concerned with health-related behaviours contributed to controlling the worldwide spread of tobacco use? The difference between the attitudes towards the DSM-IV (the standard reference work for diagnostic categories in psychiatry) classification 305.10 (Nicotine Dependence) by the psychiatric, psychological and health promotion professions provides an example of the problematic relationship of the three groups. Is tobacco use a pathology, an expression of social meaning or both? What is the function of each discipline in affecting that pathology, that society and that meaning? What weapons can each discipline supply the others in the field of tobacco control and, more broadly, public health? How can they work together in practice in medical and community settings?

The first problem for anybody contemplating an intervention in this situation is to identify where the problem lies: with the user, with the substance, or in their interaction. One common response from the health promotion field has been to blame the substance.

"Nicotine is seen as being as addictive as alcohol or heroin. It is usually the first drug used by individuals, and the last drug given up. While 90% of alcohol drinkers do not become dependent on alcohol, only 10% of nicotine users do not become dependent on nicotine. As many as 25% of the American population is nicotine-dependent, and 20% of the Californian population" (Maheu 1994, p 3).

The model here is of the drug as invader, exterminating resistance and imposing its own government (although drugs are seen as varying in their ability to impose control). The 1952 World Health Organization (WHO) Expert Committee on Drugs described those in its "addiction-producing" category as causing an irresistible need "always and in all individuals" (Krivanek 1988, p 33). At first sight, this model has the effects of virtually absolving the user from any responsibility for the addiction and sidestepping any questions about the rights of the users or the responsibilities of the suppliers.

Subsequent re-evaluations of the responsibilities of the suppliers have taken the addictive properties of nicotine as the keystone of their attempts to control the tobacco industry. The "reasonably foreseeable" nature of nicotine's pharmacological effects upon users is the legal basis for the FDA's assertion of jurisdiction over cigarettes and smokeless tobacco in America (Kessler et al 1997). The tobacco companies' historical denial of the addictive potential of nicotine has not only been an important prop supporting their argument that smoking is an act of free will (see below), but has also enabled them to avoid regulation by the FDA.

Substance Abuse and Substance Dependence

The DSM-IV (1994) distinguishes "substance abuse" from the more serious problem of "substance dependence". The DSM-IV criterion for substance abuse is a maladaptive pattern of substance use leading to clinically significant impairment or distress, as shown by three or more specified examples from behaviours described under "tolerance", "withdrawal" or "desire to control or cut down use". Criteria for substance dependence are similar but with the addition of physical tolerance for the substance, withdrawal symptoms, loss of control over consumption, a desire to quit, heavy time and social commitment and continued use of the substance despite serious physical problems.

Examples of the way American smokers fulfil the DSM-IV criteria for substance dependence or abuse are shown in Table 10.1.

Nicotine is a potent inducer of drug dependence. For example, only 33% of "self-quitters" remain abstinent for two days and fewer than 5% are successful on any given attempt to stop (Hughes et al 1992). Nicotine is a powerful positive reinforcer, completely under the control of the smoker. It produces improved concentration and mood, decreased anger and reduced weight. A bolus dose of nicotine reaches the brain 10 seconds after inhalation, producing almost instant effects. The dose can be controlled precisely by the way the cigarette is smoked and smokers soon learn to control their blood nicotine levels. Nicotine facilitates mood control by its varying impact on the brain. Under some circumstances and doses, it has a tranquillizing effect, but under other circumstances, it has a stimulant effect (Kessler et al 1997). Smokers soon learn to use nicotine to alter their moods at will. Smoking behaviours occur frequently (a pack-a-day smoker self-administers nicotine about 200 times a day) so that there are many cues for smoking (e.g. finishing a meal).

CNS Effects of Nicotine

Although nicotine dependence can occur with the use of any tobacco products, the proportion of users addicted and the time it takes both depend on two factors: the amount of nicotine available and the speed with which it reaches the brain. Rapidly absorbed nicotine has a greater impact on the brain. The action of the drug on the hypothalamus helps people cope with stress (Slade et al 1995). At the start of the habit, small doses of nicotine have the desired results, but steadily increasing dose levels are needed to do this. In a chronic smoker, normal balance in the stress mechanisms of the brain can only be maintained by continuous nicotine intake.

TABLE 10.1 American smokers and DSM-IV substance dependence criteria and examples

A maladaptive pattern of substance use, leading to clinically significant impairment or distress, as shown by three (or more) of the following, occurring at any time in the same 12-month period.

Criteria	Examples
Tolerance: as defined by either:	
A need for markedly increased amounts of the substance to achieve intoxication or desired effect:	Most smokers escalate to one pack/day or more by age 25
Markedly diminished effect with continued use of the same amount of the substances	Absence of nausea, dizziness, etc
Withdrawal as manifested by either:	
The characteristic withdrawal syndrome for the substance	Stopping smoking produces a characteristic pattern of craving, anxiety, overeating, insomnia, reduced heart rate and dysphoria
The substance is taken to relieve or avoid withdrawal symptoms	Many smokers light up immediately after being in a smoke-free area
The substance is often taken in larger amounts or over a longer period than was intended	Most smokers do not intend to smoke five years later but, in fact, 70% continue
Persistent desire or unsuccessful effort to cut down or control use	77% of smokers have tried to stop, 55% of these have been unsuccessful despite repeated attempts and only 5–10% of self-quitters are successful.
A great deal of time is spent in activities needed to get the substance, use it or recover from its effects	Leaving worksite to smoke
Important social, occupational or recreational activities are given up or reduced because of substance use	Not taking a job due to on-job smoking restrictions
Substance use is continued despite knowledge of having a persistent or recurrent physical or psychology problem that is likely to have been caused by the substance	Many smokers have heart disease, lung cancer or ulcers but continue to smoke

Adapted from APA (1996).

If this is inaccessible, the brain's ability to release stress hormones is greatly reduced so that the endocrine system is unbalanced and the user craves more nicotine.

The existence of a small group of smokers (about 10%) who smoke five or fewer cigarettes per day (known as "chippers" or "cadgers" from their habit of borrowing cigarettes rather than buying their own) shows that addiction in nicotine-exposed people is not inevitable. It is also possible that, like other drugs, addiction does not develop until users are regularly exposed to a certain threshold level. Cotinine is a metabolic breakdown product of nicotine and blood levels are used to measure the amount of nicotine taken in. Addicted smokers have an average blood cotinine level of 300 ng/millilitre, while smokers of five or fewer cigarettes per day have average blood cotinine levels of 54 ng/millilitre. Benowitz & Henningfield (1994) argued that the reason chippers can usually give up smoking quite easily is that they are not sufficiently exposed to nicotine to become addicted to it. They produced evidence that tobacco manufacturers manipulate the level of nicotine per cigarette to maximize their addictive potential. Nevertheless the question about the factors that protect the chippers from progressing are still unknown. How have these people opted for a very low, stable pattern of use?

Nicotine's status as an addictive drug has major legal ramifications. The tobacco industry has always publicly claimed that it is not addictive and therefore anyone who smokes is choosing to do so (Glantz et al 1995). The Brown and Williamson documents show that the industry was aware of the addictive potential of nicotine over 30 years ago and designed the structure and pharmacology of its cigarettes to facilitate absorption of the drug. Anyone who uses cigarettes consistently is at grave risk of becoming nicotine-dependent, nevertheless many people never smoke and many smokers succeed in giving them up. What is it that distinguishes nonsmokers or successful quitters from those who continue to use cigarettes? Are they primarily social and cultural factors (e.g. women are less likely to smoke than men), genetic factors or psychological characteristics?

To devise practicable and effective policies for the prevention and treatment of substance abuse disorders like tobacco smoking, accurate models of addiction are required.

MODELS OF ADDICTION

Historically, addiction models have been largely based on morality, seeing excess as a sin and the primary cause of sin as weakness of the user's will. This view is popular to this day, with many people arguing that drug addicts are weak or bad people who do not deserve treatment (Leshner 1997). The medical profession's move from a moral to an illness model coincided with the rise of the psychiatric movement in the first half of the twentieth century. By the time DSM-I appeared in 1952, alcohol and drug-use disorders were categorized under "Sociopathic Personality Disturbances". This indicated that substance-use disorder was then considered a moral weakness, and as a manifestation of a deeper psychological problem, but not as a disorder in its own right. Given that the relationship between smoking and lung cancer was only then becoming scientifically undeniable, smoking was not seen as a sufficiently damaging disorder to be placed with heroin and cocaine use.

By the time DSM-III, in 1980, finally separated substance use and dependence as pathological conditions, it was clear that tobacco was a greater killer than any illegal substance and that its use was not, in the narrow sense, rational, particularly when information on its hazards had been public knowledge for two decades. While DSM-III mentioned that social and cultural factors contribute to the onset and continuation of abuse and dependence, this edition also emphasized pharmacological criteria of tolerance and withdrawal. This emphasis is consistent with Rogler's view that DSM-III marked a shift from a psychodynamic approach to mental illness to one more compatible with traditional medical models (Rogler 1997). The appearance of dramatic physical symptoms when drug use is abruptly ceased is often taken to mean that the drug concerned is particularly serious or dangerous.

If, however, it was the presence of tolerance and withdrawal symptoms that differentiated substance use, abuse and substance dependence, this introduced problems in practice. Substance-use behaviour was not always consistent with theoretical criteria. Addictive and dangerous drugs do not necessarily produce severe physical symptoms when they are withdrawn; crack cocaine and amphetamine produce few physical symptoms (Leshner 1997). In humans, most drug users do not become abusers or dependent (Koob & Le Moal 1997). Many factors including social context of use, route of administration, genetics, and life events influence the progression from drug use to addiction. The importance of the social context of addiction was shown by the relative ease with which the heroin addiction of the returned Vietnam war veterans could be treated. They returned to an environment almost totally different from the one where they had first become addicted. The absence of the conditioned environmental cues meant they were far less likely to relapse than addicts first exposed to heroin in America (Leshner 1997).

Behavioural and Physiological Aspects

DSM-III-R (1987) was thus revised to give the behavioural aspects of substance-use disorders equal weight to the physiological components. The shift from essentially pharmacological criteria to largely behavioural criteria also shifted the balance away from psychiatrists, who as doctors were experts on drugs, towards psychologists, who could claim comparable or greater expertise on behaviour. Psychologists' movement into the substance abuse treatment has gone furthest in smoking. A representative work such as Frances & Miller's (1991) *Clinical Textbook of Addictive Disorders* cites psychology journals more often than psychiatry journals in only two of its 22 chapters—those on tobacco and behaviour therapy.

Tobacco control is also the concern of general medicine. An examination of 118 original research-oriented articles in the journal *Tobacco Control* 1992–1997, where the university affiliations of the authors could be determined, revealed that 78% came from the faculties of medicine, public health, or epidemiology, with only 4% coming from psychiatry, 8% from psychology or behavioural science, and 8% from health promotion or education. Professional divisions between psychology and psychiatry may have little impact on the field at large. Conversely, an electronic search of *Psychological Abstracts* showed steady growth of interest, with zero articles in 1972, four in 1982 and 408 in 1992. Heroin and cocaine remain in the province of psychiatry. This division may also reflect the tendency noted by Ross & Pam (1995), where "certain disorders" tend to be regarded as less severe, less biological in nature, and therefore more suitable for the treatment efforts of psychologists and social workers. The criterion by which these illnesses were selected as the primary property of psychiatry "was solely one of symptom severity" (Ross & Pam 1995, p 104).

Heredity and Environment

The move towards behavioural explanations for substance use coincided with contrary medicalizing movements towards genetic and pharmacological explanations.

"Although environmental factors may be important determinants of cigarette use, there is strong evidence that the acquisition of the smoking habit and its persistence are strongly influenced by hereditary factors. Of particular significance are studies of identical twins, which show that when one twin smokes, the other tends to smoke. This is not the case in nonidentical twins. The absence of these similarities in a control population of nonidentical twins suggests a strong biogenetic component in smoking behaviour" (Blum et al 1996, p 37).

Several large-scale population studies have now been conducted investigating genetic vulnerability for substance dependence (e.g. Bierut et al 1998). One question of interest is whether there is a general vulnerability or whether it is substance-specific. Bierut et al studied the drug use and dependence patterns of 1212 alcoholics and their 2755 siblings and found that siblings of addicted smokers had an elevated risk of being addicted smokers themselves. Despite the presence of a genetic contribution, however, it was the siblings' own characteristics (e.g. birth cohort—younger siblings were less likely to begin smoking) that were the strongest influences on their probability of becoming an addicted smoker. After controlling for other explanations of clustering within families (e.g. addicted probands supplying siblings with drugs), Bierut et al concluded that the genetic vulnerability was specific rather than general. Availability influences the chance of a person trying a substance; something more is required for dependence or addiction to develop.

The pharmacological model argues that persistent substance use and associated behavioural indicators of dependence are due to changes in the brain that motivate repeated, compulsive use of the substance (e.g. Kessler et al 1997). Observable effects of chronic drug use on the brain have been identified at all levels: molecular, cellular, structural and functional (Leshner 1997). Differences found in addicted brains include changed metabolic activity, gene expression and responsiveness to environmental cues, particularly those associated with drug use. Some lasting brain changes are common to many different drugs, while others are specific to one drug only. This model proposes that, for most people addicted to any substance, addiction is a chronic relapsing condition, so that the most reasonable expectation is a reduced level of drug intake with periods of abstinence.

No model of addiction, moral, genetic or pharmacological, can explain common observations about drug use. In most European countries and America, women are markedly less likely than men to smoke and tertiary-educated women are the least likely of all women to smoke (Kendrick & Merritt 1996). It is by no means clear how gender and education interact with moral or genetic tendencies towards addiction.

Although only 5–10% of "self-quitters" stop smoking permanently on any given attempt, the percentage of Australian men who smoke has fallen from 72% in 1947 to 24% in 1992 (Gray 1992). As most people stop smoking without outside help, either they persist and ultimately learn how to succeed or they are more effective in helping themselves than most doctors believe. Again, it is unclear how weak-willed amateurs whose brains have been permanently changed by chronic exposure to nicotine find the fortitude to overcome their addiction.

The inadequacy of available models of addiction means that predictions about human behaviour cannot be based on them. In turn, research into developing treatment programs must be ad hoc and piecemeal. Observation of the usage patterns of nicotine reveals that smoking behaviour interacts with many other behaviours and characteristics of the users. One of the most important of these is the issue of comorbidity.

COMORBIDITY AND ENVIRONMENT

Nicotine dependence is associated with other psychiatric conditions. DSM-IV notes that "Nicotine Dependence is more common among individuals with other mental disorders" (APA 1994, p 244). To some extent this correlation was in DSM terms artefactual; substance abuse correlated with antisocial personality because substance abuse was one of the criteria for a diagnosis of antisocial personality. Depending on the population studied, from 55% to 90% of individuals with other mental disorders smoke, compared with 30% in the general population. Other conditions were often seen as confounders, to be removed either mathematically or behaviourally to enable an uninterrupted concentration upon the disorder of interest.

Despite the emphasis in the pharmacological model on environmental cues to dependent behaviours, the settings in which the behaviour occurred were regarded as little more than sources of noise in the data. One study, for example, reported the irritating difficulties in conducting a scientifically rigorous trial of cigarette price elasticity in Sarajevo during its siege by the Serbs (Creson et al 1996). The assumption was that in life, as in statistics, medical interventions would work if only these confounders could be removed, and the problem was that the world in which the interventions were to be carried out was made up almost entirely by confounders.

Treating comorbidity as worthy of study in its own right, Patton et al (1996) found that smoking positively correlated with depression and anxiety among teenage Australians. Subjects reporting high levels of depression and anxiety were twice as likely to be smokers after the potential confounders of year level, sex, alcohol use and parental smoking were controlled for. This association was particularly marked amongst the girls. The authors suggested that teenage girls might smoke as self-medication for depression and anxiety. Such a pattern of nicotine use would be reasonable, given many smokers' self-admitted use of the drug to manage their moods (see above). Moreover, smoking correlated with the use of other drugs and other risk behaviours.

"Strong interrelationships in drug use were found, with a pattern of association between smoking and drinking consistent with a mutual elevation of risk. Frequent use of tobacco and alcohol had a high risk for associated marijuana use" (Patton et al 1996, p 228).

Such an approach pointed away from regarding single diseases or conditions as the core concern of the psychologist or psychiatrist, towards the general situation of the person—the context, cultural and physical, in which these activities were an outcome of these behaviours. Attending to the context suggests that interventions would be more effective if they were directed at groups of people or towards an environment.

HEALTH PSYCHOLOGY

Moving away from individual therapy would, however, involve a considerable redirection of psychology. The rapidly expanding field of health psychology emerged in America during the late 1970s in response to the growing emphasis on lifestyle change to reduce health risks. In 1978 the American Psychological Association set up a Division of Health Psychology (although it took Australia until 1998 to follow suit).

Social Class and Health

Four books entitled *Health Psychology* were published in the 1970s, and 20 in the decade after that. The emphasis has consistently been much directed towards the psychology of the individual, with most attention being given to behavioural factors, e.g. Type A behaviour and heart disease. Social psychology was rarely considered relevant. Consider three representative American health psychology textbooks written between 1987 and 1991 (Feist & Brannon 1988; Genest & Genest 1987; DiMatteo 1991). Although Feist and Brannon do mention social disadvantage, none of these books contains a full analysis of the impact of social class upon health, including the ways that belonging to a higher social class facilitates good health and belonging to a lower social class impairs it. None referred to the Ottawa Charter definition of health, none discussed the wider health promotion movement, and all covered the tolerance/withdrawal model of nicotine addiction in detail (while also emphasizing such microsocial factors as peer pressure). Discussion of the relationship between health psychology and health promotion was limited to the contribution that psychology could make to improving educational initiatives and dealing with client motivations rather than in advocating for broader social policy change.

The absence of class analysis is particularly felt in the study of smoking behaviours. Upper-class smokers were the first to give up cigarettes (Doll et al 1994) and higher social class has become ever more strongly associated both with nonsmoking and better life expectancy over the past 25 years. The difference between life expectancy of the highest and lowest social groups is increasing in all countries where the impact of social class on health is seriously studied. Rejection of smoking amongst upper-class people is a major contributor, but there are many other lifestyle factors that contribute to this worrying trend (see below). This phenomenon was first remarked upon in Biblical times: "For unto every one that hath shall be given, and he shall have abundance: but from him that hath not shall be taken away even that which he hath" (Matthew 25: 29), but comparatively little research into the exact mechanisms of the impact of social class on health has been carried out. Is it, for example, something in the experience of being an underdog that reduces the health of the people low in the hierarchy, or is it the pleasure of wielding power over others that promotes the health of the ruling class?

ENVIRONMENTS AND POPULATIONS

Once the wider context is admitted to the debate it can be seen that the available models are inadequate to explain the observed prevalence of smoking and non-smoking. Public health, and with it health promotion, now enter the picture, bringing with them an emphasis on causation that goes beyond the individual. These disciplines work with population, and identify differences between social groups. It has become clear that there is a strong socioeconomic status gradient to smoking rates, and a link between disadvantage and disease that has been largely ignored in past American studies.

"The one social factor about which there can be no argument is social class, but until recently researchers in public health have not studied social class. Everyone knows that the lower people are in socioeconomic status—however defined—the higher are the rates of virtually all diseases and conditions. In spite of this universal recognition, almost nothing is known about the reasons for this phenomenon. The list of possible explanations is long and well known. It includes poverty, bad housing, unemployment, poor nutrition, inadequate medical care and low levels of education. We do not know the relative importance of these various factors because we do not study social class. Social class is of such overwhelming power that we in our research typically hold it constant so that we can study other things. If we did not, it would swamp all other factors and we would not be able to see the role of any other issues. In consequence, we know virtually nothing about the various subcomponents associated with social class" (Syme 1997). Social class can also become a holdall into which all variance is disposed of, and much work in social epidemiology is necessary to distinguish its components.

European work, notably the long-term follow-up study of British male doctors (Doll et al 1994), was always more frank about the relationship of social class to illness. Doll et al charted the moment in British history when smoking became "non-U", with enormous benefits to the health and longevity of the upper classes. What no one has attempted to explain is the continuing popularity of smoking amongst the poorest of the poor and its association with the increasing socioeconomic gradients in coronary heart disease and lung cancer.

INTERVENTIONS

Failed Interventions

Following the recognition that social factors were significant in health behaviours, it became clear that neither interventions based on traditional models of disease and addiction nor those based on health psychology-oriented lifestyle change appeared to be having the desired effect. A new research fashion arose for multiple intervention trials, in which a wide range of hazardous behaviours, including smoking, would be targeted. The major population intervention trials used the full resources of contemporary psychological and psychiatric theory: Bennet & Hodgson (1992), for example, concluded that "Most of the major programs have been explicitly premised, at least in part, on the models..." (p 38) of Bandura (1997) (social learning theory), Abramson et al (1978) (attribution theory), Becker (1974) (health belief theory), and Rogers (1983) (diffusion theory). Despite this weight of academic theory, these programs produced no major effects on behaviour.

Perhaps the most famous of the failed interventions was the Multiple Risk Factor Intervention Trial (MRFIT) beginning in 1971 and ending in 1981 and intended to reduce the death rate from coronary heart disease in America by getting men in the top 10% risk group in the country to change hazardous behaviours. A massive screening of 400 000 men in 22 cities located men at high risk from serum cholesterol level, cigarette smoking and high blood pressure. After three screening exams, 6000 men were randomized to intervention in MRFIT clinics while another 6000 men, chosen at random, were sent back to their own doctors with a report on their risk factors. This trial cost US $180 million and involved the most expensive, ambitious and intensive processes ever tried anywhere. Every clinic had trained counsellors who worked very closely with each participant for six years. None the less, the trial failed. Six years later, the men in the special intervention group did not achieve a lower death rate from coronary heart disease than men in the control group.

Relatively few in the special intervention group (SI) changed their behaviour to lower their risk. While 42% of the men stopped smoking after six years, for example, 58% continued. Other changes were even less marked: only half of the men with hypertension had their blood pressures under control by the end of the trial, and there were almost no changes made to their diet.

One explanation for the failure of MRFIT is that the SI men did not change their behaviour enough: another is that men in the control group (C) changed too much. The control group went through three screening exams and knew they were in the top 10% risk group in the nation. Denied admission to the special intervention group, many simply changed their behaviours on their own. As many C group men shared workplaces with the SI men, they were privy to the medical recommendations given the SI men. This important phenomenon suggests that providing people with information is not a waste of time, and underlines the importance of the way information is transmitted. In MRFIT, the C men provided with personalized and relevant information about their health, but then forced to find their own solutions, did as well as the SI men.

After the MRFIT failure, many public health programs explored community intervention programs. If individuals would not change their behaviour, perhaps campaigns could succeed by changing their communities. In America, the National Cancer Institute set up a nationwide series of Community Intervention Trials for Smoking Cessation, or COMMIT. In these projects, business and government leaders were involved, with a local captain on every block of the targeted research area. The nationwide COMMIT studies involved over 10 000 heavy smokers in 11 intervention cities. A matched group of another 11 cities served as the control group. In the intervention cities, the goal was to create a social climate that did not support tobacco use, and efforts were made to implement smoke-free policies at work sites and elsewhere in the community, provide a newsletter and other information, offer training to people to become smoking counsellors, and so on.

At the end of this massive and very expensive nationwide trial, there was no difference in the quit rate among heavy smokers between the intervention and control communities (approximately 18% quit in both communities). Among light to moderate smokers, 31% quit in the intervention cities while 28% quit in the control communities (Bauman et al 1999). This observation suggested an existing tendency to stop smoking, driven by forces external to the intervention, but in no way enhanced by it.

The Health of the Organization

With the wisdom of hindsight it can be seen that the problem even with interventions such as COMMIT has been that insufficient attention has been paid to the place of the psychology of organizational change in community development. There are two approaches to community-wide social change: a gradual process of the accretion of small, inexpensive changes and a more rapid, but more expensive, approach involving large-scale changes.

Relatively small changes in organizational structures can change smoking behaviour. Following Justice Morling's 1991 ruling in the Australian Federal Court that the Tobacco Institute of Australia had been guilty of misleading the public about the dangers of passive smoking, many employers banned smoking at work for fear of civil actions against them (Allen 1998). These bans, costing nothing, enforce relative tobacco abstinence for several hours per day. The need to leave a workstation in order to go outside and smoke makes the habit less convenient and the result is lower consumption (Borland et al 1991). Self-reported daily smoking by moderate and heavy smokers fell by about 25% after worksite bans were introduced, and this was stable over a six-month follow-up period. Over the next two years, 5% of Telecom employees (twice the population rate) stopped smoking completely. The steady spread of smoke-free zones throughout the community puts increasing pressure on smokers, both to defer or stop smoking and to consider the health of others. Nonsmokers cease to be inured to the stench of stale tobacco smoke and are liable to object when they encounter it. The existence of smoke-free zones and the acceptance of the smoke-free concept empowers nonsmokers to ask for consideration.

By contrast, the 1986 Ottawa conference that defined health promotion as the process of enabling people to increase control over and to improve their health, called for an integrated program of public policy, community action, the development of personal skills, and the creation of healthy environments. They called for effective community power that determined the course of the program—setting priorities, making decisions, planning strategies and implementing them to achieve better health. At the heart of this process is the empowerment of communities to control their own endeavours and destinies. The aim of interventions was to use the work of community organizations within the project to build capacities for change that could be employed to meet their other priorities. "Improvements in health status are believed to come about primarily from gaining more power over the policy environment rather than simply gaining more knowledge about health behaviors" (Wallack 1994).

Syme (1997) has found that it is possible to enhance people's abilities to control their own destinies—or, at least, to be confident about the likelihood that they can solve problems and to be creative in thinking about ways to do this. By empowering such people, we may improve well-being.

Other evaluations of interventions to empower communities to resist erosion by alcohol have found a more mixed health outcome from strengthening the native culture. Petoskey et al (1998) worked with a Chippewa community and found that participation in tribal ceremonies was linked to cigarette, marijuana and alcohol use for males and to cigarette use for females. While this is hardly surprising, given the ancient social role played by tobacco in American Indian culture, how do we know that people will choose healthy outcomes if they are free to do so? It is likely that most of them would, but in fact we cannot be sure. Whatever the role played by the delights of power in the longer lifespans of upper-class Europeans, a large majority of them have rejected smoking.

Health-Promoting Settings

When even such interventions as COMMIT, interventions that recognized the social correlates of smoking, appeared to do little good, the health promotion field faced a crisis. The resolution of that crisis has led psychology, psychiatry, and health promotion into new areas. Antonovsky's (1996) work on salutogenesis and the "sense of coherence" and Syme's work on the importance of a sense of control have increased the complexity of what was once seen as the simple delivery of an uncomplicated message on the evils of tobacco.

The unsuccessful mass health promotion measures discussed above did have a common factor: their community involvement did not confer community control. While the direction of modern health promotion is largely into the unknown, the role of the community should be investigated and enhanced, in order to create supportive environments for people to exercise informed choices about their health.

CONCLUSION

This chapter has briefly outlined and identified some of the deficiencies in current models of addiction, describes some of the difficulties in designing large-scale intervention programs based on them, and suggested alternative intervention approaches.

The creation of truly supportive environments would call on organizational psychology to map organizational change strategies that would ensure that any improvements would be sustainable. The new approach to health promotion will require also a blurring of professional boundaries to incorporate not only public health, psychology, and psychiatry but also social epidemiology and semiotics.

A realignment of effort in this direction will require a reconsideration of the nature of a psychological or psychiatric "disorder". If the intervention is to be targeted to the perceived societal concern, it cannot be structured around an invariant medico-legal set of diagnostic criteria. "Nicotine dependence" must be deconstructed to recognize its implications for the mechanisms of social control. Members of both professions need to accept that current models of addiction to any drug offer very little that is useful to either research or intervention. This acceptance will entail a recognition that neither profession has very much in the way of practical suggestions with which to combat one of the major health issues of our time. While more effective models of substance use or abuse are being developed, the most humane approach to people currently using nicotine to regulate their moods might be to provide long-term maintenance options for the drug which do not require them to inhale large amounts of carcinogenic smoke.

REFERENCES

Abramson L, Seligman M and Teasdale J: Learned helplessness in humans. *J Abn Psychol* **87**: 49–74, 1978.
Allen F: *Health Psychology: Theory and Practice.* Allen and Unwin: Sydney, 1998.
Antonovsky A: The Salutogenic Model as a theory to guide health promotion. *Health Promotion International* **11**: 11–18, 1996.

APA (American Psychiatric Association): *DSM-I*: *Diagnostic and Standard Manual of Mental Disorders*, *1st Edn*. APA: Washington, DC, 1952.

APA (American Psychiatric Association): *DSM-III*: *Diagnostic and Standard Manual of Mental Disorders*, *3rd Edn*. APA: Washington, DC, 1980.

APA (American Psychiatric Association): *DSM-III-R*: *Diagnostic and Standard Manual of Mental Disorders*, *revised 3rd Edn.*, revised APA: Washington, DC, 1987.

APA (American Psychiatric Association): *DSM-IV*: *Diagnostic and Standard Manual of Mental Disorders*, *4th Edn*. APA: Washington, DC, 1994.

APA (American Psychiatric Association): Practice guidelines for the treatment of patients with nicotine dependence. *Am J Psychiatry* **153**: (10S) Supplement, 131, 1996.

Bandura A: *Social Learning Theory*. Prentice-Hall: Englewood Cliffs, NJ, 1977.

Bauman KE, Suchindran CM and Murray DM: The paucity of effects in community trials: is secular trend the culprit? *Prev Med* **28**: 426–429, 1999.

Becker M: The health belief model and personal health behaviour. *Health Education Monographs* **2**: 324–508, 1974.

Bennet P and Hodgson R: Psychology and health promotion. In R Brunton and G Mac-Donald (Eds) *Health Promotion: Disciplines and Diversity*. Routledge: London, 1992.

Benowitz N and Henningfield J: Establishing a nicotine threshold for addiction: the implications for tobacco regulation. *N Engl J Med* **331**: 123–125, 1994.

Bierut L, Dinwiddie S, Begleiter H, Crowe R, Hesselbrock V, Nurnberger J, Porjesz B, Schuckit M and Reich T: Familial transmission of substance dependence: alcohol, marijuana, cocaine and habitual smoking: a report from the collaborative study on the genetics of alcoholism. *Arch Gen Psychiatry* **55**: 982–988, 1998.

Bird E and Podmore U: Children's understanding of health and illness. *Psychology & Health* **4**: 175–185, 1990.

Blum K, Cull J, Braverman E and Comings D: Reward Deficiency Syndrome. *Am Sci*, March–April, 33–42, 1996.

Booker S: *The Usefulness of General Theories of Addiction*. Department of Psychology, University of Sydney: Sydney, 1994.

Borland R, Owen N and Hocking B: Changes in smoking behaviour after a total workplace smoking ban. *Aust J Pub Health* **80**: 130–134, 1991.

Breslau N, Kilbey M and Andreski P: DSM-III-R nicotine dependence in young adults: prevalence, correlates and associated psychiatric disorders. *Addiction* **89**: 743–754, 1994.

Camp D, Klesges R and Relyea G: The relationship between body weight concerns and adolescent smoking. *Health Psychol* **12**: 2224, 1993.

Creson D, Schmitz JM and Arnoutovic A: War-related changes in cigarette smoking: a survey study of health professionals in Sarajevo. *Subst Use Misuse* **31**: 639–646, 1996.

DiMatteo R: *The Psychology of Health, Illness and Medical Care*. Brooks Cole: Pacific Grove, CA, 1991.

Doll R, Peto R, Wheatley K, Gray R and Sutherland I: Mortality in relation to smoking: 40 years' observations on British male doctors. *BMJ* **309**: 901–911, 1994.

Feist J and Brannon L: *Health Psychology: An Introduction to Behavior and Health*. Wadsworth: Belmont, CA, 1988.

Fishbein M and Ajzen I: *Belief, Attitude, Intention and Behavior: An Introduction to Theory and Research*. Addison-Wesley: Reading, MA, 1975.

Fishbein M, Middlestadt S and Hitchcock P: Using the theory of reasoned action as a framework for understanding and changing AIDS-related behaviors. In di Clemente R and Peterson J (Eds) *Preventing AIDS: Theories and Methods of Behavioral Interventions*. Plenum Press: New York, 1994.

Frances RJ and Miller SI: *Clinical Textbook of Addictive Disorders*. Guilford Press: New York, 1991.

Genest M and Genest S: *Psychology and Health*. Research Press: Chicago, IL, 1987.

Glantz S, Barnes D, Bero L, Hanauer P and Slade J: Looking through a keyhole at the tobacco industry: The Brown and Williamson documents. *JAMA* **274**: 219–224, 1995.

Gray N: Active and passive smoking. *Med J Australia* **156**: 826–827, 1992.

Hughes J, Gulliver S, Fenwick J, Cruser K, Valliere W, Pepper S, Shea P and Solomon L: Smoking cessation among self-quitters. *Health Psychology* **11**: 331–334, 1992.

Kendrick J and Merritt R: Women and smoking: an update for the 1990s. *Am J Obstet Gynecol* **175**: 528–535, 1996.

Kessler D, Barnett P, Witt A, Zeller M, Mande J and Schultz W: The legal and scientific basis for FDA's assertion of jurisdiction over cigarettes and smokeless tobacco. *JAMA* **277**: 405–409, 1997.

Koob G and Le Moal M: Drug abuse: hedonic homeostatic dysregulation. *Science* **278**: 52–58, 1997.

Krivanek J: *Addictions*. Allen & Unwin: Sydney, 1988.

Leckie J: The effects of informational intervention on state anxiety and satisfaction in patients undergoing bone scan. *Nuclear Med Communi* **15**: 921–927, 1994.

Leckie J: The role of psychology within health promotion. In M Wilkinson (Ed) *Proceedings of the International Health Promotion Conference: Where Social Values and Personal Worth Meet*. Brunel University: London, 1995.

Leshner A: Frontiers in neuroscience: the science of substance abuse: addiction is a brain disease and it matters. *Science* **278**: 4547, 1997.

Maheu M: Nicotine dependency treatment: new opportunities for psychologists. *Psychological Association Newsletter* **3**: 1–4, 1994.

Maheu M: Nicotine dependency treatment: new opportunities for psychologists. *Psychology Magazine* (web), 1996.

Matthew 25: 29. *The Holy Bible, King James Version*. Broadman and Holman Publishers: Nashville, TE, USA.

Patton G, Hibbert M, Rosier M, Carlin J, Caust J and Bowes G: Patterns of common drug use in teenagers. *Aust J Public Health* **19**: 393–399, 1995.

Patton G, Hibbert M, Rosier M, Carlin J, Caust J and Bowes G: Is smoking associated with depression and anxiety in teenagers? *Am J Public Health* **86**: 225–230, 1996.

Payne S: Lay representations of breast cancer. *Psychology and Health* **25**: 111–118, 1990.

Peto R, Lopez A, Boreham J, Thun M and Clark H: Mortality from tobacco in developed countries: indirect estimation from national vital statistics. *Lancet* **339**: 1268–1278, 1992.

Petoskey E, van Stelle K and de Jong J: Prevention through empowerment in a Native American Community. In J Valentine, J de Jong and N Kennedy (Eds) *Substance Abuse Prevention in Multicultural Communities*. Haworth Press: New York, 1998.

Robinson J and Pritchard W: The role of nicotine in tobacco use. [Review]. *Psychopharmacology* **108**: 397–407, 1992.

Rogers E: *Diffusion of Innovation*. Free Press: New York, 1983.

Rogler L: Making sense of historical changes in the Diagnostic and Statistical Manual of Mental Disorders: five propositions. *J Health Soc Behav* **38**: 9–20, 1997.

Rosenstock I: Historical origins of the Health Belief model. *Health Education Monographs* **2**: 328–335, 1974.

Ross C and Pam A: *Pseudoscience in Biological Psychiatry*. John Wiley: New York, 1995.

Slade J, Bero L, Hanauer P, Barnes D and Glantz S: Nicotine and addiction: the Brown and Williamson documents. *JAMA* **274**: 225–233, 1995.

Stroebe W and Stroebe MS: *Social Psychology and Health*. Open University Press: Birmingham, UK, 1995.

Syme SL: Individual vs. Community interventions in public health practice: some thoughts about a new approach. *Health Promotion Matters* **2**: 1–4, 1997.

Touyz S, Blaszczynski A, Digiusto E and Byrne D: The emergence of clinical psychology departments in Australian teaching hospitals. *ANZJ Psychiatry*, **26**: 554–559, 1992.

Wallack L: Media advocacy: a strategy for empowering people and communities. *J Pub Health Policy* **15**: 420–436, 1994.

West R: Nicotine addiction: a reanalysis of the arguments. *Psychopharmacology* **108**: 408–416, 1992.

11

Teaching, Training and Research: Future Directions

Bruce S. Singh
Royal Melbourne Hospital, Melbourne, Australia

and

Paul R. Martin
School of Psychology, University of New England, Armidale, Australia

INTRODUCTION

Profound changes have occurred in both psychiatry and psychology in the past two or three decades with respect to the domain of professional practice on the one hand, and the associated models of health and illness, training programs and research agenda, on the other. The most noticeable have been the shift towards a biopsychosocial perspective, and a corresponding divergence away from an exclusive focus on "mental illness" to a broader interest in health and illness generally.

This chapter is concerned with a number of issues of relevance to teaching, training and research in the integrated medical practice:

1. Training psychiatrists and psychologists to function in medical settings. This section will be concerned with mechanisms whereby the biopsychosocial perspective can be incorporated into the generic training of all psychiatrists and psychologists as well as the specific training available in liaison psychiatry, and clinical and health psychology.
2. How psychiatrists and psychologists can contribute to the training of medical practitioners (both GPs and specialists), as well as of other health professionals involved in the medical setting (e.g. social workers, physiotherapists). The role that liaison psychiatry and health psychology can play in educating specialists in secondary and tertiary medical settings will also be highlighted.
3. Research into psychological, psychiatric and psychosomatic factors as they affect medical settings. This section will give an overview of opportunities for

Psychology and Psychiatry: Integrating Medical Practice.
Edited by J. Milgrom and G. D. Burrows © 2001 John Wiley & Sons, Ltd.

psychological research on medically ill populations and some of the practical and methodological issues which affect such research.

THE TRAINING OF PSYCHIATRISTS

Psychiatry is a medical speciality which grew up separately from other medical specialties. Its origins were in the asylum system which had been created specifically for the care of those members of society who suffered from a major mental illness. Its traditions and links with medicine did not really become formalized until this century, when psychiatry entered the realm of general medicine through the incorporation of psychiatric units into general hospitals and psychiatry came to be recognized more and more as a legitimate medical discipline.

The effect of this medical background is evident in the attention that psychiatric training bodies, and national organizations of psychiatrists, give to the medical origins of the discipline. This is reflected in the requirements in regard to internship and mandatory general residency experience before embarking on formal psychiatric training, the specification of training experiences within a general medical setting for psychiatric trainees, and the enunciation of knowledge that trainees of psychiatry are expected to have about medical conditions and their relationship to psychiatry, and finally on the role of psychiatrists in consultation-liaison roles in general hospitals.

Different Colleges put different emphases on these requirements. For example in the mid-1970s the American Psychiatric Association deemed it inappropriate that trainees going into psychiatry should require a mandatory internship. This decision caused immense controversy and was finally repealed, but reflected the ambivalence in which medicine has been seen by psychiatric practitioners and the similarly ambivalent attitude of medical practitioners towards psychiatry. In the past two decades, psychiatry has re-emphasized its links with medicine through the particular emphasis on biological psychiatry and biological research into mechanisms that might underpin the major psychiatric disorders. The so-called medical model has been strongly reaffirmed and psychiatrists are now legitimate parts of both the medical school curriculum as well as an essential part of the service in many general medical settings around the world. Similarly, the growth of consultation-liaison psychiatry has led to its increasing acceptance by the medical profession as a legitimate sub-speciality of psychiatry and widespread demand for services that psychiatrists can provide to the medically ill.

In Australia, training of psychiatrists is conducted by the Royal Australian and New Zealand College of Psychiatrists (RANZCP), which has recently celebrated its fiftieth anniversary. Since 1967, the College General Council has approved By-Laws to govern the training and examination for Fellowship of the College, and has updated these requirements on three occasions to accord more closely with the College philosophy on training, and prevailing clinical psychiatric practice. The College has established a comprehensive training program that involves a broad range of mandatory training experiences, reflecting the view that trainees need to have experience in a variety of settings and clinical practice.

The program for postgraduate training in psychiatry requires successful completion of a minimum of five years full-time or equivalent part-time training. The emphasis that the College places on its relationship to medicine is highlighted throughout the period of training. The College specifies that anyone entering training must have spent at least two years equivalent full-time as a medical officer. They state that this includes the mandatory intern year, but suggest that the second year is necessary to gain sufficient maturity and experience as a medical practitioner prior to the commencement of speciality training. It is recognized that experience in a wide variety of fields of medical practice is a valuable background to psychiatric specialization. This is not a mandatory requirement for training in many other parts of the world, where the minimum one year of internship is often seen as sufficient.

The College also specifies that in the first three years of training, the candidate will spend a period of six months in a consultation and liaison psychiatry service of a hospital offering such a service. This experience may be obtained in Child Psychiatry, Psychogeriatrics or other sub-speciality placement, provided there is sufficient breadth of experience. The term Consultation-Liaison Psychiatry is taken to mean a sub-speciality of psychiatry concerned with clinical service, teaching and research at the interface of psychiatry and medicine. The clinical service should include provision of formal psychiatric consultations to nonpsychiatric physicians and medical workers as well as informal professional contacts; liaison in this context implies a regular contact with a given service and its clinical team and patients. The College also specifies that a mandatory case history, so-called Liaison Case History, must be submitted within four weeks of completion of the rotation. Suitable clinical problems for presentation include those demonstrating the psychiatric complications of organic disease or treatment, psychological reactions to physical illness, the somatic presentation of psychiatric illness, somatic complications of psychiatric illness and psychosomatic disorders.

Where possible, the case should demonstrate aspects of the scope of liaison psychiatry, such as sensitizing physicians and nurses to the psychosocial aspects of patient care, prevention of the development of psychiatric problems in the physically ill, their early detection and treatment, mediation of conflict between patients and staff, and education of nonpsychiatrist clinicians and staff.

Trainees must demonstrate that they have been primarily responsible for the assessment and management of the patient in this setting. The presentation should include an account of the clinical features of the patient's medical and psychiatric problems, and of the setting in which they are treated. Trainees should make it clear that they saw the patient as a ward consultation or as part of a specific liaison placement. In addition to focusing on interventions with the patient and his/her family, management should highlight the trainee's interaction with the referring service. The trainee should demonstrate an awareness of issues such as the importance of factors leading to facilitation or hindrance of referral of patients in this setting, difficulties of assessment and case definition, the need to communicate recommendations clearly to the consultee, and what factors influence whether recommendations are put into effect by the consultee.

A further demonstration of the commitment to general medicine is the requirement that the trainees demonstrate their competency in general medicine during their third year of training, in order to demonstrate that they have maintained their skills in the clinical assessment of medically ill patients. The requirements for this examination are quite specific in that trainees expect that they will be examined on the general medical aspects of a long case, and the psychosocial aspects as they relate to that case. The trainees spend an hour with the patient, in which they are expected to conduct their clinical interview and physical examination, and then are examined for half an hour, to demonstrate relevant physical science to the examiner on the case that they have seen. The College specifies the requirements that it expects of trainees:

> Trainees will be examined on the general medical aspects of a long case. In addition, psychosocial aspects will be examined as they relate to the case. The trainee will spend one hour with the patient, and after a fifteen minute period to consider the case, will be examined for half an hour. The trainee will usually be expected to demonstrate relevant physical signs to the examiners on the case that he/she has seen.
>
> The examination will be conducted in the third year of training. It is anticipated that trainees will sit for the written examinations within twelve months of the general medicine examination. The clinical case will be discussed with at least two examiners, one of whom shall be a senior physician. The other examiner shall be a member (or co-opted member) of the Committee for Examinations.

The College has also developed a Fellowship Curriculum, where it specifies the attitudes, knowledge and skills that it requires of trainees. The curriculum was developed by a sub-committee chaired by one of the authors of this chapter. Of particular relevance to medical practice is the section on attitudes to colleagues and other mental health professionals, where it is stated that trainees should develop a positive attitude and respect for the knowledge and skills of their own psychiatric colleagues, and other medical colleagues and health professionals.

Under knowledge objectives, criteria are specified as follows:

> By the completion of training, trainees should be knowledgeable about general medical and surgical conditions. Higher levels of knowledge, tempered by maturity and experience, are expected in those areas of general medicine which particularly relate to psychiatric practice.

In particular, trainees should be able to demonstrate knowledge of:

> The presentation, investigation, diagnosis and treatment of medical conditions, particularly in those areas which relate to psychiatric practice.
>
> Further investigations which are necessary to confirm or reject diagnostic hypotheses and to aid the patient's management.
>
> The basic principles involved in the management of significant medical illnesses.

All quotations reproduced from RANZCP (1995) by permission.

The interaction between medical and psychiatric disorders.

The psychosocial and cultural aspects of medical illness and the significance to patients and their families of both the illness and its treatment.

The College again is very specific in regard to skills:

By the completion of training, trainees should be able to competently assess patients for the presence of medical illnesses. Higher levels of skill, tempered by maturity and experience, are expected in those areas of general medicine which particularly relate to psychiatric practice.

In particular, trainees should be able to:

Elicit a thorough, accurate and organized medical history relating to all systems of the body.

Perform a proficient physical examination of all systems of the body and competently elicit and recognize signs indicative of the presence of illness.

Interpret and integrate the history and physical findings and formulate an appropriate differential diagnosis.

Specify and interpret laboratory, radiological and other further investigations appropriate to clarify the differential diagnosis and to aid the patient's management.

In both assessment and management, recognize the interrelation between physical illness and psychiatric disorder.

Recognize with a high level of expertise, symptoms and signs of physical illness which may arise as complications of psychiatric treatments.

Recognize with a high level of expertise, symptoms and signs of those physical illnesses which may be more directly associated with psychiatric disorders.

Demonstrate competence in the practice of consultation liaison psychiatry including:

- the psychiatric assessment of medically ill patients
- the management of psychiatric disorders in medically ill patients
- effective communication with non-psychiatric medical and other health professionals
- the ability to grasp, and effectively deal with, the psychological issues which often surround the referral and psychiatric management of patients in medical settings.

THE TRAINING OF PSYCHOLOGISTS

Whilst responsibility for the training of psychiatrists in Australia lies with their professional association (RANZCP), responsibility for training psychologists is vested in the universities. The Australian Psychological Society (APS) plays an important role in the accreditation of the university courses, and professionals in the field contribute to training, but the courses leading to professional qualifications are offered within the higher education sector. Training in psychology begins with a four-year degree that provides a broad education in the discipline of psychology. Many graduates of these programs do not progress to further training in psychology, choosing instead to use the degree as a generalist qualification for careers in areas that are related to psychology, such as positions in personnel, marketing, welfare and education. Those who opt for careers in psychology follow either an academic route by enrolling in a Doctor of Philosophy (PhD) or a professional route by enrolling in a Master of Psychology (MPsych), Doctor of Psychology (DPsych) or a program that combines doctoral level research training with professional training (Clinical PhD or Combined MPsych/PhD) (Martin 1996).

Psychology recognizes a number of professional specialties and 20 years ago it could have been said unequivocally that the relevant specialty for this chapter was clinical psychology. Clinical psychology as an area of professional practice began around the end of the nineteenth century in the USA and in the second decade of the twentieth century in Australia. Clinical psychology as we know it today, however, is a post-Second World War phenomenon.

In the late 1970s, the professional specialization of health psychology began to evolve. The reasons for the emergence of health psychology are complex but include a dissatisfaction by some psychologists with the field of clinical psychology. Criticisms offered of clinical psychology included not paying enough attention to healthcare systems and policy, and too great a focus on: mental health as opposed to physical health; illness and dysfunction rather than health; assessment and treatment as opposed to health promotion and disease prevention; and working with individuals, couples, families and groups rather than workforces, communities and populations. Health psychology was established to redress the balance.

The relationship between clinical and health psychology is controversial, with each of the following models suggested: (a) two independent specialties; (b) one a subspeciality of the other; and (c) clinical health psychology as a specialty at the interface of clinical and health psychology (Milgrom & Hardardottir 1995). One of the authors has argued that as the fields have grown, the overlap between clinical and health psychology has increased, and that no one has been able to define the two fields in ways that clearly differentiate them (Martin 1997). A high proportion of health psychologists are clinical psychologists—about 30% in the UK and 50% in the USA. Nevertheless, the APS recently established a College of Health Psychologists to join the existing eight Colleges, one of which is the College of Clinical Psychologists. This chapter will consider both clinical and health psychology but not other professional specialties in psychology, even though some are relevant to medical practice, in particular, clinical neuropsychology and counselling.

The minimum training for qualification as a clinical or health psychologist is a four-year degree in psychology, followed by a two-year masters degree in the specialty area, followed by two years of professional practice under the supervision of a member of the relevant APS College. Professional psychologists require a doctoral degree for independent practice in the USA, and there has been a marked increase in Australian doctoral programs during the last decade. Currently in Australia, training in clinical psychology is offered via 29 MPsych programs, 10 DPsych programs and 14 Clinical PhDs or Combined MPsych/PhD programs (Martin 1998a). Courses specifically devoted to health psychology are new in Australia, although all of the clinical programs should have content identified as health psychology, since health psychology is a "core area of study" for clinical training according to the accreditation guidelines of the APS College of Clinical Psychologists.

The APS College of Health Psychologists has recently drawn up course accreditation guidelines and has suggested that "Health Psychology may be viewed as falling on a continuum anchored at one end by principles of psychology applied to health promotion and public health, and at the other, by psychology applied to the care of the physically ill. For convenience, the College has identified two broad areas of Health Psychology representing respective ends of the continuum, 'health promotion' and 'clinical health psychology'" (APS College of Health Psychologists 1998). There is overlap between the suggested content of clinical and health psychology programs but the guidelines for courses in health psychology include much content that is particularly related to working in medical settings such as:

- Biological, psychological and social determinants of health and illness
- Epidemiology of Australian population groups
- Basic physical systems
- Health beliefs and attitudes
- Systems approaches relevant to health
- Stress, stress management, coping and social support in health and illness
- Models of health care
- Processes of acute and chronic illness, and seeking medical care
- Developmental issues in acute and chronic illness
- Communication in health settings
- the patient–practitioner relationship
- Trauma, disability and rehabilitation.

Increasingly, psychologists training in clinical and health psychology are receiving specialized information to make them particularly relevant to general medicine. For example, cognitive-behavioural techniques have been tailored to treat particular symptoms accompanying medical disorders (e.g. nausea) and additional strategies have been developed to maximize effectiveness in the medical setting (e.g. use of handouts and self-help material to help prepare patients for hospital procedures). Psychometric tests have likewise been adapted for hospital settings with the development of scales such as the recovery locus of control (Partridge & Johnston 1989), the hospital anxiety and depression questionnaire (Snaith & Zigmond 1994) and measures of health beliefs (Leventhal et al 1984; Leventhal et al 1997). Pain management is a particular specialty as it is a central component of many medical complaints, and psychological techniques have been refined for the management of both acute and chronic pain. Furthermore, as psychology is a proponent of evidence-based practice, training tends to be continually informed by research developments in treatment outcome and in the needs of the health-care system. Thus clinical health psychologists have adapted their general skills to be more pertinent to a busy clinical setting (such as brief succinct report writing or one-session interventions) and graduates are looking beyond the one-to-one intervention to the wider system (e.g. patient–doctor communication and health promotion).

Professional training in psychology, at least in Australia, is based on the scientist-practitioner model. The fundamental premise of this model is that practitioners should not only be trained to base their practice on the available research evidence; they should also be trained in applied research and evaluation methodology, so that they can contribute to the development of new knowledge (Barlow et al 1984). In fact, as the various health professions have expanded their domains, leading to greater overlap in expertise, many have argued that it is psychologists' advanced training in research and evaluation methods that most distinguishes them from the other health-care professions.

The training programs have three components weighted as follows by the APS: coursework (40–50%); placements (25–30%); and research (20–30%). Up to a point, the three components teach about relevant theory and data, train practical skills, and research skills, respectively, but the components are more integrated than this simplistic analysis would suggest. The coursework component, for example, covers theories, models and research findings, but also includes much training in practical skills. Students watch videos of experienced clinicians in action, engage in role-plays and other class exercises, and practise tasks such as intake interviews, diagnostic assessments, test administration and therapeutic techniques. Lectures are given predominantly by university staff of whom the majority must be practising clinicians, but guest lectures are contributed by psychologists who work in diverse settings and other health-care professionals, including psychiatrists. Assessments of this part of training are very varied and include written assignments (literature reviews, reports, responses to ethical vignettes, etc.), exams (conventional and take-home), observation of work with clients (direct or indirect), and vivas. The coursework component does much to prepare students for the other two components and consequently dominates the early stages of training.

The placement component involves four or more placements, one of which is completed in the university clinic whilst the remainder are completed outside the university in settings such as various types of hospital (e.g. general, psychiatric, children's, women's, rehabilitation), community clinics (e.g. mental health, sexually transmitted diseases, sexual assault), corrective service facilities, alcohol and drug agencies, disability services (intellectual and physical), and so forth. A recent development is for placements to be based in primary care settings. The internal placement is usually completed first and students receive intensive individual and group supervision from university staff. Staff observe students working with clients either by watching sessions through a one-way screen or, more commonly, by watching videotapes of sessions. For each hour a student sees a client, one hour of supervision is provided.

The external placements must provide students with the experience of dealing with a wide range of client problems (acute and chronic), across varying age ranges (child, adult), settings (inpatient/outpatient, community), and use of a variety of clinical skills (assessment, treatment, and professional). All placements must be

supervised by appropriately qualified psychologists. Assessment of student performance on placements is always the responsibility of university staff but in the case of
external placements, this assessment is based on detailed, structured reports submitted by the psychologists who supervised the students during the placement, and
work diaries completed by the students. Just as the coursework component does
more than teach about theory and research, the placement component does more
than train practical skills. Hence, a critical aspect of placements is the supervised
reading that students undertake in support of their work with clients (e.g. reading
articles and chapters related to the presenting problems of the clients, and the
assessment and treatment techniques that they are using).

Training in the coursework and placement components of postgraduate psychology programs involves exposure to a number of different theoretical frameworks for
assessment and treatment. Consistent with the scientist-practitioner model and the
current emphasis on evidence-based medicine, however, all students are provided
with in-depth training in the theory and practice of cognitive-behavioural assessment and therapy.

For the research component, students must complete a research project of direct
relevance to clinical or health psychology. Supervision is provided by university staff,
and it is common for professionals from outside the university to be involved as co-
supervisors. The research has to be written up in the form of a thesis, although thesis
requirements vary from university to university with some requiring the format of a
conventional thesis (i.e. describing all aspects of the research in considerable detail)
whilst others have opted for a journal-style, manuscript format. Assessment of the
research component is based on examination of the thesis, which must involve at
least two examiners.

The most significant developments in professional psychology training in Australia in recent years have been the increase in the number of programs and the shift
from masters level programs to doctoral level programs, discussed above. Other
significant developments include the establishment of more specialist programs, such
as the programs in child clinical psychology or in health psychology at the University
of Melbourne. Another innovation has been to utilise modern teaching technologies
such as computer-based clinical consultation in which expert or knowledge-based
systems are used to assist in assessment and treatment planning, and simulation of
the encounter between the health-care provider and the client in which the computer is programmed to take the role of the client (Bloom 1992). Also, some
professional psychology programs, such as the MPsych and DPsych in clinical and
health psychology at the University of New England, use web-based teaching to
support their coursework component.

THE TRAINING OF OTHER HEALTH PROFESSIONALS

Psychiatrists and psychologists can play a particular role in the training of other
health professionals in order to improve their management and provide integrated

medical care. In this section, a number of programs currently under development are described which demonstrate how formal university programs have been implemented to cater for the increasing interest and need for training in the psychiatric aspects of general practitioners and other trainees. These programs are essentially based on the model that the psychiatrist has an understanding of the total biopsychosocial approach to the patient and is an expert in the holistic assessment of their problems. This, however, is combined with a considerable knowledge about normal development and the psychological reactions to illness.

The discipline of Consultation-Liaison Psychiatry has taken a particular interest in this re-education of other medical professionals. Various models for how these services can operate have been developed. One of the key models was the liaison psychiatry program developed by George Engel in Rochester, New York, which was intended to sensitize physicians to the psychosocial aspects of their patients. This involved activities by psychiatrists with specific units, in which they participated in the active management of the patient and educated the staff in regard to the psychosocial aspects of the condition. It was seen to be particularly important in certain so-called "high-risk" or high-stress wards such as the Intensive Care Unit, the Oncology Unit, the Burns Unit, Orthopaedic Wards, and so forth. A considerable body of knowledge has now accumulated on the psychological reactions of patients suffering such disorders and on the techniques that are available to assist both patients and staff.

A second model has been that of the consultation psychiatrist who is available for consultations on medical inpatients and outpatients in order to support medical staff in the assessment and ongoing management of these patients, where the interactions between their medical condition and other disorders are clear. Psychiatrists have become valuable members of Pain Clinics and have assisted in the treatment of various chronic disorders such as diabetes, rheumatoid arthritis, ulcerative colitis, asthma, and so forth. A number of journals have developed over the years which record the activities of such practitioners, including *General Hospital Psychiatry* and *International Journal of Psychiatry and Medicine*, to name just two.

The role of psychiatrists working with general practitioners has been a much more problematic one. Psychiatry as a medical specialty has remained relatively isolated from general practitioners. Its concepts have overlapped very little with the patients seen in general practice as a result of the so-called "filters" which determine the types of patients that eventually are referred to psychiatrists (Goldberg & Huxley 1992). Thus, psychiatrists end up seeing only a small proportion of patients who present or are treated in general practice. In recent years, there has been increasing attention as to how psychiatrists can assist general practitioners, as well as modify their concepts. The World Health Organization has taken a particular interest in this interface and so has the Australian Government as part of the National Mental Health Strategy. A document highlighting some of the issues has been published in recent years (Joint Consultative Committee in Psychiatry 1997).

In response to this initiative, various forms of development of educational programs have occurred. In addition, there has been a great emphasis on community surveys of psychiatric disorders as they present to general practitioners or in the community. The development of a Graduate Certificate in General Practice Psychiatry, which has been developed jointly by the University of Melbourne Department of Psychiatry and the Monash University Department of Psychological Medicine, as well as the relevant Community Medicine Departments of those two universities, is an example of the educational programs that are available. These cover various fields including general psychiatry, child and family psychiatry, transcultural psychiatry, community psychiatry, hypnosis and cognitive-behavioural treatment.

Whilst the training of psychologists in Australia is largely accomplished through university departments of psychology, the contribution of psychology to training other health professionals has occurred mainly through psychologists employed by other university departments. Medical schools, for example, employ psychologists in departments of psychiatry/psychological medicine, and sometimes in other medical departments or in departments of behavioural science. Such appointments result in contributions to teaching the medical curriculum but also in training psychiatrists and other health professionals (as in the case of training general practitioners described above). One of the authors, for example, held an appointment in a rehabilitation unit based in a university department of orthopaedic surgery; this unit acted as a national demonstration centre that provided courses for general practitioners, occupational therapists, physiotherapists and nurses.

In addition to this route for psychological input into training health professionals, psychologists in university departments of psychology, and psychologists working in hospitals and other health settings, are often asked to contribute lectures or series of lectures into training programs for medical practitioners, occupational therapists, physiotherapists, social workers, dietitians and speech therapists.

Psychologists working in medical settings contribute to the training of other health professionals in a number of ways, one of which is training in behavioural management principles. An extreme example of such training is to establish wards in which the interactions between staff and patients follow operant conditioning principles, whereby patients are "rewarded" for behaving in accordance with predetermined goals and not rewarded for behaving inappropriately. This approach has been used across a range of problems including schizophrenia, eating disorders, and chronic pain. A second example is provided by training staff in how to increase the compliance of patients with instructions such as when to take their medication, when to practise their exercises, and how to change their diet. Sometimes psychologists develop treatment protocols but then train other staff in how to carry out the protocols once the efficacy of the approach has been established. An example involving one of the authors of this chapter was treating "needle phobias" on a Renal Ward. Different approaches were explored and then the nursing staff were trained in the most effective method. Psychologists employed in medical settings also teach health professionals via providing counselling services and crisis debriefing.

RESEARCH INTO PSYCHOLOGICAL FACTORS IN MEDICAL SETTINGS

The case for increased research activity with respect to psychological and behavioural factors in medical settings is stimulated by both empirical and conceptual advances. With respect to the former, research has demonstrated that at least nine of the ten leading causes of death in developed countries are related to behaviour and lifestyle (Sexton 1979). Behaviour, and associated thoughts and feelings, that are linked to health and illness include: eating and drinking; exercising and activity levels; cigarette smoking and alcohol consumption; substance abuse (recreational drugs and overuse of prescription medications); engaging in safety-related behaviours (e.g. wearing seatbelts, using condoms); exposure to hazardous conditions such as the sun and dangerous chemicals; and stress, depression, anger and hostility (McGinnis & Foege 1993). Examples of links between behaviour and illness include diseases of the heart which are related to eating excessive animal fats and calories, smoking cigarettes, inadequate physical activity, and certain personality traits such as excessive hostility. Lung cancer is related to smoking cigarettes, breast cancer to excessive dietary fat intake, and melanoma to sun exposure. Cerebrovascular disease is related to smoking cigarettes, and excessive consumption of calories and dietary sodium. Motor vehicle accidents are related to nonuse of seat belts and to consumption of alcohol.

The conceptual stimulus comes from adoption of the biopsychosocial model which is based on the assumption that health or illness is a consequence of the interplay between biological, psychological and social factors (see Chapter 2 for a detailed discussion of the model). The model asserts that macrolevel processes, such as stress and depression, and microlevel processes, such as cellular disorders and chemical imbalances, interact to produce a state of health or illness. The implication for researchers is that they must consider the operation of biological, psychological and social processes simultaneously, measuring all three classes of variables, or they must make assumptions about variables not measured (Taylor 1995).

To illustrate this point, one of the authors has developed with colleagues a biopsychosocial model of postnatal depression (Milgrom et al 1999). This model includes: biological factors such as the biological substrate of personality traits that act as vulnerability factors for postnatal depression, and low oestrogen levels after birth that can precipitate postnatal depression; psychological factors such as the role of childhood family experiences and the stress-mediating variable of coping style; and social factors such as the vulnerability factor of poor marital relationships and the cultural context that creates the unrealistically positive beliefs of motherhood that can be so dysfunctional. An implication of this model is that researchers either need to take a broad set of measures or make assumptions. For example, if a study exploring the relationship between stress and postnatal depression only measures variables within the psychosocial domain, then the assumption has to be made that the biological conditions necessary for postnatal depression to occur are present.

Driven by the biopsychosocial model, and findings demonstrating links between psychological and behavioural factors on the one hand, and illness and health on the other, research in the field of health psychology has grown exponentially in recent years. An index of this expansion is provided by the development of new journals. The first journal in health psychology was founded by the Division of Health Psychology of the American Psychological Association in 1982 (*Health Psychology*) and the second by the European Health Psychology Society five years later (*Psychology and Health*). In the last three years of the twentieth century, four new major international health psychology journals have been established: *Journal of Clinical Psychology in Medical Settings*, *British Journal of Health Psychology*, *Journal of Health Psychology*, and *Psychology, Health and Medicine*.

In addition to the studies demonstrating links between behaviour, cognition and affect, and health and illness, studies have shown that interventions that focus on the former can impact on the latter. Spiegel et al (1989) demonstrated, for example, that metastatic breast cancer patients randomly assigned to a one-year group coping intervention program lived on average twice as long as controls. Similarly, Fawzey et al (1993) showed that malignant melanoma patients who underwent a six-week coping intervention that enhanced active problem-orientated coping, were less likely to have a recurrence or to have died of their cancer when compared with a control group. Friedman et al (1986) reported that a stress-management program for Type A behaviour reduced the risk of recurrent myocardial infarction. Stress-management programs offered to men at the time of testing for HIV infection have been found to enhance immune defences as well as reducing the distress caused by positive tests (Antoni et al 1991).

Research has demonstrated the value of other types of psychological intervention in medical settings. Meta-analytic reviews have shown, for example, that preparing people psychologically for surgery may lead to reduced distress in hospital and to more rapid recovery (Johnston & Vogele 1993). Meta-analytic reviews of the psychological management of pain testify to the effectiveness of this approach (Malone & Strube, 1988). Interventions combining a number of behavioural and educational techniques have demonstrated a relative improvement in compliance with medication regimens of 40–50% (Haynes et al 1987). Meta-analytic reviews have also shown that psychological interventions in medical settings result in cost savings, with 85% of studies reporting a decrease in variables such as inpatient days, cost/year/patient, outpatient visits, prescriptions, X-rays and laboratory visits (Mumford et al 1984).

Where will research into psychological factors in medical settings go from here? Current research fields are at different stages of development. In the areas cited above, the value of psychological interventions has already been demonstrated. Many questions still remain unanswered, however. For example, little information is available about why interventions have achieved positive results, a non-trivial question if we are to further enhance the efficacy of these interventions and make them more cost-effective. Also, most of the research has been carried out in universities and teaching hospitals, and it is not clear whether health-care professionals in the field can be trained to implement the interventions with equal success to the developers of the interventions.

Other fields of research are at an earlier stage of development. For example, much research has been carried out on medical decision-making and the findings make a strong case that decisions may not always be optimal and that, with the application of developing methods, they can be improved (Ayton et al 1997). Nevertheless, demonstrations of improved decision-making as a consequence of intervention have yet to be reported. Another example is provided by the issue of how health professionals should break bad news to their patients. A literature is emerging on this topic which provides clear guidelines but the guidelines have not been subjected to empirical evaluation (Mohr et al 1999).

Clues to directions for future research can be gleaned from funding opportunities. Currently, governments around the world seem prepared to make additional funds available for health and medical research, particularly biomedical research with an emphasis on biotechnology. In Australia, for example, following a review of health and medical research in 1999 (Wills 1999), the federal government made a commitment to doubling the budget of the National Health and Medical Research Council (NHMRC) over the next five years. At the same time, NHMRC is negotiating with a commercial investment fund for the fund to invest substantial sums of money in health and medical research. These developments should increase the amount of research being completed and will shape up the type of research being carried out. For example, NHMRC has made it clear that it wants to concentrate its funding, that is, support fewer but larger research projects/programs. Related to this point, NHMRC has emphasized the value of multi-disciplinary research. Earlier in this section it was argued that an implication of the biopsychosocial model was that researchers had to either measure biological, psychological and social processes simultaneously, or make assumptions about variables not measured, and changes in funding will (appropriately) encourage the former approach.

With respect to content areas, the field of stress research appears to be on the verge of a major expansion. As studies show more and more links between stress and stress-moderating variables such as coping and social support on the one hand, and illness and dysfunction on the other hand, the pressure increases for us to understand the multiple cognitive-behavioural and physiological pathways that link these phenomena (Steptoe 1991). An indicator of the increased efforts in this field is the extra funding made available to the Office of Behavioral and Social Sciences of the National Institutes of Health in the USA in 1999, to establish five new "Mind–Body Centers", for which the predominant theme is research on stress and disease.

Improvements in technology will stimulate growth in some research areas. Telehealth and telepsychiatry, for example, have been around for many years (Baer et al 1997) but recent developments in the telecommunications industry have created new opportunities. Some health professionals see telemedicine as having the capacity for providing health services to people living in rural and remote areas who are currently underserviced, but although such services have become established in some regions, very little research has been carried out with respect to the effectiveness of services delivered in this mode.

Developments in the booming field of biomedical/biotechnological research referred to above will stimulate psychological research. For example, much money is currently going into supporting research in the field of genomics. This research raises a host of psychological questions. Assuming that in the next decade or so, DNA testing will enable us to inform people of the illnesses of which they are most at risk, will this lead to people altering appropriate health behaviours? As we learn more about the biological bases of similarities and differences between people, how will this affect our perceptions of ourselves?

A CASE FOR COLLABORATION

We would argue that there is a need to develop more collaboration and cooperation between psychologists and psychiatrists, in particular, but also between other health professionals, in the domains of both training and research. With respect to training, each health profession is evolving with little input from other professions. The resulting developments have advantages both to patients and to the professions, but may lead to a far from optimal and integrated health-care system. Many of the changes amount to professions extending their boundaries, which in turn results in less differentiation between the professions. Taking psychology as an example, psychologists in the USA have been pushing for some years for hospital privileges and prescription privileges on grounds such as continuity of care, and cost-effectiveness. Psychologists have been granted hospital privileges so far in over 20 states in the USA (Ludwigsen & Albright 1994), and psychologists can prescribe medication in certain settings (e.g. Indian Health Services and Department of Veteran Affairs), and states are expected to start passing legislation granting prescription privileges to psychologists in the near future (Deleon et al 1991). At another level, health psychologists argue for the importance of including in the curriculum, training in the systems of the body as they believe that this is necessary if psychologists are to work with patients suffering from physical disorders. Clearly, these developments result in overlap with other professions, in particular, the medical profession. Other professions have followed similar paths. Psychiatrists, for example, have increased their training in the cognitive-behavioural approach, which has been the corner-stone of clinical psychology for the past 20 to 30 years. Occupational therapy has evolved from a profession that focused on occupying patients usefully between treatment to a profession that perceives itself as having a broad range of assessment and therapeutic skills. Nurses no longer simply assist doctors and take care of patients; instead they are also entering the realm of therapy.

Associated with the above developments, the training period of most health professions has lengthened. If one accepts that there are limits to how much can be accomplished in training, however, then the new directions are achieved at a cost to previous core activities. The additional training necessary, for example, for psychologists to prescribe drugs may impact on their skills in psychological assessment and treatment.

It is difficult to see how a more coordinated approach to the future of training the different health professions can be accomplished as none of the professions will be prepared to "wind the clock back" and none of the professions will accept being dictated to by any other profession. The establishment of working groups across professional organizations such as the RANZCP and APS might be a good start. Also, training programs inviting members of other health professions to join their coordinating committees would add new perspectives.

With respect to research and scholarly activities, there are, of course, impressive instances of collaboration between health professions, of which this volume is a good example. Nevertheless, much more is needed. In the field of headache research, for example, the number of studies evaluating pharmacological approaches is in the thousands and the number of studies evaluating psychological treatment approaches is in the hundreds. Studies comparing treatment in these two modalities, and studies evaluating treatments that combine the two modalities, are limited to less than ten, however (Martin 1998b). Similar statements could be made about many other research areas.

The case for collaboration between clinical and health psychologists and psychiatrists seems particularly compelling as both have a central interest in the mental life of individuals: how they think, feel and behave. Both professions have moved away from a narrow focus on mental illness to a broad interest in health and illness. Psychiatrists bring to the collaboration their medical training and psychologists bring to the collaboration their more in-depth knowledge of psychological science.

Increased collaboration in research should be less contentious and therefore easier to achieve than increased collaboration in training. As with training, working groups established across professional associations may stimulate developments. Conferences provide one avenue for collaboration. Currently, some professional societies hold conferences that are not open to members of other professions, a policy that runs counter to facilitating collaboration. Perhaps setting up symposia and workshops at conferences jointly sponsored by more than one professional association would be a useful strategy. Establishing journals sponsored by more than one professional society would facilitate greater collaboration although a recent attempt to found an electronic journal by the American Psychological Association and American Psychiatric Association collapsed in acrimony (Seligman 1998). A more modest step would be special issues of journals with joint sponsorship.

As a final point, collaboration in Australia may be enhanced by some of the structural changes currently taking place in universities. Specifically, a combination of universities reorganizing departments/faculties into larger units, and psychology departments moving out of arts faculties, has resulted in a number of psychology departments relocating to faculties/divisions of biomedical sciences/health sciences/medicine. Two recent examples are the departments of psychology at the Universities of Melbourne and Adelaide that have shifted into medical faculties. These developments augur well for new research and teaching synergies in health.

CONCLUDING REMARKS

In conclusion, features of the training of psychiatrists and psychologists prepare them well for working in medical settings. Developments in the training programs of both professions over the past two decades have raised the standard of relevant knowledge and skills. Nevertheless, there is a danger of increasing overlap and duplication unless the professions can develop a more co-ordinated, integrated approach.

Possibilities for research into psychological factors in medical settings in the next decade are excellent, as a consequence of increased funding for health and medical research. Bodies such as NHMRC have traditionally shown a bias towards funding biomedical research (Martin 1999), however, so that psychiatry and psychology will have to plan strategically to gain their share of the increased funding. A key to succeeding in this endeavour is likely to be in planning ambitious, large-scale, multi-disciplinary research programs.

REFERENCES

Antoni MH, Baggett L, Ironson G, August S, LaPerriere A, Klimas N, Schneiderman N and Fletcher MA: Cognitive-behavioural stress management intervention buffers distress responses and immunologic changes following notification of HIV-1 seropositivity. *J Consult Clin Psychol* **59**: 906–915, 1991.

APS College of Health Psychologists: *Course Approval Guidelines for Membership of the APS College of Health Psychologists.* APS: Melbourne, 1998.

Ayton P, Wright G and Rowe G: Medical decision-making. In A Baum, S Newman, J Weinman, R West, and C McManus (Eds): *Cambridge Handbook of Psychology, Health and Medicine*, pp 294–297. Cambridge University Press: Cambridge, 1997.

Baer L, Elford R and Cukor P: Telepsychiatry at forty: what have we learned? *Harvard Review of Psychiatry* **5**: 7–17, 1997.

Barlow DH, Hayes SC and Nelson RO: *The Scientist-Practitioner: Research and Accountability in Clinical and Educational Settings.* Pergamon: New York, 1984.

Bloom BL: Computer assisted psychological intervention: a review and commentary. *Clin Psychol Rev* **12**: 169–197, 1992.

Deleon PH, Fox RE and Graham SR: Prescription privileges: psychology's next frontier? *Am Psychologist* **46**: 384–393, 1991.

Fawzey FI, Fawzey NW, Hyun CS, Elastoff R, Guthrie D, Fahey JL and Morton DL: Malignant melanoma: effects of an early structured psychiatric intervention, coping, and affective state on recurrence and survival 6 years later. *Arch Gen Psychiatry* **50**: 681–689, 1993.

Friedman M, Thoreson CE, Gill JJ, Ulmer D, Powell LH, Price VA, Brown B, Thompson L, Rabin DD, Breall WS, Bourg E, Levy R and Dixon T: Alteration of type A behavior and its effect on cardiac recurrences in post myocardial infarction patients: summary results of the recurrent coronary prevention project. *Am Heart J* **112**: 653–665, 1986.

Goldberg DP and Huxley PJ: *Common Mental Disorders—A Biosocial Model.* Routledge: London, 1992.

Haynes RB, Wang E and da Mota Gomes M: A critical review of interventions to improve compliance with prescribed medications. *Patient Education and Counselling* **10**: 155–166, 1987.

Johnston M and Vogele C: Benefits of psychological preparation for surgery: a meta-analysis. *Ann Behav Med* **15**: 245–256, 1993.

Joint Consultative Committee in Psychiatry: *Primary Care Psychiatry—The Last Frontier.* AGPS: Canberra, 1997.

Leventhal H, Benyamini Y, Brownlee S, Diefenback M, Leventhal E, Patrick-Miller L and Robitaille C: Illness representations: theoretical foundations. In Petrie KJ and Weinman JA (Eds): *Perceptions of Health and Illness*, pp 19–45. Harwood Academic Publishers, 1997.

Leventhal H, Nerenz K and Steele J: Illness representations and coping with health threats. In Baum A, Taylor SE and Singer JE (Eds): *Handbook of Psychology and Health, Vol IV: Social Psychological Aspects of Health*, pp 219–252. Lawrence Erlbaum: Hillsdale, NJ, 1984.

Ludwigsen KR and Albright DG: Training psychologists for hospital practice: A proposal. *Prof Psychol: Research and Practice* **25**: 241–246, 1994.

Malone MD and Strube MJ: Meta-analysis of non-medical treatments for chronic pain. *Pain* **34**: 231–244, 1988.

Martin PR: Training in clinical psychology. In PR Martin and JS Birnbrauer (Eds): *Clinical Psychology: Profession and Practice in Australia*, pp 52–76. Macmillan: Melbourne, 1996.

Martin PR: Health and clinical psychology: Redefining the domains. Paper presented at the World Congress on Psychosomatic Medicine, Cairns, 1997.

Martin PR: Generalist and specialist training in clinical psychology in Australia. In AN Wiens (Ed): *Volume 2: Professional Issues*, pp 209–220. In AS Bellack and M Hersen (Eds): *Comprehensive Clinical Psychology*. Elsevier Science: Oxford, 1998a.

Martin PR: Headache. In DW Johnston and M Johnston (Eds): *Volume 8: Health Psychology*, pp 529–556. In AS Bellack and M Hersen (Eds): *Comprehensive Clinical Psychology*. Elsevier Science: Oxford, 1998b.

Martin PR: You are what you do: health and behaviour in the Lucky Country. Inaugural Public Lecture. University of New England: Armidale, Australia, 1999.

McGinnis JM and Foege WH: Actual causes of death in the United States. *JAMA* **270**: 2207–2212, 1993.

Milgrom J and Hardardottir D: Clinical health psychology: a speciality in its own right. *Bull Aust Psychol Soc* **17**: 13–18, 1995.

Milgrom J, Martin PR and Negri L: *Treating Postnatal Depression: a Psychological Approach for Health Care Practitioners*. John Wiley: Chichester, UK, 1999.

Mohr C, Milgrom J, Griffiths M and Nomikoudis K: Breaking the bad news: Dilemmas in shared decision making in medical practice. *Aust Psychologist* **34**: 1–4, 1999.

Mumford E, Schlesinger HJ, Glass GV, Patrick K and Cuerdon T: A new look at evidence about reduced cost of medical utilization following mental health treatment. *Am J Psychiatry* **141**: 1145–1158, 1984.

Partridge C and Johnston M: Perceived control of recovery from physical disability: measurement and prediction. *Br J Clin Psychol* **28**: 53–59, 1989.

RANZCP (Royal Australian and New Zealand College of Psychiatrists): *Fellowship Curriculum: A Curriculum for the RANZCP Fellowship Training Program*. RANZCP: Melbourne, Australia, 1995.

Seligman MEP: A big step backward. *American Psychological Association Monitor* **February, 2**: 1998.

Sexton MM: Behavioral epidemiology. In OF Pomerleau and JP Brady (Eds): *Behavioral Medicine: Theory and Practice*, pp 3–21. Williams & Wilkins: Baltimore, MD, 1979.

Snaith RP and Zigmond AS: *The Hospital Anxiety and Depression Scale*. Nefer-Nelson: Windsor, UK 1994.

Spiegel D, Bloom JR, Kraemer HC and Gottheil E: Effect of psychosocial treatment on survival of patients with metastatic breast cancer. *Lancet* **ii**: 888–891, 1989.

Steptoe A: Psychobiological processes in the etiology of disease. In PR Martin (Ed): *Handbook of Behavior Therapy and Psychological Science: An Integrative Approach*, pp 325–347. New York: Pergamon, 1991.

Taylor SE: *Health Psychology (3rd edn)*. McGraw-Hill: New York, 1995.

Wills PJ: *Health and Medical Research Strategic Review*. Commonwealth of Australia: Canberra, ACT, 1999.

12

The Future of Psychology and Psychiatry in the Medical Centre

Jeannette Milgrom and Graham Burrows

*Departments of Psychology and Psychiatry, University of Melbourne, and
Austin & Repatriation Medical Centre, Melbourne, Australia*

and

Steven Schwartz

Murdoch University, Murdoch, Australia

The preceding chapters have demonstrated the significant contributions of psychologists and psychiatrists in the provision of mental health treatment, as an integral part of patient care in the medical centre. Our increased awareness of the role of psychological factors in illness has also highlighted the need for ongoing research continually to expand our knowledge base and guide the appropriate practice and training of psychologists and psychiatrists. This chapter considers professional issues for psychology and psychiatry as their place in medical treatment becomes increasingly consolidated, and reviews the following issues.

- The role of the psychologist and psychiatrist in the multidisciplinary medical treatment team, and their ability to influence the organization and the health-care system
- Ethical issues, together with a consideration of quality assurance activities and staff burnout
- Adapting to the hospital of the future
- Demonstrating the value of mental health treatments: are psychology and psychiatry worth paying for?

Psychology and Psychiatry: Integrating Medical Practice.
Edited by J. Milgrom and G. D. Burrows © 2001 John Wiley & Sons, Ltd.

SECTION A CONSOLIDATING THE ROLE OF PSYCHOLOGY AND PSYCHIATRY IN MEDICAL TREATMENT

Jeannette Milgrom and Graham D. Burrows

THE MULTIDISCIPLINARY TEAM: WORKING IN LIAISON WITH MEDICAL AND OTHER COLLEAGUES

Historically, consultation-liaison (C-L) psychiatrists established the importance of having a "liaison" role in the medical setting through regular attendance at ward meetings and developing relationships with ward staff. More recently, psychologists stressed the importance of doctor–patient communication, and how these principles extend to professional–professional communication, as the relationships between staff are seen to affect patient care. A major goal of the liaison role is to facilitate communication and staff relationships and this best occurs by becoming part of the multidisciplinary treatment team (Milgrom et al 1996).

Inevitably in the medical setting, a large number of professionals are involved in the care of any one patient. The cast may include medical (consultant, registrar, intern), nursing (nurse manager and rostered staff) and allied health (psychologist, social worker, physiotherapist, chaplain, occupational therapist) professionals. In order to provide sensible patient care, multidisciplinary team meetings to determine how a patient should be treated are usually held. This forum provides an opportunity for the various professionals, including the psychologist and psychiatrist, to clarify their roles and provide interdependent and integrated treatment plans. By meeting regularly together, different professionals get to know each other, learn to respect each other's professional contributions and relate at a more informal level. Effective two-way communication means that mental health professionals can provide psychological input to the medical process to assure quality and holistic care, and that relevant medical information is in turn imparted to them by the physician to assist diagnosis and treatment plans.

The relationship of the psychologist and psychiatrist with nursing staff is often central to successful liaison services. Nurses are usually aware of the day-to-day details of a patient's behaviour, historical details, interpersonal reactions and family issues. As a result, they are commonly in the best position to initiate referrals, observe changes and become involved in treatment programmes. However, it is important also to involve consultant physicians and their registrars in the referral process to achieve true integrated medical practice. This can be difficult due to time pressure, which may lead to a tendency not to involve medical staff; this is a risky procedure which results in psychological processes being considered secondary to mainstream medical management. Another reason for bypassing some members of the team may be due to their focus on medical management only, and because of this, a continuing role is to educate other staff about which referrals are most appropriate, and the many manifestations of psychological distress.

Clarification of how the roles of the psychologist and psychiatrist are different from each other and from those of other members of the health team is an ongoing process (see Chapters 4 and 5 for an earlier discussion of these issues). Role overlap often needs discussion, and the goal is to maximize skills available to the treatment team, so that a social worker with family therapy skills may complement a psychologist with cognitive-behavioural skills. Shared skills need to be differentiated from specialist expertise pertinent to a particular discipline. In addition, as the team has a complex and often unspoken hierarchy of helpers, from doctors to nurses to clerical staff, a major hurdle is often learning how to navigate through established lines of communication. To function well and form good working relationships, psychologists and psychiatrists must recognize and adapt their ways of working to the methods of operation of the institution, and be sensitive to the unwritten rules of conduct, and the role relationships among various members of the treatment team. This is an ideal chance for psychologists and psychiatrists to utilize their understanding of interpersonal interactions and how systems operate. At times they also need to challenge traditional hierarchies. Multidisciplinary teams are therefore not without conflict, and as strategies to resolve conflict fall well within the skills of psychology and psychiatry, it is a case of continually keeping in mind a systemic perspective and dealing directly with team issues to manage these tensions. In addition, in order to be maximally effective, the psychologist and psychiatrist must look carefully at their own roles, and develop a collaborative rather than a parallel or overlapping relationship.

Major challenges to the continuing role of psychology and psychiatry on the liaison team are the economic pressures facing the health system. These threaten to reduce services to a consultation and referral process, since the liaison role is time-consuming and therefore expensive. Nevertheless, it is important not to abandon the liaison role because it is essential, serving a number of functions in addition to the educational and communication roles. It allows an opportunity to troubleshoot at any level of the ward where a difficulty may be occurring. For instance, patient distress may actually be a function of staff behaviour, as in the case of a young quadriplegic boy who bit and spat at staff, who in turn were ambivalent and inconsistent in his management (Milgrom & Green 1990). Similarly, intervention may need to be directed at ward practices, such as making certain that patients understand the procedures that are to be performed. A presence on the ward also allows for interventions to be tailored to the culture of the particular organization and perhaps even to challenge some cultural practices. This organizational role of psychology and psychiatry is further elaborated below.

THE PSYCHOLOGIST'S AND PSYCHIATRIST'S ROLES IN INFLUENCING THE ORGANIZATION

Is it appropriate for psychologists and psychiatrists to use their skills to influence the organization they find themselves in? Should they "infiltrate" the organization and coax it to act in the humane function for which it was set up in the first instance, since at times this aim is lost because of economic pressures? Butcher & McPherson (1983) urged mental health professionals to draw upon their psychological knowledge in order to understand the workings of the institutions within which they were employed, as a means of improving the efficacy of their interventions. This still remains a challenging area for the psychologist and psychiatrist, but they are in an ideal position to move beyond the constraints imposed by the dynamics within organizations, and the distinct status and executive hierarchies (Milgrom & Green 1990). By redefining their relationships with others, they can increase therapeutic options according to the principles of "systems consultation", described some time ago by Wynne et al (1986, p 6). This approach explicitly attempts to consider the multiple contexts or systems of the presenting problem, and from this viewpoint consider the alternatives available for problem resolution. The consultant takes a "meta" position, and assesses the systemic relationships and patterns surrounding the presenting problem. For example, a "difficult" patient may be symptomatic of conflict between staff and family carers about "who knows what is best" for that patient. Alternatively, the problem facing a patient may be overwhelming for staff and result in avoidance of interaction. This may suggest that the consultant at times needs to engage in a staff intervention rather than succumbing to the traditional tendency to surrender the meta position and treat the "difficult" patient. A further danger of "joining" the individual as the focus of the therapeutic system, lies in the accompanying expectations and constraints which require "curative" action (Wynne et al 1986, p 10). It is as if the psychologist and psychiatrist are asked to "fix" the patient and take the responsibility for facilitating change and the action required.

Systems consultation, by contrast, often normalizes seemingly abnormal behaviour, uncovers underlying dynamics and utilizes a collaborative relationship between all staff, rather than deriving from a hierarchical helper–helpee relationship. The referring person, such as a nurse, is supported in using her own decision-making skills, building upon healthy resources and competencies, particularly capabilities for problem-solving, self-direction and autonomy. The quality of patient care can be improved by this type of interdisciplinary communication and co-ordination of treatment of the individual patient.

In summary, a systems consultation approach stresses the need to view individual patient referrals from multiple viewpoints and to ensure flexible shifts in roles and activities, so that at times the psychologist and psychiatrist take an organizational role, which may include:

- Staff counselling or mediation
- Organizational trouble-shooting, e.g. tackling absenteeism
- Policy-making, e.g. corporate code of ethics, patient management
- Bioethics and ethical issues, e.g. end-of-life decisions.

Each of these potential roles raises further issues. For instance, is it appropriate for the liaison psychologist or psychiatrist to engage in staff counselling, bearing in mind issues of confidentiality and the effect that this intervention may have on ongoing working relationships? At the Austin & Repatriation Medical Centre, the psychologist/counsellor does not work in other areas of the hospital. Whilst psychologists and psychiatrists working on wards often find themselves trouble-shooting problems for specific staff groups who referred a patient, it is important to remember that their objectivity may be influenced by their relationships with team members. Moreover, the use of a systems approach for change can at times threaten well differentiated hierarchies and unbalance the organizational system (Haley 1975).

On balance, however, this broader role of psychology and psychiatry is usually productive and facilitated by an understanding of organizational culture, which can be a powerful asset not only in knowing how to behave, but how to intervene, facilitate change and improve organizational performance. Situations such as the following may strongly differentiate various hospitals and influence styles of operation and ward management:

- University presence in teaching hospitals is a significant stimulus for constant review of standards. How does this influence how much priority is given to patient care versus research and training?
- Organizational structures vary widely between hospitals. Do employees identify with the organization as a whole rather than with their particular field of expertise? How does this influence staff relationships?

Armed with a good understanding of organizational culture and a systemic approach, the mental health professional is in a strong position to make an impact on the medical setting in a way that ultimately benefits patient care.

ADAPTING PSYCHOLOGY PRACTICE TO THE MEDICAL SETTING

Whilst psychiatrists have had extensive exposure to the medical setting in their training, psychologists have been required to adapt and supplement core psychology skills with training relevant to working in a medical environment. In the past, "Newly qualified psychologists often experienced culture shock on moving from an academic milieu which emphasized the intricacies of a dyadic model of intervention into the 'real world' of an organization or institution" (Sinnott 1985). Specialized training in clinical health psychology is now including not only basic knowledge of medical jargon and issues, but exposure to health systems and the unwritten rules of conduct. Belar (1980) suggested that in addition to the basic repertoire of clinical skills, the psychologist in a medical setting needs to be skilled in time efficiency, succinctness in written reports and clarification of referral questions. Additional skills in staff training, crisis management, and dealing with organizational issues are also useful.

The checklist below gives examples of behaviours that are useful for treating psychological problems in a way that is consistent with the rules of the medical setting (Milgrom et al 1996).

- *Be aware and respect the rules of conduct.* It is vital to understand organizational dynamics and to be respectful and sensitive to role relationships of other team members.
- *Be clear and brief.* Clarity of communication is essential both for oral and written reports. Focus on the case problems and treatment goal; be succinct; do not use jargon.
- *Make it practical.* It is helpful to staff to be direct about practical suggestions that follow from psychological assessment.
- *Do your homework.* Familiarity with medical procedures, side-effects and medication is important, not to interpret results, but to be able to converse and seek advice from medical colleagues.
- *Know your limits.* It is important to know your limits. Acknowledging areas you do not know about and asking advice, aids credibility.
- *Respond quickly.* Patients' condition may deteriorate rapidly, they may be discharged or a decision regarding their care may be made within 24 hours. Spending the weekend writing up a report may be generating an archive.
- *Educate colleagues.* Not all units of the hospital are psychologically minded. This can result in frustration in establishing new services. Be aware that you will need a long-term approach, physical presence at team meetings and rapid, accurate feedback on management of psychological problems, the effectiveness of intervention, and relevance to medical management.

Another important adaptation necessary for psychological practice is acceptance of the medical model, involving a focus on medical diagnosis, treatment and hospitalization. More recently, the medical model has begun to broaden, and recognize the role of social context and the mind–body interrelationship. As this biopsychosocial model of illness is being increasingly accepted (Sarafino 1994), psychologists are finding themselves less likely to experience a conflict between psychological and medical approaches to treatment. Positive working relationships with medical team members are a function of respecting the other professionals' approach, contributions and competencies in the context of a complex model that provides a framework for understanding how medical and psychological factors interact.

WHOM TO REFER TO: PSYCHIATRIST OR PSYCHOLOGIST?

The problems presenting to psychology and psychiatry are broad and include a range of referrals such as:

- Patient difficulties in dealing with pain, the diagnosis or hospitalization
- Behavioural, emotional or psychiatric difficulties
- Poor compliance to medical treatment
- Issues in patient–staff communication
- Preparation for aversive investigations or procedures such as surgery
- Support of staff in dealing with the stresses of daily hospital life, including issues of death, grieving, and general patient management.

This book has attempted to demonstrate the complementary nature of the two professions. There are enormous advantages to the treatment team of having available both a psychologist and a psychiatrist, and these were described in Chapter 4. Other chapters have outlined similarities and differences between psychology and psychiatry. As both psychologists and psychiatrists accept referrals directly, it is important to be aware that whilst there may be considerable overlap in the use of treatment approaches between these professionals, depending on an individual's specialist training, the following differences usually emerge:

- Psychiatrists prescribe and specialize in psychotropic drug therapies which may be used as the sole treatment approach or as part of a complementary therapeutic management programme. Psychiatrists are also experts in understanding interactions between medical disorders and psychiatric conditions, and in differential diagnoses and psychopathology.
- Psychologists have received extensive training in research and evaluation and have greater expertise in providing complex cognitive-behavioural therapy and formal assessment (behavioural, cognitive and intellectual).

These differences mean that when selecting a treatment of choice for a particular target symptom (e.g. sleep difficulty), a number of approaches can be considered (e.g. cognitive-therapy for anxiety or sedatives). It is important for the C-L psychiatrist and psychologist to work together in order to enhance optimal therapeutic effects. To work productively as part of the liaison team, psychology and psychiatry must be clear about their respective contributions. For example, a patient with a medical phobia may have high anxiety arousal and avoidance behaviours. Prescribing anxiolytic medication prior to commencing a psychological treatment such as systematic desensitization may help the patient utilize psychological treatment due to the rapid reduction in anxiety. Collaboration is also required in order to prevent iatrogenic problems resulting from mixed messages to the patient. There are many cognitive-behavioural interventions that can be used with the physically ill patient (e.g. Horne et al 1986) but it is important to make sure psychotropic medication is not counterproductive to the psychological treatment, e.g. often it is important that the patient take responsibility for treatment through psychological means rather than relying on medication for the change as this does not result in skills development and lasting change. As a team, psychology and psychiatry can go a long way towards integrating their principles and practice in medical practice. A potential outcome is a high standard of diagnosis and treatment as problems are considered from all perspectives—social, psychological and psychiatric.

NEUROPSYCHOLOGY

Psychologists and psychiatrists refer not only to each other, but increasingly to specialists within their own field. Whilst this book focuses on the role of the clinical health psychologist, psychology is expanding its specialty areas at a rapid rate. Twenty years ago, the same psychologist would often conduct both clinical treatment and cognitive assessment for possible brain dysfunction. Today, as our knowledge base and evaluation tools expand, neuropsychology is its own area of expertise and the clinical health psychologist commonly refers on for detailed assessments (Sweet et al 1991). Clinical neuropsychologists have training in neuroanatomy, neuropathology and brain–behaviour relationships and are often core members of teams in psychiatry, neurology, aged care and medical units, as well as providing consultancies to other areas of the hospital. Neuropsychologists utilize a range of both standardized and neurobehavioural measures to investigate specific areas of brain function. These may include tests of attention, learning and memory, language, visual-spatial abilities, sensory processes, motor abilities and high-level executive functions in addition to assessment of general intellectual ability and academic achievement. The patient's test performances will be evaluated and interpreted in the context of their developmental, personal and medical history and in conjunction with careful clinical observation. By utilizing their expertise in test interpretation and their in-depth knowledge of neuropsychological syndromes, the neuropsychologist is able to formulate hypotheses that assist in the differential diagnosis of brain dysfunction. Common questions the neuropsychologist is asked to answer include: Does the patient have evidence of higher cortical dysfunction? If so, is the locus of dysfunction diffuse or focal? Which hemisphere/lobe is affected? Is the pattern of test performance consistent with a particular disorder/diagnosis? What are the practical consequences of any neurological impairment? What are suggestions for remediation? How does the disease affect functioning over time?

Neuropsychologists continue to make more sophisticated contributions to medical practice, both by developing more effective methodologies and in expanding our understanding of brain function. Indeed, there are today subspecialty areas within the neuropsychology profession, including paediatrics, geriatrics, neuropsychiatry, stroke/neurology and rehabilitation. For further reading about the history of neuropsychological assessment and the specific application of neuropsychology to the medical patients, several excellent texts exist, e.g. Walsh & Darby (1999), Lezak (1995), Touyz et al (1994).

PSYCHOLOGY AND PSYCHIATRY DEPARTMENTS

We have already described how the psychologist and psychiatrist are part of a multidisciplinary team. Each health professional in the team may also belong to a department, and there are distinct advantages to a departmental structure which allows psychologists and psychiatrists to lobby and place themselves centrally in the organization, to assure their continued relevance to medical practice.

For example, The Austin Hospital in Australia formed an independent Clinical Psychology Department in 1978, which at the time was an unusual situation. A Rehabilitation Psychology section was later added following amalgamation with a nearby rehabilitation hospital. Soon after, amalgamation with a Repatriation hospital brought a veteran focus. More recently the Department changed its name to Clinical and Health Psychology to reflect its increasing specialization. The development of a Department has meant that about 20 psychologists who have similar clinical interests can meet regularly and exchange ideas, as well as stimulating, supporting and challenging each other. It has meant that psychologists can sharpen their skills with peer support and engage in ongoing professional development, shape developing services and tackle new issues that arise, from a psychological perspective. For example, given limited resources, psychologists may decide that providing a pain clinic across various medical units is better than selecting one unit to service. In Australia, psychologists in hospitals do not yet have privileges to admit or discharge patients. However, they do coordinate and provide psychological care, write and sign treatment plans, and re-refer for medical, consultation and other non-medical services, as needed. Affiliations with universities also provide an ideal opportunity for training of graduate psychology students. At the Austin & Repatriation Medical Centre a joint University of Melbourne Department of Psychology position of Professor/Director was established which provided the opportunity to develop a joint Doctor of Psychology in Health. This Doctorate training programme was designed to equip future graduates with skills needed to contribute maximally to the health system, providing a training venue immersed in the medical system. A particular challenge for psychologists in this Department, has been the trend for specialist disciplines to assume a secondary role in the organization and the evolution of "business units". These units (e.g. a surgical unit) are often medical in nature but may have psychologists attached as part of the multidisciplinary group reporting to a non-psychology manager. This has advantages in terms of teamwork but it is more difficult for psychologists to continue to develop specialist skills. The ideal scenario is forming loyalties and developing clinical accountability within the multidisciplinary team, as well as relating professionally within a Department of Psychology.

Psychiatry departments have a similar role to that described for psychology departments, and although they have evolved similarly, they often have a more established history. Mainstreaming of psychiatric patients into general hospitals has introduced another complexity. One of the interesting challenges for consultation-psychiatry is their dual identity—are they part of the acute hospital or part of psychiatric services?

Different departments may be grouped together into clinical services. The Psychiatry and Psychology Clinical Service Unit at the Austin & Repatriation Medical Centre was established in recognition of the importance of integrated mental health services to health care, and subsumes a number of departments including Adult Psychiatry, Psychology, Child Psychiatry, Community Psychiatry and Veteran Psychiatry (see Figure 12.1). The Heads of the departments are accountable to the Director of the Psychiatry and Psychology Clinical Service Unit for major policy and budget issues, whilst managing day-to-day issues internally.

In order to understand the place in the hierarchy of Clinical Services Units, it is of interest to understand the typical organizational structure of a general hospital. The chart shown in Figure 12.2 begins with a single point of management, the Chief Executive Officer who is responsible for six directorates. In turn, each Director is responsible for a variety of areas. For example, the Executive Director of Medical Services represents clinical services including Medicine, Surgery, Allied Health and Psychiatry and Psychology, as well as other portfolios such as health information. The Directors of clinical services are responsible to The Executive Director of Medical Services who reports to the Chief Executive Officer, who in turn reports to a Board of Management. Typically, Board members are not engaged in the day-to-day running of the hospital, and are generally appointed by the State Minister for Health. They are often chosen to bring a range of skills and perspectives, including medical, legal, financial/business and community. They are charged with fulfilling the objectives of the hospital with responsibilities to the funding body (the hospital may be private or public), the community, and the patients.

A number of key meetings are held regularly at all levels of the organization to bring together information and recommendations in a two-way communication process. Thus, maintaining a place in the hospital system is a complex process and involves competition with the demands of many other departments, as well as requiring the support of numerous people up the hierarchy.

Hospitals in turn have to negotiate for resources and service profiles, as they operate within the national health-care system. In Australia, hospitals generally interface through State Health Departments, and there are numerous separate branches, e.g. Acute Health, Psychiatry, Youth and Family. To complicate things further, State Health Departments have to maintain good relationships with national authorities, who provide 50% of their health funding.

An example of the difficulties encountered is the funding of mental health services to medical patients. Is it the Health Department or the Director of Psychiatric Programmes or the Director of Acute Health who is responsible? In practice, whilst C-L psychiatry and psychology provide services in both areas, there is a risk of falling between the two in terms of financial support.

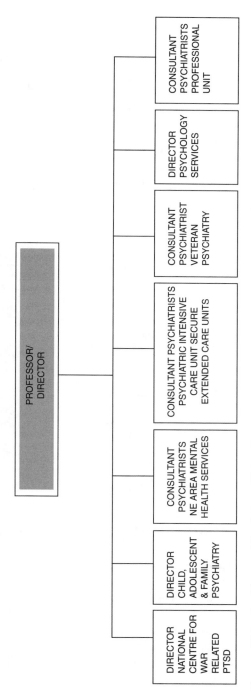

Figure 12.1 Psychiatry and Psychology Clinical Services Unit

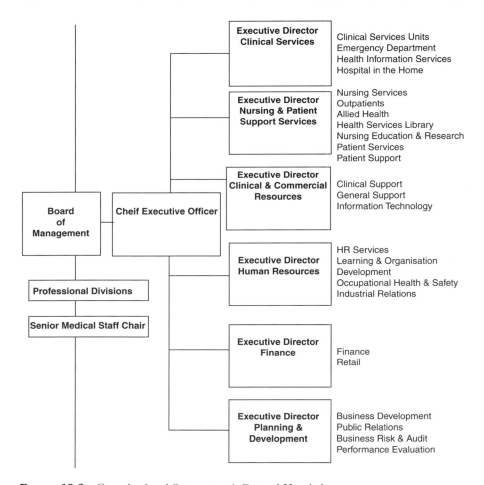

FIGURE 12.2   Organizational Structure—A General Hospital

SECTION B   PROFESSIONAL ISSUES IN A MEDICAL ENVIRONMENT

Jeannette Milgrom and Graham D. Burrows

A critical issue is to make sure that what psychologists and psychiatrists are doing is worthwhile, of the highest standard that resources and opportunities permit, and to take into consideration the ethical implications of what they and their colleagues do. Procedures need to be developed to ensure that this occurs. In addition, psychologists and psychiatrists need to be aware of how not only themselves but different health-care professionals are affected by their work environment. There are widespread reports of job stress amongst health-care workers, with suicide rates for doctors twice as high as for the general population (Editorial, *The Lancet*, 1994). It is important for psychologists and psychiatrists to be able to offer interventions for preventing and combating these deleterious effects.

QUALITY IMPROVEMENT

In recent years, health professionals have been asked to be increasingly accountable in what they do and to demonstrate procedures for maintaining high standards of patient care and efficient and cost-effective services. Successful treatment outcomes need to be demonstrated. Effectiveness of strategies developed are tested against outcome measures. Outcome measures may include: number of patients seen; waiting list; diagnostic groups; number of appointments; number of treatment goals met; number of physical symptoms; length of hospital admissions and use of medical services; rating on patient self-report of outcome; rating on referral source satisfaction. Analysis of outcome also requires rigorous collection of data on what sorts of patients were assessed and treated and often includes information, presenting problems, diagnosis, length and type of therapy, numbers of patients entering treatment and patient/referral source satisfaction. A feedback loop allows poor results on outcome measures to be considered to plan new strategies for standards of care. This is achieved by case conferences, audits, planning days, reviews of statistics and staff meetings.

ETHICS

With the growing acceptance of the biopsychosocial model of health and illness, psychiatrists and psychologists are working together in hospitals and medical centres to provide psychological intervention. These hospitals and medical centres which deal daily with dependent and vulnerable people have a duty to ensure that the services they offer are governed by ethical principles, and that those who offer service within them, as well as the recipients of these services, are fully aware of these principles.

Ethics has been defined as "the study and philosophy of human conduct, with emphasis on the determination of right and wrong; the basic principles of right action" (Funk & Wagnalls 1963). Rapid advances in medicine over the past decades have introduced great complexity into ethical considerations. There are now many journals devoted to these issues, as well as articles appearing in established journals. A good text for examination of issues of importance in medicine and psychiatry is Bloch & Pargiter (1999). Professional codes of ethics usually explicate the morality already accepted by the profession, but the codification of ethics by professional societies serves to promote self-scrutiny as well as awareness of issues where morality may be in question.

The basic professional Code of Ethics is the Hippocratic Oath, which defines the goals of medicine as firstly beneficence and the absence of maleficence, to preserve patients' confidences, to resist exploiting them sexually, and to refrain from procedures beyond their expertise. "Not only must the physician be prepared to do his duty, but the patient, the attendants and the external circumstances must conduce to the cure" (Lloyd 1983).

As Bloch & Pargiter conclude in their chapter on "Codes of ethics in psychiatry", "... they [codes of ethics] can no longer be relegated to a footnote in the exercise of a profession" (Bloch & Pargiter 1999, p 101). For instance, since the therapist–patient relationship tends to place therapists in a position of power, and patients in a dependent position, members of professional societies such as those representing Psychiatry and Psychology have power to influence others, rendering them vulnerable to exploitation. Any such exploitation is unethical and completely unacceptable. The Codes of Ethics adopted by these societies serve as a basis to investigate possible violations of accepted practice and to impose sanctions.

In the Australian Psychological Society's "Code of Ethics" (APS 1999) the psychologist is provided with firm guidelines concerning procedures ranging from assessment of clients, relationships with clients including confidentiality and maintaining boundaries, to providing services on the Internet and ethical considerations in teaching and research. For example, Section B, Item 9 makes explicit that "Sexual relationships between members and current clients must not occur. When a therapeutic procedure entails some level of physical intimacy with a client, informed written consent must be obtained from the client or the client's legal guardian prior to the introduction of that procedure." Furthermore, general principles of *responsibility, competence and propriety* are expected to operate in all situations (APS 1999). On the other hand, in setting up a code for psychiatrists, the Ethics Committee of the Royal Australian and New Zealand College of Psychiatrists (RANZCP) noted that for psychiatry, it was desirable to permit latitude in professional judgement, while ensuring that ethical considerations are rigorously adhered to (Bloch & Pargiter 1999, p 95).

The Principles and Code of Ethics of the RANZCP (RANZCP 1992) as given here lists the essentials of the psychiatrist's duty to patients.

1. Psychiatrists shall have respect for the essential humanity and dignity of each of their patients.
2. Psychiatrists shall provide the best possible psychiatric care for their patients.
3. Psychiatrists shall hold information about the patient in confidence.
4. Psychiatrists shall obtain consent from the patient before undertaking any procedure or treatment.
5. Psychiatrists shall not allow the misuse of their professional knowledge and skills.
6. Psychiatrists shall continue to develop their professional knowledge and share this knowledge with colleagues and other relevant health professionals.
7. Psychiatrists shall share the responsibility of upholding the integrity of the medical profession.

8. Psychiatrists conducting clinical research shall adhere to those relevant ethical principles embodied in national and international guidelines.
9. Psychiatrists in their societal role shall strive to improve the quality of psychiatric services, promote the just allocation of these services and contribute to the education of society regarding mental health.

At the Austin & Repatriation Medical Centre (A&RMC), the Patient Care Ethics Committee has developed a Corporate Code of Ethics to ensure that the highest ethical standards will apply to all its activities. In brief, the A&RMC will be guided by the following Statement of Values and Principles submitted by the Patient Care Ethics Committee:

- The inherent dignity of each and every human being
- The autonomy of the individual
- The exercise of care and compassion
- The practice of justice, fairness, honesty and integrity
- The striving for excellence
- The advancement of knowledge and learning
- The proper stewardship of resources.

In the expansion of this Statement, the issue of collaboration between the various professions engaged in clinical treatment and care receives attention, noting that sharing of information and decision-making is in the best interests of the patient.

Two disparate instances where ethical considerations are an important concern illustrate the issues involved: solid organ transplantation and human gene research.

The practice of solid organ transplantation depended originally on cadaveric organs; since these have always been in short supply, organ allocation raises ethical issues (Kefalides 1999). Further ethical problems arise when organs from healthy individuals (not always a blood relative or spouse) are donated to recipients. In the case of living-donor organ transplantation, traditional professional ethics are being re-evaluated and "replaced by more complex modes of moral reasoning" (Gutmann & Land 1999). A number of articles have appeared on guidelines for human organ transplantation (e.g. WHO 1991; Neuberger & James 1999).

Many and complex problems are also developing from human genome research which is proceeding to elucidate gene function. In the not-distant future it should be possible to develop drugs "with specificity for each human genotype", and thus minimize side-effects (Bosch 1998). But concerns are expressed about the use of genetic information in a discriminatory fashion. The identification of the Huntington's gene has had results of mixed benefits. Some of those at risk prefer not to be tested, rather than risk knowing for certain that they carry the deleterious gene. In epidemiological gene research, fears are expressed that with the difficulty of maintaining anonymity, ethics and privacy will be breached (Horner 1998; *Scientific American* 2000).

In all the problems listed above, assisting in coping with difficulties and fears encountered by patients will be the province of psychiatrists and psychologists. In addition, some ethical issues confront psychologists and psychiatrists in particular, and these are discussed in the ensuing sections.

Confidentiality

Over the past decades, the previously paternal aspect of the doctor–patient relationship has been transformed to a more equal partnership. Part of this change has resulted from the doctor's duty to inform the patient of the nature of the proposed treatment and the risks and benefits involved. "Informed consent" of the patient is thus obtained. A further duty of care involves the patient's right to confidentiality, although it is generally accepted that colleagues may share information. Exceptions to confidentiality must be noted when obtaining informed consent.

During psychotherapy, in particular, intimate and sometimes distressing information may be revealed. Both psychiatrists and psychologists must respect the confidentiality of information obtained from clients in the course of their professional duties. They may reveal such information to others only with the consent of the person or the person's legal representative. However, in those unusual circumstances where failure to disclose may result in clear risk to the client or others, they may disclose minimal information necessary to avert risk (see Tarasoff 1974). Patients and clients must be informed of the legal and other limits of confidentiality.

Psychiatric ethics do not preclude informing family members of a patient's intent to commit suicide, but psychiatrists also need to inform patients that their own actions have jeopardized confidentiality. Many ethical dilemmas concerning confidentiality have also arisen from the AIDS epidemic (e.g. Seawright & Pound 1994; Weinstock 1988).

Power Imbalance and Maintaining Boundaries

The paternalistic aspect of the doctor/therapist–patient relationship has changed for a more equitable one, but the power inequality cannot be overcome. There still remains some of the former awe of the priest-like therapist who will relieve the troubled patient/client of severe mental or physical pain. A power imbalance is also generated between therapist and patient by transfer of confidential information in psychotherapy. Because of this power imbalance, ethical problems are often raised when therapists blend their professional relationship with a client with another kind of relationship, which may impair the objectivity and/or judgement of the psychiatrist or psychologist. Proper boundaries provide a foundation for professional relationships by fostering a sense of trust and safety for the patient or client, and the belief that the professional will always act in the latter's best interests. The point, however, has been made that too rigid boundaries may not "allow the therapist to interact with warmth, empathy and spontaneity within certain conditions that create a climate of safety" (Gabbard 1999, p 143).

Sexual Exploitation

The issue of sexual exploitation has become more prevalent recently, possibly because of the rise of feminism and women's empowerment. The true prevalence is unknown, but studies which have surveyed psychiatrists, psychologists and social workers have found no difference in prevalence between the three (Gabbard 1999, pp 145–6). The history and ambivalent ethics of this all-too-human problem is discussed by Chodoff (1999, p 52) and also Epstein (1994).

Hazards in Diagnosis

As with sexual exploitation, social trends can exert an influence on the practice of psychiatry and psychology. The diagnosis of "recovered" or "repressed" memory was prevalent in the early 1990s to explain symptoms or behaviours in terms of childhood trauma, especially sexual abuse. In many instances this resulted in criminal charges or lawsuits, and a great deal of harm resulted to families of patients, to the patients themselves, and to the professions involved. In some cases diagnoses were shown to be baseless, as suggestions by therapists appeared to have resulted in the "recovery" of memories supporting the diagnoses. This phenomenon to some extent occurred in the effort to reduce sexual abuse of children, but unsound diagnostic methods were used in the search for abuse (Reich 1999, p 217). Therapists need to be aware that diagnosis, while a powerful tool, has limitations. Perceptions of behaviour and theories of causation have their fashions; these can permit diagnoses to be swayed by current schools of thought and the prevailing cultural climate.

Ethical Aspects of Psychotherapy

Despite their diversity, the ethical principles are common to all forms of therapy. Codes of practice of the psychotherapies in the United Kingdom contain sections on "the responsibility of practitioners to match therapy to patient need, to respect confidentiality, not to exploit patients sexually or financially, and to receive supervision and continuing education" (Holmes 1999, p 241). More than in any other form of therapy, the psychotherapies depend on the doctor–patient (therapist–client) relationship. Overstepping boundaries becomes easier, jeopardizing the neutrality the therapist should maintain for good practice. Moreover, psychotherapy patients may be more vulnerable because of their backgrounds which have led them to seek help. Regulation by means of ethical guidelines serves to "lend respectability to the profession", and also assists the practitioner in making difficult decisions by viewing contentious issues in public, e.g. the repressed memory controversy, and the pathology or non-pathology of homosexuality (Holmes 1999, p 241).

The Ethics of Resource Allocation and Managed Care

In the allocation of limited resources for health care, impairment of mental health in general is at a disadvantage compared with physical disorder and yet, it causes diminished quality of life equal in severity to any chronic illness. The Oregon priority-setting process demonstrates what happens when mental health conditions compete with physical ones such as diabetes, rather than as a block (Garland 1992; Sabin & Daniels 1997). The final ranking depended on severity of impact of conditions and effectiveness of treatment. The Oregon example supports the contention that mental health conditions should not be disadvantaged in competing for resources with medical and surgical conditions. With the inevitable limitation of health-care resources, how can a fair and equitable distribution be attained? Daniels & Sabin (1998) have proposed four necessary conditions to be met:

- Resource allocation policies and limit-setting conditions must be publicly accessible.
- Comprehensible and plausible explanations for allocations should be available, together with how decisions about the best "value for money" for the population are arrived at.
- A mechanism for dealing with challenges and disputes can be an agent for change if necessary, together with an opportunity for educating clinicians and the public about the validity of the decisions. If convinced of "fairness", people find them more acceptable even if unpleasant.
- Fourthly, there must be voluntary or public recognition of the process that allocates mental-health resources, to ensure that the first three conditions are met (Daniels & Sabin 1998; Sabin & Daniels 1999).

Efforts to manage health care with greater efficiency began with health maintenance organizations (HMOs), corporate organizations of selected physicians and hospitals providing a set of services to enrolled members usually for a predetermined premium with a number of conditions attached for both patients and clinicians. This procedure fundamentally altered the function of doctors from protecting a patient's welfare to balancing their health needs against cost control (Iglehart 1992). Eventually this progressed to the current system of managed care, which increasingly brought clinical decision-making under the authority of managed care organizations (MCOs) (Geraty 1995).

The current revolution in organization and financing of health care has effects not only on economic values, but also on human values. How do these changes relate to traditional assumptions about professional/medical ethics? The quality of health care has been compromised by its transformation to an industry. Where the doctor/ therapist–patient relationship was an essential part of the healing process, professionals such as psychiatrists and psychologists have become merely providers, and patients the recipients, of technology (Dyer 1999, p 72). In the process of changing medicine from a profession to a trade, in place of a human service it has become a marketable commodity which has only succeeded in lowering costs without adequately addressing quality of service or distribution and allocation of resources (Dyer 1999, p 72).

Daniels & Sabin (1998) comment on the ethical implications of accountability in proposals to reform managed care. Firstly, market accountability requires that consumers should be informed of the limits of availability of care, with the assumption that consumers will agree to and accept the limits. This demands a considerable degree of education of patients and clinicians about the need for limits. It will not be an easy task to explain why an expensive pharmacotherapy or procedure, which may be successful, is not available because resources are already stretched to the limits. What then happens to informed consent?

In all the problems listed above, psychiatrists and psychologists have a central role to play in ethical decision-making of resource allocation, whether it involves their own practice or that of their colleagues. As the Austin & Repatriation Medical Centre has been a leader in liver transplantation in Victoria, Australia, our liaison team has been involved with this work since its beginning (Moore et al 1991). The sharing of information and decision-making between psychiatrists, psychologists and other health workers on our liaison team as set out in the Austin & Repatriation Medical Centre's Corporate Code of Ethics has proved an essential component of efficient practice.

BURNOUT

Maslach & Jackson (1981) define burnout as "a syndrome of emotional exhaustion and cynicism that frequently occurs among individuals who do 'people work' of some kind." Emotional exhaustion, the development of negative and cynical attitudes towards work, and a tendency to evaluate oneself and one's work performance negatively are regarded as key symptoms. Factors which may contribute include the workload, physical environment and confrontation with unpleasant tasks. For health professionals, there are also responsibility and ethical issues, and the continual need for upgrading of skills and knowledge. Burnout is described as well in non-people-centred occupations, where high workload, pressure for speed, monotony and physical environmental stressors can be contributing factors.

As noted in Chapter 4, page 116, professional burnout can be minimized by acknowledging clinician needs and concerns with patient care, helping them cope with issues of control and ambiguity and providing social support (Maslach 1982; 1997). Stebnicki (2000) suggests a framework for dealing with the "empathy fatigue" which results from the emotional stress on rehabilitation counsellors. Burnout in clinical staff in community mental health agencies was measured by Webster & Hackett (1999) using the Maslach Burnout Inventory. The authors discuss implications for prevention of burnout in mental-health professionals. Fallowfield & Jenkins's (1999) work with oncology departments suggests insufficient training in communication skills as a major factor contributing to stress, lack of job satisfaction and burnout. This factor, an area where the skills of psychologists are of particular value, probably applies to many other areas in health care.

Finally, caretakers of relatives with Alzheimer's disease, chronic illness or psychiatric illness are also subject to burnout because, like health professionals, they shoulder the burden of care and can suffer emotional exhaustion. Preventive intervention involves identification of potential stressors, and teaching methods of coping for those who are likely to be experiencing an ongoing subjective burden.

In the "non-people-oriented" workplace, education is a key tool in the management of stressors, not forgetting that the individual has a duty of self-care, and assumption of personal responsibility (Turner et al 1995). A complete publication devoted to theories of organizational stress (Maslach 1998) includes an article entitled, "A multidimensional theory of burnout" by Maslach, the originator of the Burnout Scale, and provides a review of the topic.

SECTION C THE HOSPITAL OF THE FUTURE
Jeannette Milgrom and Graham D. Burrows

These are times of change, and many hospitals are altering their names to "medical centre" to emphasize new directions. The "hospital of the future" is already taking shape, with reduction in the breadth of services, focus on limited core acute services with fast throughput, and other roles traditionally associated with hospitals managed out in the community (Braithwaite et al 1994). Other changes vary depending on locality and may include the privatization of outpatients departments and internal restructuring of hospitals as a number of "business units". Under this arrangement, multidisciplinary business units are grouped together to provide a service (e.g. Surgery) with control over their budget. At the same time, many hospitals are being grouped together into networks, with network Chief Executive Officers.

The major impetus to this review of health systems is the escalating health cost. Currently, casemix is the funding model used in Australian hospitals as a way of improving cost-effectiveness and patient throughput (Eagar & Hindle 1994). Under this funding agreement, hospitals are paid a fee to cover costs of patients as determined by a casemix formula, which estimates the level of services required for each Diagnostic-Related Group (DRG). Patients are classified into a DRG and, for each class, the hospital is reimbursed a specific amount of money, regardless of the actual services provided or number of bed days.

THE HOSPITAL OF THE FUTURE: WHAT WILL THIS MEAN TO PSYCHOLOGY AND PSYCHIATRY?

Casemix funding, coupled with the business unit structure, may create a major crisis for the funding of psychology and psychiatry in acute health. A major argument will need to be mounted to convince the Government authorities to fund C-L psychiatry and clinical health psychology, as the major diagnosis may not be psychiatric (Simpson & Cotton 1995). Furthermore, even if casemix makes provision for allied health services, it will be important to convince individual business unit managers to spend the money on, for example, psychologists, rather than extra medical sessions or physiotherapy. Use of casemix funding will depend on the hospital's priorities.

The business structure may also disempower professional groupings so that professionals are dispersed throughout the hospital without having a major political voice. At the Austin & Repatriation Medical Centre, psychologists in Acute Health are part of a centralized Psychology Department, whereas those in Psychiatric Services are part of their business unit, e.g. Child and Adolescent Psychiatry.

The reduction of outpatient services may also have a major effect on psychology and psychiatry practice, which traditionally have provided services in this area. On the other hand, the differences between public and private health may blur. It could also be argued that in a time of change, opportunities are presented. Psychology and psychiatry may benefit from this crisis, which calls for a review of traditional services, and strengthen their position in the health field due to their relevance in reducing costs. This will depend on their ability to play the political system and retain their professional identity in the new structure.

PLAYING THE POLITICAL GAME AND INFLUENCING HEALTH POLICY

In order for psychology and psychiatry to provide services in hospitals, funding must be available. Competition for the health-care dollar means that an involvement in hospital politics and in framing the current health-care policies, together with marketing of their skills are necessary. Psychologists and psychiatrists, particularly those in more senior positions, have an opportunity to make a distinctive psychological contribution to the planning process. For example, membership of various hospital committees, representation through Clinical Service Unit Directors, written submissions to the Health department and keeping up-to-date with changes in policy are all important activities. In addition, psychologists must be more pro-active in providing health-related research which can be incorporated into the planning and delivery of health care, not only to make the case for enhanced psychology service provision, but to contribute to innovative service developments and reviews of the general health system.

Professional bodies also need to become increasingly political to assist in the development of psychology in hospitals. The American Psychological Association (APA) is notable for its activity in this area, not only by preparing informative letters and reports on the functions that psychologists are capable of performing in hospital settings, but also seeking seats on influential planning bodies and at times entering into a direct confrontation. For example, the APA made a public statement that, "It is inappropriate, costly, and exclusionary to require a licensed physician to be responsible for overall care to patients for mental health treatment, when that care does not include medical interventions for which a physician has unique and specified expertise" (Zaro et al 1982). The APA has also been influential in convincing the National Institutes of Health to change their research funding priorities to include research on behaviour and health. All these activities must rely on careful arguments based on research to advocate for the ideal size and nature of a psychological service in a hospital. This may include arguments based on a number of parameters which were described by Milgrom et al 1996:

- *The prevalence of a disorder.* Studies claiming that about one-third of patients presenting to medical practitioners have significant psychological problems are powerful arguments for the development of mental health services (e.g. Cummings 1991). However, since services are often only developed when "need" is expressed as "demand" or when consumers seek help, these prevalence statistics need to be used to create a demand. Even more powerful are arguments about lifestyle behaviours contributing to the major killers in western society (cancer, coronary disease and cerebrovascular accidents).
- *Service norms.* The British Psychological Society, amongst others, had recommended an ideal service norm of one clinical psychologist per 25 000 population (Trethowan report 1977). A later review of clinical psychology services concluded that senior-grade psychologists should constitute half of all existing positions (MAS 1989). There is enormous variation across the UK, US and Australia in the match between these "ideal" norms and reality. A similar situation exists for clinical psychiatry, where arguments based on benchmarking often reflect practical constraints rather than a realistic estimate of need.
- *Current government strategic directions.* Awareness of current directions for health services is essential. For instance, in recent years Health and Community Services Victoria, Australia (1994) advocated decentralized care for the mentally ill from psychiatric hospitals to general hospitals. This changed the role of psychologists and psychiatrists in hospitals from a focus largely on patients who are physically ill to a dual focus to include those with psychiatric disturbances.
- *Where the money is.* Planning needs to take into account where the money is and the attitude of individuals who control the money (Debelle 1995). For instance, homeless youths may be an important government agenda and developing adolescent services becomes more likely at such a time. Similarly, a focus on national priority health problems such as cancer and cancer prevention is likely to be a catalyst for the contribution of psychological services and research in this area.

- *Costs and outcomes.* The yearly expenditure on health care is enormous and growing. In the United States, expenditure grew from 27 billion dollars in 1960, representing 5.3% of Gross National Product, to 752 billion dollars in 1991, representing 13.2% of Gross National Product (Taylor 1995). Expenditure was expected to rise to 15% of Gross National Product in the year 2000 (Kaplan et al 1993). This alarming escalation may be an impetus to psychology and psychiatry if they can demonstrate a positive effect on health costs. The bottom line is that it is useful to demonstrate benefits of psychological and psychiatric treatment programmes in terms of the low cost of these programmes and the monetary savings gained as a result of positive treatment outcome (Yates 1980). Psychologists and psychiatrists need to demonstrate that patients bog down the medical services as a result of inadequately managed psychological issues such as anxiety, stress, pain, sleep disturbance, depression, interpersonal and habit difficulties. Since many patients presenting to medical practitioners have significant emotional problems, if these are treated by the appropriate mental health professional it is likely to reduce return outpatient visits, and may also result in improved adherence to treatment. A full discussion of economic analyses is found on page 323 of this chapter.

EVIDENCE-BASED INTERVENTION OR QUALITY OF CARE?

The evidence that psychological intervention can improve emotional well-being is well established in some areas. There is now an extensive body of literature on the effectiveness of cognitive-behavioural therapy techniques for problems such as anxiety and depression (Dobson & Craig 1996). This is particularly relevant as there is an increased appreciation that an important outcome following medical illness is quality of life. However, evidence of the effectiveness of psychological intervention in affecting broader outcomes, including disease progression and prevention, remains mixed (see review in Chapter 2).

As discussed in Chapter 2, objective verification of outcomes is increasingly being expected of practitioners, thereby increasing the demand for psychological interventions to be validated empirically. There is a need for further research to answer questions such as:

- Which particular type of intervention is most effective? For instance, we need better data to assess the benefits of drug versus cognitive-behavioural therapy treatment, against efficacy in treating particular conditions, and therapy time required to produce symptom relief. Medication has a rapid effect whereas therapeutic strategies such as cognitive-behavioural therapies are also efficient and effective and result in less relapse of symptoms. Is this the case for all conditions?
- What outcomes change?

- What is the comparative success of various health professionals?
- Have medical centres reduced the use of other medical services and kept costs down by the employment of psychologists and psychiatrists?

Despite the increasing evidence of the role of psychological factors in physical illness and disease, many studies are uncontrolled and research demonstrating that psychological intervention can affect disease progression is still inconclusive. Nevertheless, due to escalating health costs, interest has focused on the existing cost-effectiveness of psychological intervention. A number of studies provide evidence for a decrease in medical utilization with mental health treatment (e.g. inpatient days; cost/year per patient; outpatient visits, prescriptions including analgesia, X-ray and lab visits following psychological treatment). Treatment has been mixed and included emotional support, instruction, short-term psychotherapy, counselling or family therapy, relaxation training, psychiatric consultation or a mixture of these interventions (Devine & Cook 1983; Groth-Marnat & Edkins 1996; Milgrom et al 1994; Schlesinger et al 1983).

The last section of this chapter provides a detailed analysis of the question: Are psychology and psychiatry worth paying for? Nearly ten years ago Lorion (1991) made a call which is only beginning to be responded to: "psychology (and psychiatry) as a scientific and applied discipline have a unique responsibility to participate in the pursuit of strategies that reduce the nation's health care needs." The final section deals with the vexed question, given our current knowledge base, how do we measure the value of mental health treatment?

SECTION D   MEASURING THE VALUE OF MENTAL HEALTH TREATMENTS[1]
Steven Schwartz

For some time, psychologists and psychiatrists have been calling on governments, health maintenance organizations and health insurers to provide more generous benefits for the treatment of psychological disorders. Yet, these health "funders" continue to resist. Their arguments are mainly financial. Many mental health treatments, especially psychotherapy, are expensive. Moreover, they are often open-ended in duration. Insurers find it difficult to budget for treatments that can go on indefinitely. On the other hand, professionals argue that mental health treatments save more money than they cost. By getting people back to work, by preventing even worse illnesses, psychological and psychiatric treatments are considered (by their champions at least) as ways to save money. The goal of this section is to analyse this claim. Taking the point of view of those who pay for health care

[1]   Earlier versions of this paper appeared in the *Bulletin of the Australian Psychological Society* and *Psychologically Speaking*. The paper was produced with the assistance of grants from the Australian Research Council and the National Health and Medical Research Council.

(insurers, governments), the evidence for the cost-effectiveness of mental health treatments will be examined and some recommendations made about how those in the field could demonstrate to insurers that more generous payments for psychological and psychiatric treatments are justified.

PRESSURE ON HEALTH BUDGETS

Health budgets are under pressure and the public is demanding greater value for their health dollars (Schwartz 1999). To get the best value for our health dollars it makes sense to spend them where they do the most good. But where is that? We do not have enough outcome studies to tell (Schwartz 1995; 1997). Mental health expenditures must compete with heart transplants, rehabilitation, drugs, high-tech medical equipment, new hospital beds, immunization programmes, and, of course, other expenditures such as schools, roads and prisons. Somehow mental health must be seen by health funders as equal to if not more important than competing demands for resources. Health funders are calling for increasing levels of proof of the efficacy and effectiveness of mental health interventions before they agree to pay for them.

WHAT IS MENTAL HEALTH TREATMENT AND WHO ARE THE PROVIDERS?

The first step in deciding whether to pay for mental health treatment is to define precisely what we mean by psychological and psychiatric treatment. It turns out that this is not easy to do. Mental health treatments include drugs, electroshock, hospital milieu, and a broad range of "psychotherapies" that seem to include any treatment designed to give people insight into their behaviour or teach them new ways of behaving. In other words, the definition of what constitutes mental health treatment is so broad that health funders may be asked to pay for anything from a highly structured behaviour therapy programme to a friendly chat over coffee. This situation stands in stark contrast to most medical treatments. With the advent of "diagnostic related groups", medical treatments have become specific and standardized (Gold et al 1996), although it should be said that some medical interventions remain quite vague. Health funders will remain resistant to reimbursing mental health treatments until we can specify just what these treatments are, who they are for, and what outcomes we expect them to produce.

Once we have decided what mental health treatment is, and who is likely to benefit from it (and by how much), we must then answer a second question: Who are the providers? At present, there appear to be an enormous number of potential providers of mental health treatments. In addition to psychiatrists and psychologists, a large number of people claim to be psychotherapists (just check the local business telephone directory). Should all of these people be eligible for reimbursement? This would be quite expensive. Health funders could never afford it. If only some providers will be reimbursed, then how do health funders decide which ones? Should health-care reimbursement go only to medical doctors? Should psychologists be included? What about social workers, psychiatric nurses, counsellors? In the past, reimbursement policies were dependent on guild membership. Medical doctors, sometimes psychologists, were covered by health funders, but no one else. In the future, government health funders are more likely to make their decisions based on results (who actually achieves the best outcomes) while private insurers will make their decisions on commercial grounds. If consumers want to be covered for treatment by psychotherapists, naturopaths, and hypnotists—and they are willing to pay premiums for such coverage—then their services will be reimbursed. In either case, there will need to be some definition of which professional groups are recognized mental health service providers.

DOES MENTAL HEALTH TREATMENT WORK?

Having decided what mental health treatment is, and who should be providing it, the next question health funders ask is: Does it work? Psychiatrists and psychologists have been performing treatment-outcome studies for more than 50 years, yet there is still considerable disagreement about what works and what does not work in the clinic. Part of the problem is that there is no standard measure of treatment outcome. Numerous different outcome measures exist (see Table 12.1 and Streiner & Norman 1989). A treatment may produce a benefit on one outcome measure and not on another. Does this mean that the treatment is a success? Government health-care authorities are likely to favour outcomes that lower overall health costs, such as decreased use of prescription drugs, lower absenteeism and increased productivity. Private insurers are more responsive to consumer satisfaction. This is why they offer coverage for services not covered by government health funders.

Even when outcomes are carefully specified, mental health treatment studies are often vague about what constitutes treatment. Health funders want standard treatments for specific patients. Many mental health treatment outcome studies describe their treatments in sketchy terms ("cognitive restructuring") and do not even include a treatment manual.

TABLE 12.1 Sample of mental health outcomes

Clinical outcomes	Functional outcomes
Measures of symptoms and signs, e.g. Brief Psychiatric Rating Scale	Work-related, e.g. less absenteeism, increased productivity
Measures of health-care usage, e.g. decreased use of prescription drugs	Socially related, e.g. lower divorce rates, greater marital satisfaction
Improved general health status	
High consumer satisfaction	

Outcome trials in the field of mental health (particularly studies of psychotherapy) vary from anecdotal case reports to carefully controlled studies with specially selected patients and highly motivated therapists. Controlled studies, while crucial for identifying whether a treatment works, always produce more positive outcomes that those that will be obtained in the real world of the clinic where patients are not carefully selected and clinicians vary in their abilities. In the jargon of clinical trials, mental health outcome research focuses on efficacy rather than effectiveness, and on statistical rather than clinical significance.

Moreover, mental health researchers have rarely been concerned with cost. They often seem content to show that a treatment does something, without worrying about whether it is also cost-effective. In the past, mental health treatment studies have tended to ignore cost, yet this is crucial information for health funders (Gold et al 1996). For example, if psychotherapy is more expensive than antidepressant drugs for depression, the extra expense can only be justified if psychotherapy is more effective than drugs. In recent years, costs have become part of mental health outcome research. We have found that the costs of psychological conditions can be considerable. They involve direct costs such as hospital charges, professional salaries, tests, drugs, rehabilitation and follow-up visits. They also include indirect costs such as missed work days, lowered productivity, lowered productivity of care-givers, and the costs of training replacement workers. Mental health treatment would be valuable if it reduced these costs by more than the cost of treatment. In other words, health funders trade off costs against benefits; they will pay more for treatments that yield greater benefits. Doing this requires some form of economic analysis (Drummond et al 1997).

ECONOMIC ANALYSES

Cost–Benefit Analysis

In this analysis, both the costs and benefits of a treatment are measured in dollars. The advantage of this approach is that we can make absolute judgements—either a treatment's benefits outweigh its costs or they do not. In reality, cost–benefit analyses are difficult to conduct. We can estimate costs in dollars, but to estimate a treat-ment's benefits in financial terms means putting a dollar value on outcomes such as a lower score on a depression inventory. This is often difficult to do. This is why there have been so few cost–benefit analyses in general medicine and even fewer in the area of mental health treatment.

Cost–Effectiveness Analysis

In contrast to cost–benefit analysis, a cost–effectiveness analysis does not require that the benefits be measured in dollars. Instead of money, outputs can be measured in health-relevant terms. For example, an outcome measure of psychological treatment for depression might be a score on the Beck Depression Inventory. Cost–effectiveness analysis allows us to identify which treatment produces the best outcome as measured by the Beck Depression Inventory for the fewest dollars. In other words, a cost–effectiveness analysis is designed to answer questions such as: Is psychotherapy a better treatment than drugs alone? However, unlike cost–benefit analysis, cost–effectiveness analysis cannot determine whether any treatment is worthwhile in the absolute sense (that is, its benefits exceed its costs).

Cost–Utility Analysis

This is the name given to a cost–effectiveness analysis in which the outcome measure is some measure of utility or preference for certain outcomes. One commonly used outcome measure in cost–effectiveness analyses is quality-adjusted life years or QALYs (Schwartz et al 1993; Spilker 1990).

Traditionally, medical outcomes were measured by a "survival analysis". Thus, a 50-year-old man with throat cancer who would be expected to die has life-saving surgery and lives to 75. We say that the surgery has produced 25 extra life-years. We could stop there, but we would be missing something very important. While the man clearly survived, he could no longer speak, eating was painful, and he had to breathe through a hole in his throat. In other words, the quality of his life was not the same as before his surgery. QALYs attempt to factor quality into the traditional life-year measure by expressing, in a single number, a person's trade-off between length and quality of life. Quality of life is measured on a scale that goes from 0 (dead) to 1 (perfect health).[2] The man whose surgery added 25 years to his life estimated his post-surgical quality of life as only half as good as his previous life (e.g. 0.5 on the quality-of-life scale). To measure surgical outcome in QALYs, we must multiply the years of extra life times their quality. In this case 25 extra years times a quality of 0.5 produces 12.5 QALYs. Thus, the surgery added 12.5 quality-adjusted life years to the man's life. Table 12.2 contains QALY calculations for depression.

Cost–utility analysis provides an important tool by which researchers can analyse the outcome of mental health treatments. As an example, Table 12.3 contains a

TABLE 12.2   Calculating quality-adjusted life years for depression

Type	Length		Quality	QALYs
Normal year	1	×	1	= 1.00
Year of depression	1	×	0.3	= 0.30
Death	1	×	0	= 0.00

---

[2]   There may well be quality of life situations that are worse than death such as living in a vegetative coma, but we consider death to be 0 here in order to simplify the presentation.

TABLE 12.3 Hypothetical cost–utility analysis for treating depression

Treatment	Cost ($)	QALYs	Marginal Cost–Utility ($ per QALY)
Watching and waiting	0	0.40	
Antidepressants	500	0.65	2000
CBT	1000	0.90	2000
CBT + Drugs	1500	0.99	2542

cost–utility analysis of four approaches to treating depression: drugs, cognitive-behaviour therapy, both drugs and cognitive-behaviour therapy, and just watching and waiting. (These numbers are hypothetical but close to the real figures.) As you can see from Table 12.3, many people are likely to recover from depression without treatment, although their recovery might be slow and their quality of life will be low while they recover. Recovery is faster with drugs and cognitive-behaviour therapy (CBT), which both produce more QALYs. What we are interested in is how much each treatment adds to simply watching and waiting. To examine this, we must look at the extra marginal costs incurred when we go from watching and waiting to a treatment.

For example, antidepressants produce an improvement of 0.25 QALYs, at a cost of $500, over just watching and waiting. Dividing $500 by 0.25 QALYs produces a marginal cost–utility ratio of $2000 per extra QALY. Similarly, CBT produces a 0.50 improvement in QALYs over just watching and waiting at a cost of $1000. Dividing 1000 by 0.50 also produces a marginal cost–utility ratio of $2000. At the margin, therefore, both drugs and CBT have the same cost–utility ratio of $2000. The combination of drugs and therapy produces a better outcome than either alone (0.99 QALYs), but the extra QALYs gained by adding drugs to CBT are very expensive. The extra cost of adding drugs to CBT is $500 ($1500 − $1000) while the extra gain in QALYS is 0.09 (0.99 − 0.90). This gives a marginal cost–utility value of $5556 for every extra QALY ($500 / 0.09 QALYs). By aggregating the results of many such studies, health funders can gain some idea of what outcomes they can expect from different levels of expenditure (Pettiti 1994). Health funders may be willing to fund CBT or antidepressants, as both have similar cost-utility ratios, but may baulk at paying the extra money for both in combination.

Conclusions

Early results from cost–effectiveness research bode well for mental health treatment (Dewan 1999; Sharfstein 1998). Psychiatric and psychological treatment does seem to be cost-effective. Expenditures on mental health treatment seem to result in greater worker productivity and a decrease in other health costs. Thus, it seems that mental health treatment may be justifiable on cost–effectiveness grounds. Still, certain questions remain to be answered by further research. These are:

- Which therapists are competent?
- Which patients are most likely to benefit from which treatments?
- What is the optimal length of treatment for different conditions?
- What are the best outcome measures?
- What are the costs?
- What is the cost–effectiveness and cost–utility of specific treatments for specific conditions?

CONCLUDING REMARKS AND FUTURE DIRECTIONS

Will psychology and psychiatry survive and develop in the medical setting? The turmoil that is currently generated in hospitals as a result of increasing costs has resulted in continuing changes to the health system making it difficult to predict the future. On the one hand, it is possible that we are not proficient enough at the political game and we will not be able to ensure that a medically oriented system values the input of psychology and psychiatry sufficiently to continue public funding despite the evidence emerging that we are worth paying for. Is it possible that we will take a step back in time, servicing once more mainly psychiatric patients who are being mainstreamed into hospitals or have sporadic appointments with psychologists and psychiatrists employed because of a particularly psychologically minded physician? Are we applying our skills at the root of the problem? Should we be challenging a health system that is being reorganized on economic agendas, ignoring the trauma to staff involved in the inevitable downsizing, and not primarily considering patients as people but as "throughputs" to be increased in terms of efficiency?

Our experiences to date in the field of clinical health psychology and consultation-liaison psychiatry in hospitals have given us a glimpse of the future, since the possibilities for truly holistic patient care are achievable by having active, vibrant and innovative mental health services. Our research knowledge is also expanding rapidly, providing exciting evidence of the role of psychological factors in illness and health. Our future is our own making and our new psychology and psychiatry graduates are being trained to have vision, skills and the ability to provide quality services. These future ambassadors of psychology and psychiatry will no doubt continue to educate relevant policy-makers, and increase the likelihood that this expansion will continue, towards a truly integrated medical practice.

Finally, we need to target the major difficulties of our time. Since mood disorders, including depression, are estimated to affect some 340 million people at the one time, and represent a significant co-morbid condition in medical patients, we have used this as an example throughout the book, in terms of its impact on illness and as an example in consideration of QALYs. In addition, we will describe below how we have approached the problem of depression in Australia (WHO 1997) and suggest a model for increasing the awareness in the community and the hospital of the importance of mental health treatment. One in four females and one in six males in Australia will have a depressive disorder requiring treatment in their lifetime, but surveys have shown that only 25% of people who have depression will receive treatment. Of the 75% not receiving treatment, depression may be concomitant with another illness, or may be caused by the treatment for the illness, for example by the drugs used. Between 15 and 29% of people who consult a general practitioner are depressed. Most will present with physical symptoms such as aches and pains, sleep disturbance and fatigue. About 2500 people commit suicide in Australia each year and about 60 000 more attempt suicide. In most cases depression is easily and effectively treated. The cost of untreated depression to the country is estimated at between four and five billion dollars per year. About 70% of those who commit suicide have a primary depressive disorder, undiagnosed.

In 1994 The Mental Health Foundation in Australia launched a national "Depression Awareness Campaign". Psychiatrists and psychologists collaborated with advertising people, representatives from the corporate sector, from the banking world and non-government organizations. Support was obtained from both international sources—The World Federation for Mental Health, the World Psychiatric Association—and national medical groups—the Australian Medical Association, the Royal Australian and New Zealand College of Psychiatrists, and the Royal Australian College of General Practitioners, and to 53 support organizations representing every conceivable area, including psychology. During National Mental Health Week we launched the National Depression Awareness Campaign. A "guide to overcoming depression" was published in a national magazine, and a rating scale on which people could rate themselves appeared in a newspaper on National Depression Screening Day. To influence politicians, it is necessary to influence their constituency, and since the way to do this is to go to the people, we went on to public education. We have also run interactive educational programmes for general practitioners. A further programme called "Options" was aimed at promoting better mental well-being in school and in the general community by reducing the influence of violence and by substituting non-violent coping behaviour.

To change the course of depression and its treatment, we must start early. A community education programme must start in schools. We interviewed 3700 staff, students and parents, and conducted print, TV and radio presentations all highlighting mental health issues in schools and in the community. We increased community awareness of mental health, depression and suicide, drawing attention to the treatability of mental distress, the need to take responsibility for one's own mental wellness, and the availability of education in methods of coping.

Furthermore, targeting the "Wellness Sector" will improve the health status of the entire community. As a result the Second World Congress on Stress is entitled, "Vision of Enhanced Wellbeing in the 21st Century—VIEW 21". There will be a collaboration of The Mental Health Foundation of Australia, The International Diabetes Institute, The National Stroke Foundation of Australia, The Australian Cancer Society, and The Alzheimer's Association of Australia. The VIEW 21 Network provides Mental Health Members with access to health information resources through multiple, integrated approaches, including walk-in centres, books, CDs, videos, Internet, personal computers, Multimedia kiosks, Fax and telephony devices. Information on View 21 is available through the authors.

VIEW 21 Program Levels are:

1. Wellbeing.
2. Primary prevention.
3. Self-care management.
4. Acute disease self-care management.
5. Chronic disease self-care management.

This example provides a view of the future—the relevance of intervention by psychologists and psychiatrists will become more evident both within and outside the medical centre, and every medium possible will be used to increase awareness of the relevance of psychological factors to health and illness.

ACKNOWLEDGEMENTS

Gertrude Rubinstein provided invaluable assistance in the preparation of this chapter.

REFERENCES

APS: *The Australian Psychological Society Code of Ethics*. The Australian Psychological Society Ltd: Melbourne, 1999.

Belar CD: Training the clinical psychology student in behavioral medicine. *Prof Psychol* **11**: 620–627, 1980.

Bloch S and Pargiter R: Codes of ethics in psychiatry. In Bloch S, Chodoff P and Green SA (Eds): *Psychiatric Ethics*, 3rd edition, pp 81–103. Oxford University Press: Oxford, 1999.

Bosch X: Geneticists discuss ethics of human genome project. *Lancet* **352**: 1448, 1998.

Braithwaite J, Vining RF and Lazarus L: The boundaryless hospital. *A NZ J Med* **24**: 565–571, 1994.

Butcher D and McPherson I: The organisational context of clinical practice. *Bull Br Psychol Soc* **36**: 45–48, 1983.

Chodoff P: Misuse and abuse of psychiatry. In Bloch S, Chodoff P and Green SA (Eds): *Psychiatric Ethics*, 3rd edition, pp 49–66. Oxford University Press: Oxford, 1999.

Cummings NA: Arguments for the financial efficacy of psychological services in health care settings. In Sweet JJ, Rozensky RH and Tovian SM (Eds): *Handbook of Clinical Psychology in Medical Settings*. Plenum: New York, 1991.

Daniels N and Sabin J: The ethics of accountability in managed care reform. *Health Affairs* **17**(5): 50–64, 1998.

Debelle P: Modern hospital management based on the survival of the fittest. Taking care of business. *The Age* 13, 1995.

Devine EL and Cook TD: A meta-analysis of effects of psychoeducation interventions on length of post-surgical hospital stay. *Nursing Res* **132**: 267–274, 1983.

Dewan M: Are psychiatrists cost-effective? An analysis of integrated versus split treatment. *Am J Psychiatry* **156**: 324–326, 1999.

Dobson KS and Craig KD (Eds): *Advances in Cognitive-Behavioral Therapy*. Sage Publications: Thousand Oaks, CA, 1996.

Drummond MF, O'Brien BJ, Stoddart GL and Torrance GW: *Methods for the Economic Evaluation of Health Care Programs*, 2nd edition. Oxford University Press: New York, 1997.

Dyer AR: Psychiatry as a profession. In Bloch S, Chodoff P and Green SA (Eds), *Psychiatric Ethics*, 3rd edition, pp 67–79. Oxford University Press: Oxford, 1999.

Eagar K and Hindle D: *Casemix in Australia: An Overview*. Department of Human Services and Health: Canberra, ACT, 1994.

Editorial: Burnished or burnt out: The delights and dangers of working in health. *Lancet* **344** (8937): 1583–1584, 1994.

Epstein R: *Keeping Boundaries: Maintaining Safety and Integrity in the Psychotherapeutic Process*. APA: Washington, DC, 1994.

Fallowfield L and Jenkins V: Effective communication skills are the key to good cancer care. *Eur J Cancer* **35**: 1592–1597, 1999.

Funk and Wagnalls' Standard Dictionary of the English Language, International Edition. Funk and Wagnalls Company: New York, 1963.

Gabbard GO: Boundary violation. In Bloch S, Chodoff P and Green SA (Eds): *Psychiatric Ethics*, 3rd edition, pp 141–160. Oxford University Press: Oxford, 1999.

Garland M: Justice, politics and community: expanding access and rationing health services in Oregon. *Law, Medicine and Health Care* **20**: 67–81, 1992.

Geraty R: General hospital psychiatry and the new behavioral health care system. *Gen Hosp Psychiatry* **17**: 245–250, 1995.

Gold R, Siegel JA, Russell LB and Weinstein MC: *Cost-effectiveness in Health and Medicine*. Oxford University Press: New York, 1996.

Groth-Marnat G and Edkins G: Professional psychologists in general health care settings: A review of the financial efficacy of direct treatment interventions. *Prof Psychol: Research and Pratice* **27**(2): 161–174, 1996.

Gutmann T and Land W: Ethics regarding living-donor organ transplantation. *Langenbecks Arch Surg* **384**: 515–522, 1999.

Haley J: Why a mental health clinic should avoid family therapy. *J Marriage Fam Counselling* **11**: 3–13, 1975.

Health and Community Services Victoria: *Victoria's Mental Health Services: The Framework for Service Delivery*. Psychiatric Services Division: Melbourne, 1994.

Holmes J: Ethical aspects of the psychotherapies. In Bloch S, Chodoff P and Green SA (Eds): *Psychiatric Ethics*, 3rd edition, pp 225–243. Oxford University Press: Oxford, 1999.

Horne DJdeL, McCormack HM, Collins JP, Forbes JF and Russell IS: Psychological treatment of phobic anxiety associated with adjuvant chemotherapy. *Med J Aust* **145**: 346–348, 1986.

Horner JS: Research, ethics and privacy: the limits of knowledge. *Public Health* **112**: 217–220, 1998.

Iglehart J: The American health care system: managed care. *N Engl J Med* **327**: 742–747, 1992.

Kahan JP, Bernstein SJ, Leape LL, Hilborne LH, Park RE, Parker L, Kornberg CJ and Brook RH: Measuring the necessity of medical procedures. *Med Care* **32**: 357–365, 1994.

Kaplan RM, Sallis JF and Patterson TL: *Health and Human Behavior*. McGraw-Hill: New York, 1993.

Kefalides P: Solid organ transplantation. 2: Ethical considerations. *Ann Intern Med* **130**: 169–170, 1999.

Lezak MD: *Neuropsychological Asessment*, 3rd Edition. Oxford University Press: New York, 1995.

Lloyd GER (Ed): *Hippocratic Writings*. Harmondsworth: New York, 1983.

Lorion RP: Prevention and public health: Psychology's response to the nation's health care crisis. *Am Psychologist* **46**: 516–519, 1991.

MAS: Management Advisory Service to the National Health Scheme—Review of clinical psychology services. Department of Health: UK, 1989.

Maslach C: *Burnout: The Cost of Caring.* Prentice-Hall: Englewood Cliffs, NJ, 1982.

Maslach C: Burnout in health professionals. In Baum A, Newman S, Weinman J, West R and McManus C (Eds): *Cambridge Handbook of Psychology Health and Medicine*, pp 275–278. Cambridge University Press: Cambridge, England, 1997.

Maslach C: A multidimensional theory of burnout. In CL Cooper (Ed): *Theories of Organizational Stress*, pp 68–85. Oxford University Press: New York, NY, 1998.

Maslach C and Jackson SE: The measurement of experienced burnout. *J Occup Behav* **2**: 99–113, 1981.

Milgrom J and Green S: Systems consultation in a hospital. *A NZ J Fam Ther* **11**: 11–19, 1990.

Milgrom J, Nathan PR and Martin PR: Health psychology: overview and practice in a general hospital setting. In Martin PR and Birnbrauer JS (Eds): *Clinical Psychology: Profession and Practice in Australia*, pp 191–235. MacMillan: Melbourne, 1996.

Moore KA, Jones RMcL, Hardy K and Burrows GD: Liver transplantation: The ethical debate. *J Transplant Coordination* **1**: 111–116, 1991.

Neuberger J and James O: Guidelines for selection of patients for liver transplantation in the era of donor-organ shortage. *Lancet* **354**: 1636–1639, 1999.

Pettiti DB: Meta-analysis, decision analysis, and cost-effectiveness analysis. Oxford University Press: New York, 1994.

RANZCP (Royal Australian and New Zealand College of Psychiatrists): *Principles, Code of Ethics.* RANZCP, Melbourne, Australia, 1992.

Reich W: Psychiatric diagnosis as an ethical problem. In Bloch S, Chodoff P and Green SA (Eds): *Psychiatric Ethics*, 3rd edition, pp 193–224. Oxford University Press: Oxford, 1999.

Sabin J and Daniels N: Setting behavioral health priorities: good news and crucial lessons from the Oregon Health Plan. *Psychiatric Services* **48**: 883–889, 1997.

Sabin J and Daniels N: Ethical issues in health research allocation. In Bloch S, Chodoff P and Green SA (Eds): *Psychiatric Ethics*, 3rd edition, pp 383–399. Oxford University Press: Oxford, 1999.

Sarafino EP: *Health Psychology: Biopsychosocial Interactions*, 2nd edition. Wiley & Sons: New York, 1994.

Schlesinger HJ, Mumford E, Glass GV, Patrick CZ and Sharfstein S: Mental health treatment and medical care utilization in a fee-for-service system: the onset of a chronic disease. *Am J Publ Health* **73**: 422–429, 1983.

Schwartz S: Should the government pay for psychotherapy? *Bull Aust Psychol Soc* **17**: 5–8, 1995.

Schwartz S: Is psychotherapy worth paying for? Economic analyses of psychological treatments. *Psychologically Speaking*, **July**: 2–4, 1997.

Schwartz S: Saving Australia's health care system. *Policy* **Autumn**: 3–7, 1999.

Schwartz S, Richardson J and Glasziou PP: Quality-adjusted life years: origins, measurements, applications, objections. *Aust J Publ Health* **17**: 272–278, 1993.

Scientific American: *Scientific American* special report: the human genome business. *Scientific American*: New York, 2000.

Seawright HR and Pound P: The HIV positive patient and the duty to protect: ethical and legal issues. *Int J Psych Med* **24**: 259–270, 1994.

Sharfstein SS: The high cost of spending less on care. *Psychiatric Services* **49**: 1523, 1998.

Simpson F and Cotton P: So what is casemix and what is the APS doing about it? *The Bulletin of the APS*: April: **17**, 1995.

Sinnott A: Issues in community psychology: an introduction to community psychology: a challenge for the practitioner. In Karas E (Ed): *Current Issues in Clinical Psychology*. Plenum Press: London, 1985.

Spilker B: *Quality of Life Assessments in Clinical Trials*. Raven Press: New York, 1990.

Stebnicki MA: Stress and grief reactions among rehabilitation professionals. Dealing effectively with empathy fatigue. *J Rehabil* **66**: 2329, 2000.

Streiner DL and Norman GR: *Health Measurement Scales*. Oxford University Press: New York, 1989.

Sweet J, Rozensky RH and Tovian SM: *Handbook of Clinical Psychology in Medical Settings*. Plenum Press: New York, 1991.

Tarasoff v Regents of the University of California 529 P.2D 553 (1974).

Taylor SE: *Health Psychology*, 3rd edition. McGraw-Hill: New York, 1995.

Touyz S, Byrne D and Gilandas A (Eds): *Neuropsychology in Clinical Practice*. Harcourt, Brace & Company: Sydney, 1994.

Trethowan Report: *The Role of Psychologists in the Health Services: Report of the Sub-committee*. HMSO: London, 1977.

Turner J, Meldrum L and Raphael B: Preventive aspects of occupational mental health. In B Raphael and GD Burrows (Eds): *Handbook of Studies on Preventive Psychiatry*, pp 169–183. Elsevier: Amsterdam, 1995.

Walsh KW and Darby D: *Neuropsychology: A Clinical Approach*, 4th Edition. Churchill Livingstone: Edinburgh, 1999.

Webster L and Hackett RK: Burnout and leadership in community health care. *Admin Policy Mental Health* **26**: 387–399, 1999.

Weinstock R: Confidentiality and the new duty to protect: the psychiatrist's dilemma. *Hosp Commun Psychiatry* **39**: 606–609, 1988.

WHO: Guiding principles on human organ transplantation. *Lancet* **337**: 1470–1471, 1991.

WHO: *World Health Report*. WHO: Geneva, 1997.

Wynne LC, McDaniel SH and Weber TT: *Systems Consultation: A New Perspective for Family Therapy*, pp 6, 10. Guilford Press: New York, 1986.

Yates BT: Survey comparison of success, morbidity, mortality, fees and psychological benefits and costs of 3,146 patients receiving jejunoileal or gastric bypass. *Am J Clin Nutrition* **33** (2 Suppl.): 518–522, 1980.

Zaro JS, Batchelor WF, Ginsberg MR and Pollak MS: Psychology and the JCAH. Reflections on a decade of struggle. *Am Psychologist* **37**: 1342–1349, 1982.

Index

Note: page numbers in *italics* refer to figures and tables

Index compiled by Jill Halliday